P9-ASL-864

ADVANCES IN

Otolaryngology—Head and Neck Surgery®

VOLUME 9

ADVANCES IN

Otolaryngology—Head and Neck Surgery®

VOLUMES 1 THROUGH 5 (OUT OF PRINT)

VOLUME 6

ADVANCES IN

Otolaryngology—Head and Neck Surgery®

VOLUME 9

Editor-in-Chief
Eugene N. Myers, M.D.
Professor and Chairman, Department of Otolaryngology, University of
Pittsburgh School of Medicine, Pittsburgh, Pennsylvania

Associate Editor
Charles D. Bluestone, M.D.
Professor of Otolaryngology, University of Pittsburgh School of Medicine;
Director, Pediatric Otolaryngology, Children's Hospital of Pittsburgh,
Department of Otolaryngology, Pittsburgh, Pennsylvania

Editorial Board
Derald E. Brackmann, M.D.
Clinical Professor of Otolaryngology, Clinical Professor of Neurosurgery,
University of California, School of Medicine, President, House Ear Clinic, Board
of Directors, House Ear Institute, Los Angeles, California

Charles J. Krause, M.D.
Professor, Department of Otolaryngology, Senior Associate Dean, University of
Michigan School of Medicine, Senior Associate Director, University of
Michigan Hospital, Ann Arbor, Michigan

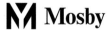 Mosby

St. Louis   Baltimore   Berlin   Boston   Carlsbad   Chicago   London   Madrid
Naples   New York   Philadelphia   Sydney   Tokyo   Toronto

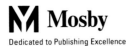

Dedicated to Publishing Excellence

Vice President and Publisher, Continuity Publishing: Kenneth H. Killion
Director, Editorial Development: Gretchen C. Murphy
Developmental Editor: Emily Veit
Acquisitions Editor: Jennifer Roche
Manager, Continuity—EDP: Maria Nevinger
Project Manager: Jill C. Waite
Assistant Project Supervisor: Sandra Rogers
Proofreading Supervisor: Barbara M. Kelly
Vice President, Professional Sales and Marketing: George M. Parker
Senior Marketing Manager: Eileen M. Lynch
Marketing Specialist: Lynn D. Stevenson

Copyright © 1995 by Mosby–Year Book, Inc.

All rights reserved. No part of this publication may be reproduced, stored in a retrieval system, or transmitted, in any form or by any means, electronic, mechanical, photocopying, recording, or otherwise, without prior written permission from the publisher.

Permission to photocopy or reproduce solely for internal or personal use is permitted for libraries or other users registered with the Copyright Clearance Center, provided that the base fee of $4.00 per chapter plus $.10 per page is paid directly to the Copyright Clearance Center, 27 Congress Street, Salem, MA 01970. This consent does not extend to other kinds of copying, such as copying for general distribution, for advertising or promotional purposes, for creating new collected works, or for resale.

Printed in the United States of America
Composition by The Clarinda Company
Printing/binding by The Maple-Vail Book Manufacturing Group

Mosby–Year Book, Inc.
11830 Westline Industrial Drive
St. Louis, Missouri 63146

Editorial Office:
Mosby–Year Book, Inc.
200 North LaSalle Street
Chicago, Illinois 60601

International Standard Serial Number: 0887–6916
International Standard Book Number: 0–8151–6267–7

Contributors

W. Benzel, M.D.
Department of Otorhinolaryngology, Head and Neck Surgery, University of Erlangen-Nuremberg, Erlangen, Germany

Derald E. Brackmann, M.D.
Clinical Professor of Otolaryngology, University of Southern California, House Ear Clinic, House Ear Institute, Los Angeles, California

Robert J. S. Briggs, M.D., F.R.A.C.S.
Assistant Otolaryngologist, Royal Melbourne Hospital, Senior Lecturer Melbourne University, Department of Otolaryngology, Melbourne, Australia

Ted A. Cook, M.D.
Associate Professor, Chief of Facial Plastic and Reconstructive Surgery, Department of Otolaryngology—Head and Neck Surgery, Oregon Health Sciences University, Portland, Oregon

Robin T. Cotton, M.D.
Professor, Otolaryngology, Department of Pediatric Otolaryngology, Children's Hospital Medical Center, Cincinnati, Ohio

H. Jacqueline Diels, O.T.R.
Facial Rehabilitation Specialist, Neuromuscular Retraining Clinic, Department of Rehabilitation Medicine, University of Wisconsin Hospital and Clinics, Madison, Wisconsin

George T. Goffas, M.D., D.D.S.
Private Practice, Facial Plastic and Maxillofacial Surgery, Birmingham, Michigan

Barry E. Hirsch, M.D.
Associate Professor, Department of Otolaryngology, University of Pittsburgh Eye and Ear Institute, Pittsburgh, Pennsylvania

Andrew J. Hotaling, M.D.
Associate Professor Otolaryngology, Head and Neck Surgery and Pediatrics, Loyola University Medical Center, Maywood, Illinois

John R. Houck, M.D.
Associate Professor, Department of Otorhinolaryngology, University of Oklahoma Health Sciences Center, Oklahoma City, Oklahoma

Heinrich Iro, M.D.
Department of Oto-Rhino-Laryngology, Head and Neck Surgery, University of Erlangen-Nuremberg, Erlangen, Germany

Herbert E. Jacob, M.D.
Assistant Professor of Critical Care Medicine, Department of Anesthesia and
Critical Care Medicine; Assistant Professor of Medicine, Division of Medical
Oncology, University of Pittsburgh, Pittsburgh Cancer Institute, Pittsburgh,
Pennsylvania

Ivo P. Janecka, M.D.
Professor of Otolaryngology and Neurology, Center for Cranial Base Surgery,
Departments of Otolaryngology and Neurological Surgery, University of
Pittsburgh, Pittsburgh, Pennsylvania

Silloo B. Kapadia, M.D.
Associate Professor, Department of Pathology, University of Pittsburgh School
of Medicine, Pittsburgh, Pennsylvania

Dewey T. Lawson, Ph.D.
Senior Scientist, Center for Auditory Prosthesis Research, Research Triangle
Institute, Research Triangle Park, North Carolina; Adjunct Assistant Professor,
Division of Otolaryngology—Head & Neck Surgery, Duke University Medical
Center, Durham, North Carolina

Jesus E. Medina, M.D.
Professor and Chairman, Department of Otorhinolaryngology, University of
Oklahoma Health Sciences Center, Oklahoma City, Oklahoma

Aage R. Møller, Ph.D.
Professor, Department of Neurological Surgery, University of Pittsburgh School
of Medicine, Pittsburgh, Pennsylvania

Stephen S. Park, M.D.
Section of Facial Plastic and Reconstructive Surgery, Department of
Otolaryngology—Head and Neck Surgery, University of Virginia Health Sciences
Center, Charlottesville, Virginia

Emil A. Popovic, M.B., B.S., F.R.A.C.S.
Assistant Neurosurgeon, Department of Neurosurgery, Clinical Neuroscience
Centre, Royal Melbourne Hospital, Melbourne, Australia

Keith H. Riding, F.R.C.S.C.
Clinical Professor, Division of Otolaryngology, Department of Surgery,
University of British Columbia; Head of the ENT Department, British
Columbia's Children's Hospital, Vancouver, British Columbia, Canada

Andrew B. Silva, M.D.
Resident, Department of Otolaryngology, Head and Neck Surgery, Loyola
University Medical Center, Maywood, Illinois

Howard A. Tobin, M.D.
Medical Director, Facial Plastic and Cosmetic Surgical Center, Abilene, Texas

Peter C. Weber, M.D.
Assistant Professor, Director, Division of Neurology/Otology, Director, Center
for Hearing and Balance Disorders, Department of Otolaryngology, Medical
University of South Carolina, Charleston, South Carolina

J. Paul Willging, M.D.
Assistant Professor, Otolaryngology, Department of Pediatric Otolaryngology,
Children's Hospital Medical Center, Cincinnati, Ohio

Blake S. Wilson

Director, Center for Auditory Prosthesis Research, Research Triangle Institute, Research Triangle Park, North Carolina; Adjunct Associate Professor, Division of Otolaryngology—Head & Neck Surgery, Duke University Medical Center, Durham, North Carolina

Robert F. Yellon, M.D.

Assistant Professor of Otolaryngology, Department of Pediatric Otolaryngology, Children's Hospital of Pittsburgh; Department of Otolaryngology, University of Pittsburgh School of Medicine, Pittsburgh, Pennsylvania

Johannes Zenk, M.D.

Department of Oto-Rhino-Laryngology, Head and Neck Surgery, University of Erlangen-Nuremberg, Erlangen, Germany

Mariangeli Zerbi, M.S.

Research Engineer, Center for Auditory Prosthesis Research, Research Triangle Institute, Research Triangle Park, North Carolina

Preface

The Board of Editors is very pleased to present volume 9 of *Advances in Otolaryngology—Head and Neck Surgery*. This volume contains more chapters and more pages than any previous volume. It also has some extraordinary chapters which are exemplary of the way that otolaryngology has harnessed technology to forge new diagnostic and treatment programs.

Examples of this advanced technology can be seen in the excellent chapter "Advances in Coding Strategies for Cochlear Implants" by Blake Wilson, Dr. Dewey Lawson and Mariangeli Zerbi, the chapter from Germany by Drs. Iro, Zenk, and Benzel entitled "Minimally Invasive Therapy of Sialolithiasis—State of the Art" and Dr. Møller's chapter, "Practical Aspects of Intraoperative Cranial Nerve Monitoring."

The chapters entitled "Congenital Perilymphatic Fistula" by Drs. Weber and Hirsch, "Recent Advances in the Treatment of Neurofibromatosis Type II" by Drs. Briggs, Popovic, and Brackmann, and "New Concepts in Nonsurgical Facial Nerve Rehabilitation" by H. Jacqueline Diels, as well as "Advances in Coding Strategies for Cochlear Implants" and "Practical Aspects of Intraoperative Cranial Nerve Monitoring" will have great appeal to those readers interested in otology/neurotology and related problems.

Those readers interested in problems concerning the pediatric population will greatly appreciate the chapters entitled "Management of Caustic Ingestion in Children" by Dr. Riding, "Gastroesophageal Reflux Disease in the Pediatric Population" by Drs. Hotaling and Silva, and "Infections of the Fascial Spaces of the Head and Neck in the Pediatric Population" by Dr. Yellon.

Several chapters describe advances in various aspects of head and neck surgery which will be appreciated by those readers interested in this area. These chapters include "Nasopharyngeal Carcinoma" by Drs. Kapadia and Janecka, "Advances in Neck Dissections" by Drs. Medina and Houck, and "The Role of Chemotherapy in the Management of Head and Neck Cancer" by Dr. Jacob.

For those readers interested in reconstructive surgery, our lead chapter in volume 9 is "Locoregional Flaps for Facial Resurfacing" by Drs. Cook and Park. This is an excellent chapter which goes into great detail about techniques for facial resurfacing following excision of various lesions. "The Extended Subperiosteal Coronal Facelift: An Improved Approach in Facial Rejuvenation Surgery" by Drs. Tobin and Goffas is another fine example of advances in this field. The chapter entitled "Reconstruction of Laryngotracheal Stenosis in the Adult" by Drs. Willging and Cotton is an extension of the well-known work of Dr. Cotton and his group on laryngotracheal reconstruction in the pediatric population.

I want to thank our reliable and creative editorial board, Drs. Charles

D. Bluestone, Derald E. Brackmann and Charles J. Krause for providing great assistance in not only selecting topics and authors but for reviewing and critiquing the manuscripts. Barbara A. Sigler, R.N., M.N.Ed., CORLN, our Editorial Coordinator, and Mary Jo Tutchko, my administrative assistant, also have been instrumental in helping to assemble this volume. Diana Dodge, our Assistant Managing Editor, has also been extremely helpful and very active in the organization of volume 9.

Eugene N. Myers, M.D.
Editor-in-Chief

Contents

Practical Aspects of Intraoperative Cranial Nerve Monitoring.

Nasopharyngeal Carcinoma.

Gastroesophageal Reflux Disease in the Pediatric Population.

New Concepts in Nonsurgical Facial Nerve Rehabilitation.

Mosby Document Express

Copies of the full text of journal articles referenced in this book are available by calling Mosby Document Express, toll-free, at 1-800-55-MOSBY.

With Mosby Document Express, you have convenient 24-hour-a-day access to literally every journal reference within this book. In fact, through Mosby Document Express, virtually any medical or scientific article can be located and delivered by FAX, overnight delivery service, international airmail, electronic transmission of bit-mapped images (via Internet), or regular mail. The average cost of a complete delivered copy of an article, including copyright clearance charges and first-class mail delivery, is $12.

For inquiries and pricing information, please call the toll-free number shown above. To expedite your order for material appearing in this publication, please be prepared with the code shown next to the bibliographic citation for each abstract.

Locoregional Flaps for Facial Resurfacing

Ted A. Cook, M.D.

Associate Professor, Chief of Facial Plastic and Reconstructive Surgery, Department of Otolaryngology–Head and Neck Surgery, Oregon Health Sciences University, Portland, Oregon

Stephen S. Park, M.D.

Section of Facial Plastic and Reconstructive Surgery, Department of Otolaryngology–Head and Neck Surgery, University of Virginia Health Sciences Center, Charlottesville, Virginia

T he resurfacing of soft-tissue facial defects remains a formidable challenge for the reconstructive surgeon. The face is the most visible area of the body yet is highly complex in its subtle curves and hollows, all working together in remarkable symmetry. Despite continued effort, those subtleties are still particularly difficult to recreate. Minute disturbances are readily noticeable and, because of this, improving facial reconstruction remains an enthusiastic effort.

The causes of facial defects are diverse, including congenital, infectious, traumatic, and neoplastic. A century ago, many horrifying facial defects arising from infectious causes were considered untreatable and were left to heal with dramatic stigmata. Restraint belts have markedly reduced the number of windshield lacerations during motor vehicle accidents, as has the institution of "shatterproof" glass. Physical assault on the streets has changed from blunt trauma and knife injuries to rapid-fire missile injuries with increasing fatalities. Defects from Mohs excisions of cutaneous malignancies are now the greatest source of defects requiring reconstructive endeavors. First developed by Frederick E. Mohs while a medical student in the 1930s, micrographic excision has become the "gold standard" for treating most cutaneous malignancies.

Historically, major surgical advances were made through military combat during World War I and II and with the introduction of antibiotics. Recent advances are being made in the biotechnology of implants, glues, and plates, as well as in the understanding of flap physiology, the dynamics of healing, aesthetic boundaries, and flap enhancement. This chapter focuses on the principles and techniques of facial resurfacing, and accents the recent advances in locoregional flaps.

PATIENT SELECTION

The goals in facial reconstruction are to restore soft-tissue coverage and functional integrity, to provide prompt healing, and to maximize aesthetic

Advances in Otolarynogology—Head and Neck Surgery®, vol. 9
© 1995, Mosby–Year Book, Inc.

balance. Identifying the "high risk" patient is critical when selecting the appropriate management of a defect. Special note should be made of to-bacco abuse, diabetes mellitus, hypertension, prior radiotherapy, and overall nutrition. Additionally, one must look closely at the integrity of the regional skin available for transfer. Multiple cutaneous malignancies are the rule rather than exception and one should avoid mobilizing "sick" skin. Some maneuvers will "burn bridges" and may hinder future recon-structive efforts. Attention should be given to the different skin textures of the face. Generally speaking, thin skin tends to camouflage incisions and local flaps more effectively than thick, sebaceous skin. Furthermore, pigmented and chronically sun-exposed skin does more poorly.

Timing for surgical repair can be utilized to good advantage. Most re-constructions are performed either immediately or within 2 days of trauma while the wound remains fresh. A delay of 7 to 10 days may at times be of benefit as the recipient bed fills with granulation tissue and thereby vascularity is enhanced. This will promote the receptiveness of the wound and also fill the depth of the defect, resulting in improved contour. When delaying wound repair, one must be conscious of wound contracture, particularly around mobile structures such as lips, alar rim, and eyelids.

Photographic documentation of all reconstructive steps is imperative. It allows critical review and may become integral in medicolegal issues. Perhaps most importantly, it provides a means to remind patients of their initial defect, to help them follow their own progress, and to aid in their psychological support.

ANATOMY

The aesthetic goal in facial resurfacing is to reapproximate skin color and texture and to camouflage incisions. This is best accomplished with the deliberate placement of incisions within natural lines of the face and such that the resultant tensions after wound repair lie along lines of maximal extensibility. Understanding the cutaneous anatomy of the face is there-fore fundamental to achieving satisfactory, lasting results.

The face enjoys a particularly generous blood supply, making it much more forgiving to many surgical principles. The subdermal plexus is a rich network of small random vessels feeding the overlying skin. This ar-cade of vessels gives rise to a greater local perfusion pressure, thereby improving the dependability of local, random flaps. Length-to-width ra-tios for flaps of the head and neck do not follow a linear relation, i.e., viable flap length does not increase linearly with increasing pedicle width. Most flaps have a relatively constant length of survival.[1] In the face, the length is enhanced because of the rich subdermal plexus and the general ability to design "axially oriented" flaps. The robust blood supply also promotes more rapid healing and results in infrequent infec-tions. Disrupted venous and lymphatic egress often cause flap congestion and lymphedema, especially in the setting of relatively vigorous arterial perfusion. Venous and lymphatic channels are randomly reestablished from the dermal level. Scarring and wound contraction may interfere with this process and predispose to chronic lymphedema. Thickening and discoloration are problems that often arise from poor venous and lymph drainage, and it is important, therefore, to design inferiorly based facial flaps whenever possible.

The dermal layer of skin derives its elastic properties from elastic fibers wrapped around collagen. This elasticity accounts for the gaping of linear wounds and the inherent contraction of full-thickness skin grafts. In the 1800s Dupuytren, and later Karl Langer, described how full-thickness circular wounds tend to become elliptical and follow a predictable linear orientation. These lines of orientation became known as Langer's lines and were in fact the earliest descriptions of lines of tension inherent in skin structure. They were designed from excised skin or from corpses as they developed rigor mortis. Many of these lines crossed natural skin creases and have now been found not to corroborate with practical experience.

Lines of minimal tension, also known as wrinkle lines, natural skin creases, or favorable skin tension lines, represent a cutaneous adaptation to a repeated action of the underlying muscle. Habitual buckling of the skin from muscle contraction causes permanent furrows in the skin. These arise independently of relaxed skin tension lines (RSTLs) and although the two usually run parallel, the lateral canthal and glabellar regions are areas of conflict (Fig 1).

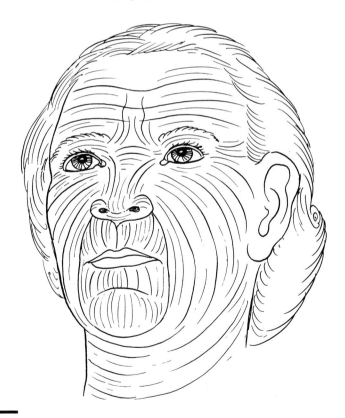

FIGURE 1.

RSTLs and lines of minimal tension. Note conflicting lines at the glabella and lateral canthal regions.

Relaxed skin tension lines, a term coined by Borges in 1962, are the lines used today to map facial incisions.[2] They are the lines of tension formed when skin is in repose and are a reflection of the intrinsic properties of the dermis. They correspond to the alignment of elastic and collagen fibers within the dermis. Unlike the lines of minimal tension (wrinkles), RSTLs are not visible on the surface in youthful skin, although most become visible with aging. They are best identified by pinching the skin and noting the furrows and ridges that form. Relaxed skin tension lines represent the constant tension on skin, even when sleeping, and thus, have the greatest influence on wound healing.

Lines of maximal extensibility represent the direction in which skin is most extensible. They generally run coaxial with muscle fibers and perpendicular to RSTLs. Locoregional flaps should be designed with the direction of greatest tension in line with the lines of maximal extensibility. All incisions should be made so that they lie parallel to the RSTLs. Incisions made in this fashion will heal with minimal scarring, whereas incisions at right angles to the RSTLs will inevitably scar more and be more visible.

Between the subcutaneous fat and mimetic musculature of the face is a broad sheet of fibrous tissue known as the superficial muscular aponeurotic system (SMAS). This plane was first described anatomically by Mitz and Peyronie in 1976.[3] It is a layer of muscular fascia with multiple fibrous septa that pierce the subcutaneous fat and adhere to the dermal layer of skin. This layer is continuous with the platysmal fibers inferiorly, the temporoparietal fascia superiorly, and the parotid fascia posteriorly. Mobilization, reorientation, and suspension of this structure provide additional support to the surrounding skin and yield more lasting results in surgery on the aging face. It may similarly be suspended during facial reconstruction and significantly helps to relieve tension.

The mimetic muscles of the face have important dynamic and functional features. In some areas they provide a majority of bulk and must be specifically addressed during reconstruction, e.g., perioral cleft repair.

Bone structure gives rise to most of the major contours of the face. Augmenting or reducing various areas can have a dramatic effect on the aesthetic balance. A variety of alloplastic and autogenous materials may be used at the bone level to change the surface contours.

The face is composed of several major aesthetic units, some separated by well-defined creases, others by gentle grooves and ridges (Fig 2). Wherever possible, incisions should be made along the borders of these aesthetic units for optimum camouflage. The nose is further broken down into nine subunits (Fig 3). Each unit has unique features best discussed individually.

SCALP

The scalp is characteristically thick, vascular, and not distensible. The skin is firmly adherent to the underlying galeal aponeurosis, which results in the lack of distensibility. The combined entity does, however, slide easily over pericranium. The blood supply is from terminal branches of the external carotid system that course superficially within the galea for some length, and enter the scalp radially from below. Venous and lym-

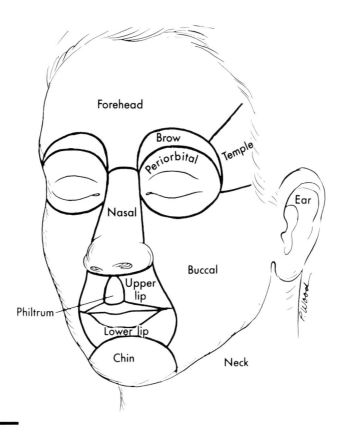

FIGURE 2.
Aesthetic units of the face.

phatic vessels conform to this same radial pattern. Long and narrow scalp flaps can be created when based on a major branch. This is beneficial because of the lack of extensibility of scalp flaps, especially when the elevation is in the avascular subgaleal plane. Galeotomies made on the underside of a flap, parallel to the axial blood supply, will improve stretch appreciably. Flaps elevated supragaleally may be more mobile, but they jeopardize the vascular supply and the hair follicles. The follicles can thus be deliberately depiliated when flaps are transferred to a nonhair-bearing region.

FOREHEAD

Forehead skin is also thick and vascular. It is firmly adherent to the underlying frontalis muscle and is one of the more active areas of facial expression, giving rise to deep furrows. The RSTLs course horizontally, but in the glabellar region they cross with the vertically oriented wrinkles from the corrugator supercilii muscles. The blood supply laterally is from the anterior branch of the superficial temporal artery, entering from each side. The medial aspect is supplied by the supraorbital and supratrochlear vessels. The supratrochlear artery is a terminal branch of the ophthalmic artery, coursing around and superficial to the corrugator muscle, deep to the orbicularis oculi, and quickly penetrating the frontalis muscle

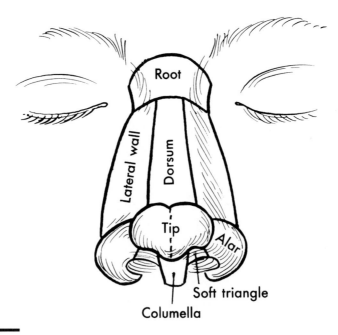

FIGURE 3.
Aesthetic subunits of the nose.

as it ascends in a superficial plane. In most elderly patients, furrows become prominent and accept incisions in an aesthetic way. Asymmetry of brow height may be disfiguring and the brows are best not mobilized.

BROW

Asymmetry or loss of brow hair-bearing tissue is readily noticeable. Hair follicles in the brow have a distinct angulation and are particularly tenuous, and even mild surgical trauma may result in permanent loss. For this reason brow tissue is never shaved and all incisions are made in a bevelled fashion parallel to the hair shafts.

EYELID

The eyelids are important cosmetic and functional structures. The skin is the thinnest in the face, devoid of subcutaneous fat and firmly bound to the underlying muscle. Eyelids heal with remarkably little scar formation, even in keloid formers. The lid serves to protect and suspend the globe while maintaining complete mobility. The tarsal skeleton and medial and lateral suspensions are critical anatomic features that must be preserved or restored during reconstruction. The underlying muscle serves to suspend the lid against the globe and assist with the lacrimal pump.

TEMPLE

Skin in the temple area is thin and freely mobile as it sits over the temporal fat pad. The "crow's feet" from the lateral canthus overlap with the oblique RSTLs. The area is bounded by three relatively fixed strutures, the lateral brow, lateral canthus and temporal hairline. The temporal branch of the facial nerve courses superficially within the SMAS and undermining in this area is fraught with danger.

NOSE

Nasal reconstruction is an exciting challenge to most surgeons because of its aesthetic and functional significance and the difficulty in recreating the natural, subtle contours. The structural foundation must provide a patent airway while maintaining flexibility. The blood supply to the skin is from the lateral nasal artery, a branch from the angular artery, and gives a tremendous arborization at the subdermal level. A rich collateral circulation exists with the columellar arteries, branching from the superior labial arteries and the infratrochlear vessels. The principles of aesthetic subunits are especially relevant to nasal reconstruction.[4] Skin over the nasal tip unit is usually quite thick and sebaceous, whereas over the dorsal and lateral subunits it tends to be thin and mobile. The nasion is covered with extremely thick soft tissues, often blunting changes in bony contour. These are important considerations when resurfacing different subunits. Vertical incisions in the exact midline, although violating the dorsal and tip subunits, are remarkably well concealed from the casual eye. Relaxed skin tension lines are poorly defined but generally run horizontally. Nasal skin is not particularly extensible despite wide undermining. Advancement from the cheek unit will distort the nasal-facial groove. For these reasons, effective nasal reconstruction must employ a large variety of locoregional flaps.

CHEEK

The cheek skin is intermediate in thickness and quite malleable. Skin grafts are rarely needed because extensive undermining will usually allow primary closure. The oblique RSTLs are helpful in many of the smaller transposition flaps, e.g., rhomboids. The plane of elevation is within the subcutaneous tissue, above the SMAS, and therefore above the facial nerve. When in the correct plane one sees the characteristic cobblestone appearance of fat. The meilolabial fold is a line of minimal tension and parallels the RSTLs of the cheek. It arises from the perioral levator muscles inserting in the dermis, just distal to the fold, and can be used to conceal large incisions. Care must be taken not to distort the fold and to provide bilateral symmetry.

LIPS/PERIORAL

The lips have important aesthetic and functional features. The blood supply comes off the facial artery as the labial, angular, and septal vessels. The skin is thick and firmly bound to the underlying muscle with minimal subcutaneous fat. Relaxed skin tension lines course radially from the stoma. Lip height, thickness, vermillion border, white roll, philtral ridges, and Cupid's bow are all important features to reestablish. Reapproximating orbicularis oris muscle is critical for function as well as to provide fullness and prevent notching. Intact sensation is necessary for oral competence. Sensory innervation is chiefly from the mental and infraorbital nerves.

CHIN

The chin is a well-delineated cutaneous structure extending in a circular pattern from the sublabial crease to the submental fold. It has very thick subcutaneous tissue which is tightly bound to the skin and results in a bulk which is difficult to restore with locoregional flaps. The prominent sublabial crease should not be violated with vertical incisions because unacceptable webbing will occur at the sulcus. The submental crease will conceal incisions remarkably well, making it a common route for procedures on the mentum and midline neck. The RSTLs run vertically. The blood supply is from the submental and inferior labial vessels off the facial artery.

NECK

Like the cheek, the neck skin is quite extensible and lends itself to primary closure with wide undermining. The blood supply is not as robust as in the face and elevation is frequently done deep to the underlying platysma for improved dependability. Branches of the facial nerve may be at jeopardy in this plane. Relaxed skin tension lines run horizontally and accept incisions well. Tissue expansion can be utilized effectively but does not work as well as at other areas, such as the scalp, since there is no underlying bone structure available.

RESURFACING

Facial resurfacing must work to restore covering and maximize camouflage while minimizing patient inconvenience. There is an extensive array of reconstructive options varying in complexity and dependability. They all have a place in facial reconstruction and the surgeon should be familiar with these techniques. We will discuss all these options briefly before describing in depth the use of locoregional flaps.

SECONDARY INTENTION HEALING

Healing by secondary intention is a simple and dependable modality which Dr. Mohs used most commonly for healing of the defects he produced. The drawbacks of prolonged wound care and wound contracture make it a seldom utilized method today. There are cases, however, where secondary healing remains the treatment of choice. Small defects on concave surfaces, such as the medial canthal area, are particularly suited for secondary intention healing. More often, large defects reconstructed with a variety of flaps develop a small portion of necrosis and slough. These areas are usually left to heal secondarily with local wound care alone before considering secondary reconstruction.

Secondary intention healing is a race between normal wound contracture and surface reepithelialization. The sooner the wound is covered and healed, the less wound contracture will result. Wound healing proceeds through four predictable stages:

1. The coagulation stage is the formation of a fibrin gel meshwork which serves as an interim framework for repair.
2. The inflammatory stage serves to debride the wound and initiate the release of chemotactic and growth factors.
3. New tissue formation is the third stage and involves neovascularization, collagen deposition, wound contraction and epidermal regeneration.
4. Remodeling is the final stage when the scar matures and softens.[5]

There is now a tremendous amount of energy focused on the pharmacologic manipulation of these components of wound healing. Angiogenic growth factors aim at expediting the healing process. Epidermal-growth factor (EGF) is perhaps the most studied factor with experience on repair of human corneal defects, epidermal ulcers, and skin graft donor sites. Platelet derived growth factor (PDGF) is a chemotactic factor for fibroblasts and smooth muscle cells. The platelet plug is the initial source of PDGF but similar compounds are later produced by macrophages and endothelial cells. There are no definitive studies on humans but there is support that topical application of EGF and PDGF to partial-thickness wounds may accelerate healing.[6, 7] Transforming growth factor-B is a cytokine which attracts fibroblasts, causing increased collagen deposition, scar formation. It also stimulates angiogenesis. It is normally produced by platelets, macrophages, and fibroblasts in all contracting wounds, but is found in excess in hypertrophic scars. Neutralizing antibody to the transforming growth factor has been injected into fresh wounds in the rat model and shown to decrease the extent of collagen deposition and scar formation.[8] Wounds containing this neutralizing antibody had a more normal histologic pattern and normal tensile strength. This is one of the more exciting agents that may prove to have great clinical utility for modulating the extent of wound contracture and scar formation while awaiting epithelialization. Recombinant human growth factor and insulin-like growth factor-1 have been shown to be diminished in patients with massive burns, and supplementation seems to augment their healing process.[9, 10] The administration and control of these proteins still need refinement but they have promising implications for the treatment of chronic nonhealing ulcers. Proteoglycans are thought to have some role in collagen regulation and are synthesized at greater levels in hypertrophic scars as compared to normal wounds.[11] Controlling this protein and understanding its biological significance remains unknown.

Growth hormones are a source of enthusiastic research with numerous experiments on the animal model using a variety of delivery systems. Their clinical application in human wound healing has not been clearly defined. No single growth factor has emerged with definitive clinical benefit for healing by secondary intention. The next frontier may use somatic gene therapy for modulating growth factor expression. A vector that codes for expression of a natural growth factor may be introduced directly into the cells of a nonhealing wound, which then magnifies selective growth factors and accelerates healing. Although gene therapy has met with some success in the animal model, it is still far from use in human clinical trials. Influencing gene expression of such potent factors may unleash uncontrolled stimulation and possible neoplastic transformation.

Corticosteroids impair wound healing by altering the local inflammatory response and inhibiting fibroblast migration. Applied topically to open wounds, they stunt both wound contracture and epithelialization, the net effect being unpredictable. Triamcinolone (Kenolog) dampens hypertrophic scar formation without weakening wound strength. It is frequently used intralesionally to treat hypertrophic scars and keloids. Systemic factors such as vitamins A, E, and C and zinc can have a positive effect on wound healing.[5] Daily multivitamins are innocuous and may be of clinical benefit. There are other areas of research looking at ways to influence natural healing. Intense and prolonged UVA radiation has been shown to adversely effect wound repair in the animal model.[12] Intense sun exposure may be another significant variable for consideration when identifying the high-risk patient. Calcium channel blockers theoretically could block contraction at the myofibroblast level but this has not proven clinically significant.[13] Fetal wound healing with the effects of amniotic fluid is a fascinating topic and remains a mystery which is presently being extensively studied. Closed incisions made in utero will mature without scar formation. Full-thickness fetal defects that are covered and shielded from amniotic fluid will heal with myofibroblasts and contraction. Excisional defects that are uncovered and bathed in amniotic fluid are devoid of myofibroblasts, do not contract, and only minimally reepithelialize.[14] Unlocking the powers of amniotic fluid will have tremendous implications in the field of wound healing and contracture. Creating a DC electric field in an open wound has shown some beneficial effect with earlier collagen deposition and normal tensile strength. It has also been shown to improve skin graft take in the rat model.[15]

Traditional wound care involves continuous moisture to prevent desiccation and expedite healing. Antibiotic ointment is frequently used in contaminated open wounds. Once the flora has diminished, however, antibiotic-free ointment works equally well. There is a suggestion that topical antimicrobial agents may be cytotoxic to fibroblasts and keratinocytes, thus adversely affecting wound healing.[16, 17] There are no in vivo studies showing impaired wound healing with antimicrobial ointments and we use them regularly. Excessive application tends to macerate surrounding normal skin and some people have a sensitivity reaction to the ointment. Microporous, semiocclusive dressings maintain a moist wound bed and require less postoperative care. The serum that accumulates under the dressing seems to provide more patient comfort, but there is some concern over local infection in the static environment. Crusting and eschar formation may serve as a "biologic dressing" but seem to impede epithelialization and leave uneven wound edges; they should be debrided and replaced with ointment.

SKIN GRAFTS

Skin grafts are a simple and dependable way to resurface. Skin grafts obtain their nutrient supply initially through direct absorption from plasma

(1 to 3 days). At this stage they are relatively deficient in erythrocytes and thus have a pale appearance. By the third day vascularity and color improves. There is some neovascularization but a majority of reperfusion is from direct ingrowth into the preexisting network of small vessels. Split-thickness grafts have better take than full-thickness grafts but have greater wound contracture, inferior protection, and poorer color match. They are usually not indicated for facial resurfacing. Full-thickness skin grafts can do extremely well and are the treatment of choice for severe defects (superficial lids, small nasal). On rare occasions, with congenital giant hairy nevi or burn patients, full-thickness skin grafts can be harvested from expanded donor sites.[18] Alternatively, the defect can be directly reduced in size by a "purse-string" closure.[19] A subcutaneous suture is placed circumferentially around the defect and as it is tied down the wound will close about 50%.

The goal in dressing a skin graft is to prevent desiccation and maintain apposition of the graft to the recipient bed. Bolsters have been traditionally used. Tie-down sutures should be placed beyond the margin of the wound in order to avoid the "crater" deformity along the graft edge. Often, simple tacking sutures of fast absorbing gut with continued moisturizing ointment will serve in place of bolsters, especially in defects with irregular contours. Fibrin glue has been used by general surgeons for hemostasis after liver biopsies. It was previously synthesized from pooled plasma and carried those inherent risks. Autologous fibrin glue can be synthesized in small quantities for use in the head and neck. It has been used with skin grafts and has shown improved take, fixation, and decreased contracture.[20, 21] It may have indications for the marginal tissue bed where the glue serves as a nutrient pool during the first few days of graft survival by plasma imbibition. At this point, however, it seems more a novel approach than practical one.

Choosing the appropriate donor site for a full-thickness skin graft is based on the desired thickness and color. Lids provide the thinnest skin. The meilolabial folds are excellent donor sites for small nasal defects. Multiple pie-crusting perforations are essential in order to allow egress of serum and blood from under the graft. These perforations should be oriented along with the RSTLs of the surrounding skin so as to mimic RSTLs of the graft. Skin grafts for facial resurfacing produce dependable and good results for many defects. Advances are being made in the area of improving fixation, take, and camouflage.

LOCOREGIONAL FLAPS

After healing by secondary intention and skin grafting, other techniques of facial resurfacing involve some form of "locoregional flaps." There are a number of different flaps available for wound closure, many of which utilize similar principles. Flap nomenclature has been inconsistent throughout the literature yet it should allow for accurate communication and identification.

NOMENCLATURE

There are four systems of flap classification, each based on different features of flaps: (1) blood supply, (2) area of origin, (3) tissue content, and

(4) method of transfer. These systems can be used interchangeably, but the terminology should be precise. The blood supply to the skin of the face comes from larger vessels in the subcutaneous tissues or deep to the mimetic musculature. Flaps containing the larger, named vessels are considered pedicled flaps and can have an indefinite length so long as that vessel is included and preserved. Axial pattern flaps are based on a linearly arranged series of small vessels in the subcutaneous plane. They usually course parallel to the underlying named vessel. Random pattern flaps are dependent on the subdermal plexus. Most teachings say there is a critical length to width ratio for these flaps, beyond which the margins are jeopardized. The face is clearly more forgiving and the length may be stretched to greater than five times the pedicle width. It is speculated that flap length survival does not follow a linear relationship to pedicle width and that flap necrosis occurs at a relatively fixed distance.[1]

The area of origin system refers to the region of the donor site with respect to the defect. Traditionally, local flaps imply the use of tissue adjacent to the defect, such as rhombic flaps. Regional flaps are those that are within the head or neck but separated from the defect by an area of intact skin. Distal flaps originate from below the clavicle and include waltzing flaps and free flaps. Recently, most flaps from within the face are considered as local flaps and those from the neck and chest (nape of neck, deltopectoral, pectoralis myocutaneous) are considered regional.

The tissue content system refers to the embryologic cell line contained in the flap. Most locoregional flaps are limited to ectodermal tissues. Muscle can be included as myocutaneous or myofascial flaps. These are infrequently needed in facial resurfacing except when bulk is desired. Composite flaps, strictly speaking, refer to all three embryologic layers, ectoderm, mesoderm, and endoderm. In practical usage, they are flaps that include cartilage or bone with skin.

The final classification system refers to the method of transfer. There are a number of terms used to describe local flaps. Translocation is the elevation and mobilization of any skin flap. This is a global term applying to all flaps. Advancement is sliding the flap in a linear direction and includes mobilization for primary closure as well as more involved flaps such as the "V-Y" advancement. Rotation flaps create an arc to their mobilization by pivoting around a point outside their base. Transposition involves elevation and moving the flap over an incomplete bridge of skin that remains undisturbed, e.g., bilobed. Interposition implies two adjacent flaps, both mobilized and crossed in order to fill each other's defect, e.g., Z-plasty. The relative positions of the transposition and interposition flaps are similar when completed. An interpolation flap crosses over an intact, complete bridge of skin, thus creating a pedicle that needs future division and inset at a second stage. This pedicle may or may not contain a named vessel and nourishes the flap until revascularization occurs from the wound bed. Island flaps are similar to interpolation flaps but the pedicle is deepithelialized and tunnelled under the bridge of skin, obviating the need for the second stage.

Distal flaps are transferred to the facial defect by either direct or indirect means. The principle of direct transfer resembles an interpolation flap but is from a distal origin and crosses more than a bridge of skin. An example is the Italian Tagliacozzi flap using a pedicled upper arm skin flap for nasal resurfacing. Indirect transfer involves a temporary carrier site for nutrient supply to the flap. The migration and "waltzing" methods are examples of this type of flap.

PRIMARY CLOSURE

Primary closure can be used for many small defects and select larger ones. Attention should be paid to meticulous soft-tissue technique and wide undermining. Standing cones are often negligible when the terminal angles are less then 30 degrees. Small cones will flatten with time, especially those in areas of elastic skin (cheek). Incisions are placed along RSTLs and advancement is done along lines of maximal extensibility. Undermining is done with the use of the scalpel and skin hooks and always continues around the apices of the wound. Undermining is avoided near mobile structures such as the lip so as to avoid distortion of natural aesthetic borders.

Many efforts focus on improving the camouflage of the resultant scar. A variety of suture materials are used but are probably secondary to strategic incision placement, eversion, and placement of edges at precisely the same level. Wound closure is done with buried, absorbable, subcuticular sutures and skin edges are reapproximated with running, locked, fast-absorbing gut sutures.

Synthetic glues have a variety of surgical applications. The cyanoacrylate derivatives are biocompatible glues with the most clinical experience. Those with a shorter side chain attached to the parent compound, in general, have a greater local toxicity, i.e., methyl- and ethyl-2-cyanoacrylate (Krazy glue) are more poorly tolerated than isobutyl- and butyl-2-cyanoacrylate (Histocryl).[22] Glues have been used for surface wound closure with no tension and appear to work well, saving operative time. Final scar appearance is probably not improved, however. There are anecdotal experiences of local reaction and extruding glue when used in buried tissues, such as stabilization of cartilage grafts during rhinoplasty.

ADVANCEMENT

Advancement flaps are those mobilized in a linear direction, either unilaterally or bilaterally. Incisions are generally parallel with RSTLs and should conform to lines of minimal tension, natural furrows, and borders of aesthetic units for better camouflage. Resultant defects are closed primarily by repeated halving. Rarely, Burrow's triangles are excised. The V-Y flap and its variations, such as the Reiger glabellar flap,[23] are popular modifications of a unilateral advancement flap.

A bipedicled flap with a relaxing incision is a form of advancement that is useful when closing a wide elliptical defect in proximity to strategic structures (Fig 4). The bipedicled flap slides to fill the primary defect, while creating a secondary defect which is both narrower and further away from important structures. This can then be closed primarily.

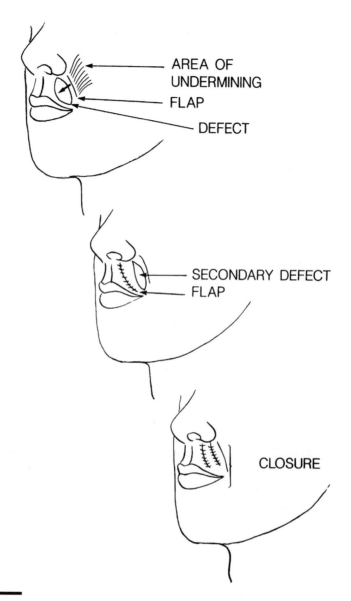

FIGURE 4.

Bipedicle advancement flap for broad elliptical defects located close to critical structures.

ROTATION

Rotation flaps pivot around a point to fill a generally triangular defect and leave a curved scar which should conform to RSTLs. The arc of the flap is usually four times the width of the base of the defect but can easily be extended as necessary. Elevation is in the subcutaneous plane creating a broad-based random donor flap. Standing cones are often eliminated by making the defect triangular in shape. The secondary defect is closed primarily by halving. Excision of Burrow's triangles on the opposite side of the flap may facilitate the rotation by suspending the flap and reducing tension but are seldom needed. Scalp defects are particularly suited for large rotation flaps but should be six times the defect because of the lack of extensibility.

The cervicofacial advancement-rotation flap is one of the most frequently used flaps for cheek resurfacing. Incisions are best concealed when in the meilolabial fold, nasal-facial groove, subciliary crease, lateral periorbital furrow, preauricular crease, and posterior neck. Special attention is made to avoid dragging the lateral canthal incision inferiorly and to preserving the sideburns and/or preauricular hair tufts. The lower lid skin is thin and elevated directly off the orbicularis oculi muscle. Skin from the lateral canthal area will replace the lid skin and is similarly elevated in the immediate subdermal plane rather than the usual face-lift plane. When necessary, the flap can extend back to include the postauricular, nonhair-bearing skin, thus creating a large bilobed cervicofacial flap.[24] This postauricular defect is then resurfaced with a skin graft or closed primarily. The cervical portion should be elevated in the subplatysmal plane for enhanced vascularity. The inferior limit can incorporate a deltopectoral flap. Generally, the arc of the flap is four times the width of the defect. Two important maneuvers are performed to suspend the cheek flap. First, a tacking stitch is placed from the deep aspect of the flap to the periosteum of the lateral orbital rim, thereby suspending the flap superiorly and releasing all tension on the lower lid. Secondly, SMAS suspension stitches are placed to suspend it to the pyriform aperature superomedially. This maneuver seems to provide a smoother contour to the cheek and may yield more lasting results.

TRANSPOSITION/INTERPOSITION

These are a versatile series of flaps which bring in local tissue, change the direction of scars, lengthen scars, and control tension on adjacent structures. Examples of these include rhombic, bilobed, Z-plasty, and meilolabial flaps.

The rhombic transposition flap is popular flap with great flexibility in that it can be designed in multiple directions around the defect. The resultant scar and tension are predictable and should be borne in mind when selecting the flap orientation. The direction of maximum tension should always align with the lines of maximal extensibility. The flap brings tissue from a single direction and tends not to distort other adjacent structures (Fig 5).

Bilobed flaps also utilize tissue from a single direction. The primary lobe should be equal in size to the defect and the secondary lobe should be half that size. The defect from the second lobe is closed primarily. The lobes are traditionally at 90 degree angles to each other but they can be blunted to 45 degrees with a triangular defect.[25] The bilobed flap should always be inferiorly based in order to minimize flap edema and late "pincushioning." In spite of this, wound contracture tends to lead to flap thickening and poor cosmesis.

The interposition Z-plasty is a common surgical maneuver used for several functions. It will break a linear scar, lengthen the central limb,

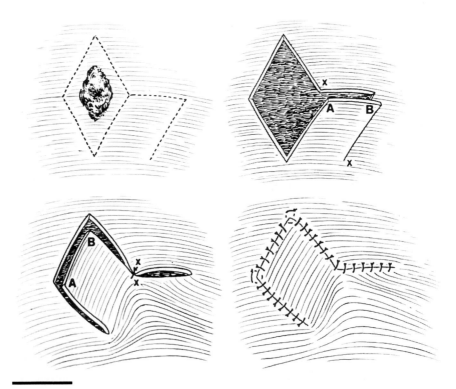

FIGURE 5.

Rhombic flap. Note direction of maximum tension at point x designed to run parallel with lines of maximal extensibility, i.e., perpendicular to RSTLs.

and fill small defects. Classically, each of the three limbs are equal in length and create equal and opposite angles. Variations on this theme are used for such maneuvers as alar interposition for vestibular stenosis.

Meilolabial flaps, when used for single stage resurfacing, often cross over an incomplete bridge of skin and cover nasal or perioral defects. Although the donor site is well hidden, the flap will inevitably blunt a natural groove as it pivots. In addition, there will be asymmetry in melar fullness and a small standing cone is created.

INTERPOLATION

Interpolation flaps cross an intact bridge of skin and are staged for future pedicle division and inset. Meilolabial flaps may be used in an interpolated fashion. They are axial flaps that are useful for lip, columellar, and nasal defects. Interpolating the meilolabial flap has distinct advantages in preserving the alarfacial groove and maintaining melar tissue and symmetry. Large scalping forehead flaps are axial flaps based on the superficial temporal and supraorbital vessels. They provide a large surface coverage but are infrequently utilized because of the unacceptable donor site scar.

The midline forehead flap is a flap frequently used in large nasal resurfacing. Its anatomic basis has been well described.[26] A precise, three-dimensional template is made using the aluminum wrapping of a suture packet. The portion of the flap that will be used for resurfacing is elevated in the subdermal plane, effectively thinning the flap during elevation. The frontalis muscle is left down and allows for more rapid healing by secondary intention and a more aesthetic donor site without the central depression. The forehead flap is often referred to as a pedicled myocutaneous flap. In fact, the layer of the flap that is utilized for coverage does not contain the supratrochlear vessels themselves. Vigorous thinning of the flap leaves it dependent on the subdermal plexus alone. The dependability of the flap is the result of an axial orientation to that vascular plexus; it is effectively an axially oriented random flap. Subtle variations in flap thickness are made during elevation to accommodate for differences in skin thickness over the nose, e.g., thick supratip and nasion skin versus thin rhinion skin. Once beyond the point where the flap is utilized for resurfacing, the dissection drops to the subgaleal plane, deep to the frontalis muscle, thus providing a vascular pedicle to the flap. This pedicle is narrowed to 1.0 cm at the orbital rim. Muscle fibers are cut in a layer-by-layer fashion in this area, taking care to be on either side of the supratrochlear vessels. The nasal defect is reconstructed after internal lining and skeletal structure are reestablished. The region of the soft-tissue triangle of the nose may be left to granulate secondarily, creating a natural appearing web. Most forehead donor sites less than 3.5 cm are closed primarily and larger defects are left to granulate.[27] A transverse incision along the hairline allows bilateral advancement flaps to assist with the closure. This hairline incision is made in a jagged fashion as a series of small W-plasty's. This tends to camouflage the incision as well as eliminate the lateral standing cones. Galeotomies close to the edges of the donor site "closing" flaps will increase the extensibility of the flaps. Pedicle division is usually done at 3 weeks postoperatively. Little additional thinning is required. Dermabrasion is done at 6 to 8 weeks. The benefit of delayed pedicle division beyond 3 weeks when free cartilage grafts are utilized has not yet been defined. For select cases, the skin of the pedicle is excised as a wedge and closed on itself, thereby completing the flap in a single stage. One can expect a fullness in the glabellar area with this maneuver. At very select times the pedicle can be deepithelialized and tunneled under the glabellar skin, effectively creating an island flap. The procerus muscle is debulked to minimize fullness in this area. Again, this completes the forehead flap in a single stage.

SPECIAL FLAP

More distant pedicled flaps can be harvested for special situations in which vascularized tissue is needed. The superficial temporoparietal facial flap is gaining wide popularity as both a pedicled and free flap. It has a dependable vascular supply that easily supports a skin graft, is easily harvested, and carries minimal bulk. It is particularly suited for such areas as skull base resurfacing and auricular reconstruction. The submental island flap has been recently described and can be applied as either a pedicled or free flap for large facial resurfacing.[28] It is based on the submental artery and includes a relatively large paddle of submental skin. Unfortunately, it is probably too bulky for most cutaneous defects of the face and appears to leave significant donor site morbidity.

REGIONAL DEFECTS

SCALP

Most scalp defects are repaired with relatively large rotation flaps. The subgaleal plane is easily lifted and provides a dependable flap. Larger defects are best resurfaced temporarily with skin grafts and later revised with serial excisions. Rapid, intraoperative tissue expansion can increase coverage by a few centimeters. Several 30 mL Foley catheters are hyperinflated in three cycles.[29] Excessive tension can cause separation and alopecia. When a large scalp defect cannot support a graft, i.e., there is no pericranium covering calvarium, either free vascularized tissue is utilized or scattered partial-thickness burr holes are made into the diploic space to promote granulation tissue, which will then subsequently support a graft.

FOREHEAD

Defects of the forehead are usually resurfaced with some form of advancement flaps based laterally. The hairline and brow position will restrict options that exert two-directional tension. Transverse incisions along the hairline are maximally camouflaged by a running W-plasty. Incisions at the hairline may be further concealed by bevelling them such that hair will grow through the nonhair-bearing side. Vertical lines in the midline are better concealed than paramedian lines.

BROW

Hair-bearing tissue can be brought in through punch grafts, strip grafts, or as a pedicled flap from the temple area. It is critical to orient the hair shafts in the same direction as the native brow hairs. In spite of this, grafted hair patches do not conceal well.

PERIORBITAL

Medial canthal defects, by nature of their concavity, lend themselves well to healing by secondary intention. The webbing which occurs conforms to concave surfaces nicely. Larger medial canthal defects can be repaired with a modified Rieger glabellar flap (Fig 6). The Rieger flap is a combination of advancement and rotation of glabellar skin that may be based on the contralateral supratrochlear vessels.

Eyelid defects can be anterior lamellar (skin and orbicularis muscle) and/or posterior lamellar (tarsus and conjunctiva). Many small skin defects can be closed primarily and should be done in a vertical orientation so as to minimize downward pull on the lid margins. Horizontal incisions clearly heal well but may cause lid edema and ectropion. Thin, full-thickness skin grafts are an effective solution to some superficial defects. Larger anterior lamellar defects are best resurfaced with cervicofacial flaps. Incisions should be in the subciliary margin and along the nasal-facial groove, although this often means expanding the original defect.

Reconstruction of full-thickness defects of the lid must also address the skeletal support and internal lining. Many of the principles for lip repair apply also to eyelid defects. Up to one-half of a lid may be repaired primarily. A lateral cantholysis and lateral canthal undermining will improve horizontal mobilization. Larger defects require special techniques. The Mustarde technique utilizes free septal composite flaps to replace the posterior lamella but depends on the cheek flap for vascular support. A tarsoconjunctival flap (Hughes flap) can be advanced from the undersurface of the upper lid, based on a conjunctival and Mueller's muscle pedicle, with staged pedicle division in 4 weeks.

TEMPLE

The temple is usually resurfaced with curvilinear advancement flaps along RSTLs. It can be thought of as an extension of the forehead area and similar principles apply. Rhombic and bilobed transposition flaps are acceptable alternatives for this region.

NOSE

The art of nasal reconstruction dates back thousands of years to India where the nose was regarded as a symbol of prestige and honor, and to where it was a common form of punishment to mutilate or amputate the nose. Our understanding of nasal reconstruction has come a long way. One must focus on the three separate layers of the nose, internal lining, structural support, and soft tissue coverage. During the reconstruction, it is important to maintain the nose in its natural functional position, specifically, with dentures and bridges in place. Internal lining must be reestablished in order to prevent subsequent contracture and notching. Options for internal lining include skin or mucosal grafts, a variety of internal nasal mucosal flaps, epithelial turn-in flaps, a separate locoregional flap, or hinging the cutaneous flap on itself. Lining may be adequate with nonepithelial tissue such as temporoparietal fascia or pericranium, especially when part of a well-vascularized flap. Replacing structural support is critical and does not aim to mimic the natural anatomic positions. Alar rim and valve areas need specific support to resist the forces of healing and contracture. Numerous materials for implantation are available, such as autogenous cartilage (conchal, septal, rib), autogenous bone (calvarial, rib, iliac crest), alloplastic (sialastic, supramid, mersilene, proplast, gortex) and irradiated homograft rib. They each have their advantages and limitations, a complete discussion of which is beyond this text.

The principle of aesthetic subunits is especially important in reconstruction of the nose. Defects that violate a substantial portion of the subunit are often extended in order to resurface the unit in its entirety. Furthermore, square corners are created leaving a more camouflaged reconstruction. Soft-tissue coverage for superficial lesions less than 1.5 cm are best reconstructed with full-thickness skin grafts harvested from the meilolabial fold region. This provides excellent color and texture match. Small rim defects (less than 1 cm) are repaired with composite ear cartilage grafts, usually in a delayed manner. Larger defects require locoregional flaps. The Rieger advancement/rotation flap lends itself to proximal nasal lesions, but when used for distal nasal defects, wound contrac-

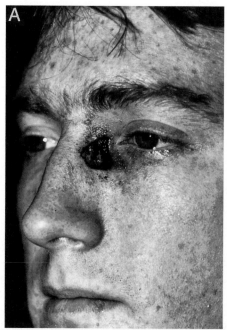

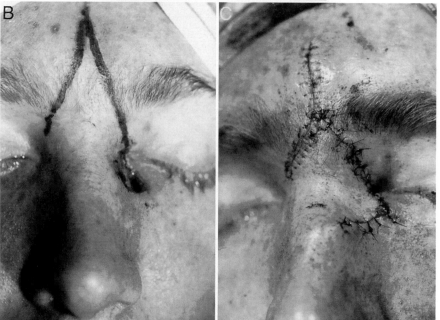

FIGURE 6.
A, medial canthal/upper nasal defect. **B,** outline of Rieger glabellar flap. **C,** advancement and rotation of flap into defect. **D** and **E,** 6-month follow-up.

(Continued.)

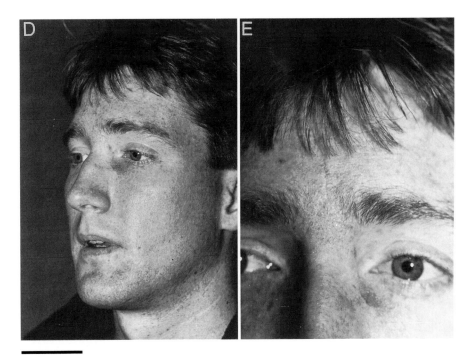

FIGURE 6 (cont.).

tion tends to cause notching or cephalic rotation. Bilobed and rhombic flaps are rarely used here because they often cross several aesthetic subunits and tend to "pincushion." Cheek advancement flaps are tempting but leave noticeable blunting of the nasal-facial groove. Interpolated flaps, either forehead or meilolabial, are the workhorses for large nasal resurfacing (Fig 7). Many defects in this region are repaired with multiple flaps, each used for a given aesthetic unit or subunit.

CHEEK

Small defects are readily closed with a large number of local advancement or transposition flaps. Whichever flap is chosen, it is deliberately designed such that resultant incisions will follow RSTLs. Larger defects are best repaired with the cervicofacial advancement-rotation flap (Fig 8). On rare occasions, a free flap is needed for thick defects, especially those involving bone.

LIP AND PERIORAL

Superficial lesions of the vermillion are resurfaced with mucosal advancement or rotation flaps from the gingival-labial sulcus. When a muscle deficit exists, however, one should convert it to a wedge defect with a three-layered, primary closure. This maintains lip height, bulk, and function. Larger defects (one-third to two-thirds) are repaired with a lip switch flap based on the labial artery, Abbe flaps or Estlander flaps (with lateral commissure involvement). Subtotal defects can be repaired with the Gilles fan flap or Bernard-Burrow-Webster flap. Currently, most major recon-

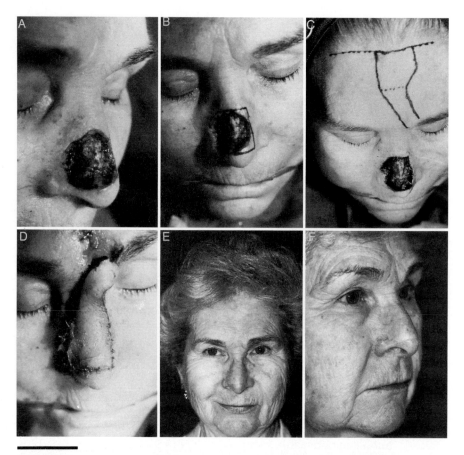

FIGURE 7.

A, nasal defect. **B,** squaring off of corners. **C,** outline of midline forehead flap based on contralateral supratrochlear vessels. **D,** forehead flap turned. **E** and **F,** 12-month follow-up.

structions utilize the Karapandzic flap, which maintains lip function and sensation. A management protocol for lip lesions and detailed operative description of the various flaps can be found.[30]

CHIN

Isolated chin defects are uncommon. Most are repaired with primary closure along RSTLs. Deep undermining and advancement is performed in an attempt to maintain bulk and projection.

NECK

A majority of neck skin defects can be closed primarily with adequate undermining. Additional tissue can be brought in from the posterior region of the neck or from the chest. Most resurfacing challenges come from metastatic neoplasms involving cervical skin. In these situations, bulk as well as cutaneous coverage is desired and musculocutaneous flaps are preferred.

COMPLICATIONS

Complications in locoregional flaps can be found early or late. Early complications refer to those that occur during the first stages of wound healing. Hematoma formation is usually a sequela to inadequate intraoperative hemostasis or the patient straining and bucking. We routinely use pressure dressings on all major flaps and do not use drains. Hematomas under the flap will not only impede neovascularization but also may release toxins that are detrimental to the flap. We recommend early evacuation once the clot is lysed. Infection is notably uncommon in the face

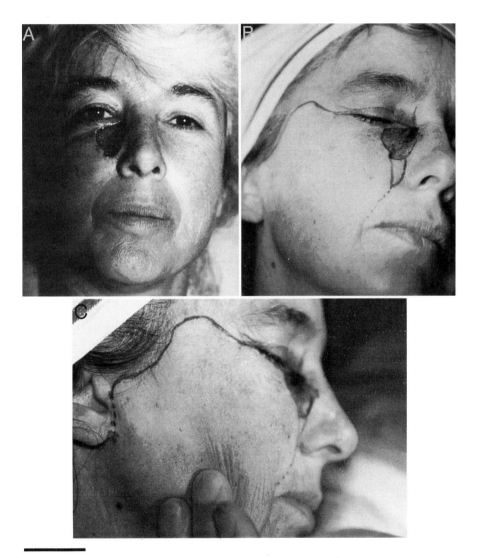

FIGURE 8.

A, medial cheek defect. **B,** inferior wedge excision along nasofacial and meilolabial groove. **C,** superior and lateral limbs of cheek flap. Note cephalic position along lateral canthus. **D** and **E,** cheek flap elevated and rotated into position. Suspension suture to periosteum of lateral orbital rim. **F** and **G,** 9-month follow-up.

(Continued.)

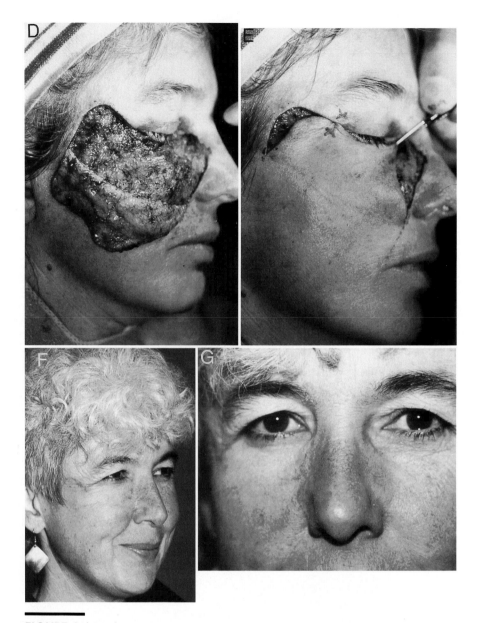

FIGURE 8 (cont.).

and is usually related to ischemic tissue or hematoma. Wound separation is the result of excess tension, inadequate sutures, insufficient sutures, or ischemia. The most nerve-wracking early complication is impending flap loss or necrosis. A number of efforts look at early detection and minimizing final flap loss. Flap enhancement is discussed additionally below. Once necrosis has occurred, the wound is managed conservatively and allowed to heal secondarily.

Late complications occur during mature scar formation. Pincushioning occurs for three reasons:

1. The natural direction of lymphatic drainage within the flap is disrupted with superiorly based flaps.
2. Venous and lymphatic egress is further blocked by a sheet of scar tissue.
3. Normal wound contracture around the periphery causes the flap to bunch together.

Corticosteroids seem to diminish this effect but excessive application will cause significant atrophy. Another late complication is hypertrophic scar formation. At times this is uncontrollable as some patients have a predisposition for such scars. Excessive tension clearly has a contributory effect. Some of the attempts at pharmacologically manipulating this process have been discussed earlier. Silcone sheeting applied topically can have a dramatic effect on hypertrophic scars, particularly in softening the texture and reducing the exophytic nature of them. The mechanism of action has not been clearly delineated, although it has achieved clinical success. Dermabrasion and scar revision are performed later as needed.

FLAP ENHANCEMENT

Tissue expansion can enhance flap coverage for a number of resurfacing problems. Conventional expansion occurs over 4 to 6 weeks and yields a lasting and dependable increase in surface area. There are disadvantages in the prolonged cosmetic deformity, obligatory two stages, and possible implant extrusion and infection. Intraoperative, rapid expansion can facilitate closure of secondary defects from locoregional flaps.[29] They expand tissue by a phenomenon termed "mechanical creep," which works primarily by two mechanisms: squeezing fluid and ground substance from the tissue and effectively dehydrating it, and recruiting adjacent tissue. Rapidly expanded flaps will promptly contract and one should not utilize such tissues for soft tissue coverage in a one-to-one fashion. In addition, the favorable physiologic response to conventional expansion is not achieved with rapid expansion, i.e., neovascularization and realignment of collagen and elastic bundles do not occur.

Surgical delay will enhance viability of locoregional flaps. It is thought that local hypoxia around the flap margins causes increased collateral vascularity and an axial orientation to the subcutaneous vascular flow. There is the obvious disadvantage of the second stage. Nonsurgical delay with suture techniques and Argon laser subdermal photocoagulation seems to provide similar results to surgical bipedicle delay and may prove clinically useful in the reconstructive armamentarium.

Pharmacologic enhancement of flap viability is a growing and exciting area of surgical experimentation; however, no conclusive protocol has been defined. Flap edema is an unavoidable sequela that compromises viability through congestion, microvascular compression, and ischemia. Steroids and nonsteroidal anti-inflammatory agents serve to minimize this edema and may improve flap perfusion and healing postoperatively. Perioperative use does not have a detrimental effect on wound maturation and strength. We routinely use 10 mg of dexamethasone preoperatively. Dextran is often used in the setting of venous thrombosis, pulmonary embolism, arterial bypass surgery, or microvascular transfer. It causes reduced platelet adhesiveness and procoagulant activity, and in the rabbit model, has been shown to reduce thrombosis at the microvascular level. This suggests that the reduced viscosity may have a beneficial effect to marginally viable flap.[31] Calcium channel blockers can serve to improve flap survival in several different ways.[32] A direct vasodilating action is observed in the microcirculation as well as in larger caliber vessels, thereby improving flap perfusion. Furthermore, calcium channel blockers have an inhibitory effect on the production of superoxide free radicals, possibly reducing ischemia-reperfusion injury. Although we are not in the habit of administering verapamil after flap reconstruction, future clinical studies may enlighten its efficacy. Pentoxifylline is a methylxanthine derivative with clinical success in patients with peripheral vascular disease and intermittent claudication. It decreases blood viscosity, improves filtration rate, and reduces platelet and erythrocyte aggregation. There are several animal studies looking at the effects of pentoxifylline on healing and viability of random and musculocutaneous flaps.[33–35] The results are conflicting. Some of the studies showing improved flap survival use much higher doses of the drug (60 mg/kg/day)[35] and others use prolonged pretreatment at 2 weeks.[36] Nonetheless, it does show promise as we await clinical trials.

Medical grade leeches (Hirudo medicinalis) are still an effective way to reduce venous congestion within a flap. They are indicated for marginal flaps that are suffering from venous congestion but have adequate arterial perfusion. They are applied directly to the flap surface and will suck venous blood and automatically detach when complete. There are obvious social and practical hurdles to overcome before wide acceptance of this technique.

Hyperbaric oxygen has an established role in salvage of radionecrosis of tissues with an obliterative microcirculation. There are financial and practical obstacles for common use but it would likely enhance the flap with impending necrosis.

Sympathetic denervation to a flap has been done in the animal model and demonstrated impaired neovascularization and possibly oxygen free radical production.[37] The precise mechanism of this is not clear but there is a suggestion that a local hyperadrenergic state arises and causes capillary vasoconstriction and ischemia. In addition, oxygen free radical scavengers exert a beneficial effect on the denervated flaps in contrast to the innervated ones, implicating free radicals in the delayed neovascularization of denervated flaps.

Theoretically, cooling the marginal flap may diminish local metabolic activity and demands. Applying ice packs to a pale flap is not common practice but may have favorable effects. We routinely apply ice to periorbital areas when they are manipulated. Conversely, heat application may enhance vascular perfusion with vasodilatation. No controlled studies in this regard have been performed.

A combination of agents may work together in a synergistic fashion. Pentoxifylline and hyperbaric oxygen have been tried.[38] Enhancing perfusion with thinning agents used in conjunction with leeches may also improve survival.

Inhalational anesthetic agents have an effect on random skin flap survival. The mechanism by which this occurs is speculative but nitrous oxide and halothane appear to have a deleterious effect as compared to isoflurane in the animal model.[39]

Autologous tissue harvested and cloned in vitro for autotransplantation and reconstruction of the head and neck is one of the more exciting advances that have been made. Epidermal cell culture has a role in major resurfacing problems, such as with near total-body burns. Fascia lata seeded with epidermal cells has been shown to promote rapid epithelialization and tissue ingrowth for full-thickness skin defects.[40] Autogenous mesenchymal tissue cultures may prove to be the implant material of the future. There is much controversy over the various implants available. Alloplastic materials are criticized for their lack of biocompatability and carcinogenic potential. Autogenous implants are associated with resorption, donor site morbidity, and warping. Cultured autogenous cartilage that grows in the predetermined, three-dimensional configuration of a template would have explosive opportunities in areas of facial augmentation and recontouring structural support.[41] It may become the tissue of choice because of its tissue compatibility and viability. The potential for growth makes it particularly attractive for microtia repair and other pediatric implantations. Additionally, it may have great applications in ossicular reconstruction and joint replacement.

CONCLUSION

Facial reconstruction dates back for millennia to the Indian forehead flap used for nasal reconstruction. In some general ways things are not that different today. Our depth of understanding and the technical details of intervention, however, continue to grow. Conservative methods of secondary healing and skin grafting have made advances in the molecular and pharmacologic manipulation of the natural healing process. Locoregional flaps are more creative and dependable than in the past. Our understanding of the dynamics of wound healing, as well as the application of sound aesthetic principles, has brought the art of facial resurfacing closer to restoring a functional and camouflaged unit. Flap enhancement, somatic gene therapy, and autologous in vitro tissue cultures as new implant materials are on the cutting edge of the next frontier in locoregional flaps for facial resurfacing.

REFERENCES

1. Milton S: Fallacy of the length-width ratio. Br J Plast Surg 57:502, 1970.
2. Borges AF, Alexander JE: Relaxed skin tension lines, Z-plasties on scars, and fusiform excision of lesions. Br J Plast Surg 15:242, 1962.
3. Mitz V, Peyronie M: The superficial musculoaponeurotic system (SMAS) in the parotid and cheek area. Plast Reconstr Surg 58:80–88, 1976.
4. Burget GC, Menick FJ: Subunit principle in nasal reconstruction. Plast Reconstr Surg 76:239, 1985.

5. Odland PB, Murakami CS: Healing by secondary intention. *Operative Tech Otolaryngol-Head Neck Surg* 4:54–60, 1993.

6. Brown GL, Curtsinger L, Jurkiewicz MJ, et al: Stimulation of healing of chronic wounds by epidermal growth factor. *Plast Reconstr Surg* 88:189–196, 1991.

7. Seppa H, Brotendorst G, Seppa S, et al: Platelet-derived growth factor is chemotactic for fibroblasts. *J Cell Biol* 92:584, 1982.

8. Shah M, Foreman DM, Ferguson MWJ: Control of scarring in adult wounds by neutralising antibody to transforming growth factor B. *Lancet* 339:213–214, 1992.

9. Kimbrough TD, Shernan S, Ziegler TR, et al: Insulin-like growth factor-I response is comparable following intravenous and subcutaneous administration of growth hormone. *J Surg Res* 51:472–476, 1991.

10. Moller S, Jensen M, Svensson P, et al: Insulin-like growth factor 1 (IGF-1) in burn patients. *Burns* 17:279–281, 1991.

11. Yeo T-K, Brown L, Dvorak HF: Alterations in proteoglycan synthesis common to healing wounds and tumors. *Am J Pathol* 138:1437–1450, 1991.

12. Ozcan G, Shenaq S, Chahadeh H, et al: Ultraviolet-A induced delayed wound contraction and decreased collagen content in healing wounds and implant capsules. *Plast Reconstr Surg* 92:480–484, 1993.

13. Larrabee WF, personal communication, 1993.

14. Ledbetter MS, Morykwas MJ, Ditesheim JA, et al: The effects of partial and total amniotic fluid exclusion on excisional fetal rabbit wounds. *Ann Plast Surg* 27:139–145, 1991.

15. Politis MJ, Zanakis MF, Miller JE: Enhanced survival of full-thickness skin grafts following the application of DC electrical fields. *Plast Reconstr Surg* 84:267–272, 1989.

16. Cooper ML, Laxer JA, Hansbrough JF: The cytotoxic effects of commonly used topical antimicrobial agents on human fibroblasts and keratinocytes. *J Trauma* 31:775–784, 1991.

17. Boyce ST, Holder IA: Selection of topical antimicrobial agents for cultured skin for burns by combined assessment of cellular cytotoxicity and antimicrobial activity. *Plast Reconstr Surg* 92:493–500, 1993.

18. Bauer BS, Vicari FA, Richard ME, et al: Expanded full-thickness skin grafts in children: Case selection, planning, and management. *Plast Reconstr Surg* 92:59–69, 1993.

19. Katz AE, Grande DJ: Purse-string closure of defects. *Operative Techniques in Otolaryngol-Head Neck Surg* 4:71–75, 1993.

20. Saltz R, Sierra D, Feldman D, et al: Experimental and clinical applications of fibrin glue. *Plast Reconstr Surg* 88:1005–1017, 1991.

21. Brown DM, Barton BR, Young VL, et al: Decreased wound contraction with fibrin glue-treated skin grafts. *Arch Surg* 127:404–406, 1992.

22. Toriumi DM, Raslan WF, Friedman M, et al: Histotoxicity of cyanoacrylate tissue adhesives: A comparative study. *Arch Otolaryngol Head Neck Surg* 116:546–550, 1990.

23. Reiger RA: A local flap for repair of the nasal tip. *Plast Reconstr Surg* 49:147, 1967.

24. Cook TA, Israel JM, Wang TD, et al: Cervical rotation flaps for midface resurfacing. *Arch Otolaryngol Head Neck Surg* 117:77–82, 1991.

25. Zitelli JA: The bilobed flap for nasal reconstruction. *Arch Dermatol* 125:957, 1989.

26. Shumrick KA, Smith TL: The anatomic basis for the design of forehead flaps in nasal reconstruction. *Arch Otolaryngol Head Neck Surg* 118:373–379, 1992.

27. Quatela VC, personal communication, forthcoming publication.
28. Martin D, Pacal JF, Baudet J, et al: The submental island flap: A new donor site. Anatomy and clinical applications as a free or pedicled flap. *Plast Reconstr Surg* 92:867–873, 1993.
29. Baker SR, Swanson NA: Rapid intraoperative tissue expansion in reconstruction of the head and neck. *Arch Otolaryngol Head Neck Surg* 116:1431–1434, 1990.
30. Cupp CL, Larrabee WF: Reconstruction of the lips. *Operative Tech Otolaryngol-Head Neck Surg* 4:46–53, 1993.
31. Rothkopf DM, Chu B, Bern S, et al: The effect of Dextran on microvascular thrombosis in an experimental rabbit model. *Plast Reconstr Surg* 92:511–515, 1993.
32. Carpenter RJ, Angel MF, Amiss LR, et al: Verapamil enhances the survival of primary ischemic venous obstructed rodent skin flaps. *Arch Otolaryngol Head Neck Surg* 119:1015–1017, 1993.
33. Hodgson RS, Brummett RE, Cook TA: Effects of pentoxiphylline on experimental skin flap survival. *Arch Otolaryngol Head Neck Surg* 113:950–952, 1987.
34. Yessenow RS, Maves MD: The effects of pentoxifylline on random skin flap survival. *Arch Otolaryngol Head Neck Surg* 115:179–181, 1989.
35. Armstrong M, Kunar DR, Cummings CW: Effect of Pentoxifylline on myocutaneous flap viability in pigs. *Otolaryngol Head Neck Surg* 109:668–675, 1993.
36. Williams PB, Hankins DB, Layton CT, et al: Long-term pretreatment with pentoxifylline increases random skin flap survival. *Arch Otolaryngol Head Neck Surg* 120:65–71, 1994.
37. Im MJ, Beil RJ, Wong L, et al: Effects of sympathetic denervation and oxygen free radicals on neovascularization in skin flaps. *Plast Reconstr Surg* 92:736–741, 1993.
38. Nemiroff PM: Synergistic effects of Pentoxifylline and hyperbaric oxygen on skin flaps. *Arch Otolaryngol Head Neck Surg* 114:977–981, 1988.
39. Dohar JE, Goding GS, Maisel RH: The effects of the inhalational anesthetic agent combination, Isoflurane-nitrous oxide, on survival in a pig random skin flap model. *Arch Otolaryngol Head Neck Surg* 120:74–77, 1994.
40. Ross UH: In vitro production and subsequent transplantation of living skin substitute in rat model. *Eur Arch Otorhinolaryngol* 249:263–267, 1992.
41. Vacanti CA, Langer R, Schloo B, et al: Synthetic polymers seeded with chondrocytes provide a template for new cartilage formation. *Plast Reconstr Surg* 88:753–759, 1991.

Minimally Invasive Therapy for Sialolithiasis—The State of the Art

Heinrich Iro, M.D.
Department of Oto-Rhino-Laryngology, Head and Neck Surgery, University of Erlangen-Nuremberg, Erlangen, Germany

Johannes Zenk, M.D.
Department of Oto-Rhino-Laryngology, Head and Neck Surgery, University of Erlangen-Nuremberg, Erlangen, Germany

W. Benzel, M.D.
Department of Otorhinolaryngology, Head and Neck Surgery, University of Erlangen-Nuremberg, Erlangen, Germany

EPIDEMIOLOGY

Among the diseases of the large salivary glands in the head and neck region, sialolithiasis accounts for more than 50% of the overall number of cases and is thus the most common cause of acute and chronic infections[1] (Fig 1). According to Rauch,[2] the prevalence of sialolithiasis is about 1.2%. Salivary calculi predominate in patients in their 30s and 40s and preferentially occur in male patients.

In our own study comprising 402 patients, however, manifestation of sialolithiasis was noted in 16 patients below the age of 20. Eighty percent of all salivary duct stones develop in the submandibular (Wharton's) duct, followed by about 20% that occur in the parotid (Stensen's) duct. A formation of sialoliths in the sublingual gland or in the smaller salivary glands is rarely observed (0% to 2%).

A simultaneous lithiasis in more than one salivary gland is uncommon,[3] although four of our patients suffered from a concomitant disease of both parotid glands (n=2) or both submandibular glands (n=2).

PATHOPHYSIOLOGY

Generalized stone development in the urinary tract, the bile duct system, and the salivary ducts has been documented in 6% to 10% of the patient population. Until now there has been no proof to corroborate the assumption that a metabolic disorder predisposes to this coincidental formation of concrements.

The clearly predominant occurrence of stones in the submandibular duct may result from the secretion of the submandibular gland being more

Advances in Otolarynogology—Head and Neck Surgery®, vol. 9
© 1995, Mosby–Year Book, Inc.

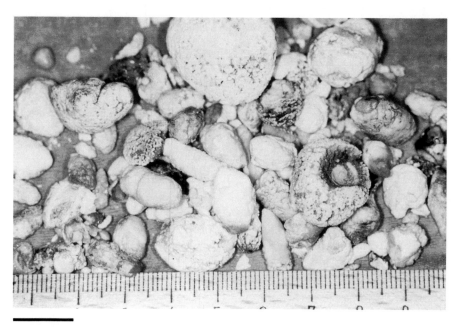

FIGURE 1.
Salivary duct calculi of different shapes, colors, and diameters.

mucinous than that of the parotid gland.[4] In addition, Wharton's duct forms an angulation in its course around the mylohyoid muscle and exhibits numerous diverticula in its distal segment. This can promote a stagnation of secretion, thus increasing the possibility of stone formation.[5] In spite of the large number of investigations on salivary gland disorders, the exact cause of sialolith formation still remains unclear. On one hand, inflammations, which may affect the colloidal equilibrium and cause subsequent gel formation ("mucoidgel") and a consecutive incorporation of inorganic material, are held responsible for the development of sialoliths.[6]

Moreover, foreign bodies could act as nuclei of crystallization.[4, 7] It is to be assumed, though, that local factors play a decisive role in lithogenesis, since only one salivary gland is affected in most cases. Solitary concrements are found in 80% of all salivary stones, whereas more than one stone is detected in the salivary duct in 20%.[2]

The composition of stones of the parotid duct differs from that of stones of the submandibular duct. While parotid duct stones are composed of up to 51% organic material and up to 49% inorganic material (the latter with a calcium contribution of 15%), the organic component of submandibular stones is only 18%, whereas the inorganic component is 82% (with a calcium contribution of 46%). The inorganic components are predominantly weddellite, whitelockite, and brushite.[8, 9]

The largest diameters of the salivary stones are in the range of 0.1 mm to 30 mm.[10] The mean diameters of stones found in our patients were 6.7 mm in the case of submandibular concrements, and 5.2 mm in the case of parotid concrements.

SYMPTOMS

The set of clinical complaints that accompanies sialolithiasis forms a typical pattern: if the duct system is partially or completely congested, colicky postprandial pain (resulting from induced secretion) and occasional very severe pain attacks, as well as swelling of the parenchyma of the affected glands, become manifest, with a variable degree of pain intensity between the attacks.[5]

If the concrement does not disappear spontaneously, an ascending retrograde infection of the duct and gland is promoted by the persisting congestion. In addition, continued retention of saliva not only leads to a dilation of the duct system but also to an increasing atrophy of the glandular parenchyma. Histologically, the changes occurring in the final stage of this chronic obstructive sialoadenitis are similar to those observed in gland atrophy caused by instrumental duct ligation or occlusion by a protein solution.[11, 12]

DIAGNOSIS

In general, the classification of clinical findings in patients presenting with sialolithiasis is typical: during examination and palpation a distinct

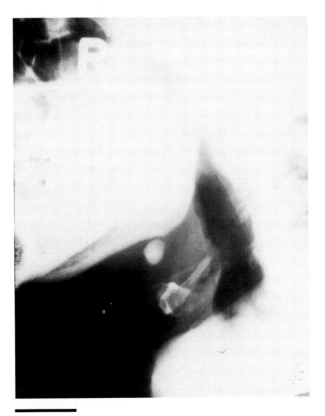

FIGURE 2.
Conventional roentgenogram of a sialolith of the right submandibular gland.

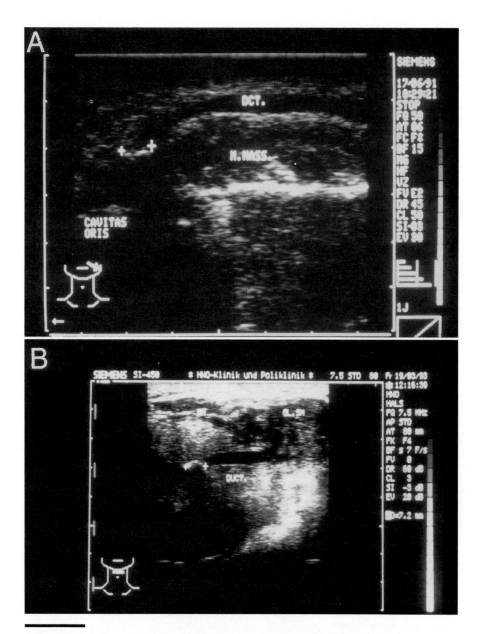

FIGURE 3.
A, sonographic image of a parotid duct stone (+. . .+, 6.6 mm in diameter) in the vicinity of the orifice of Stensen's duct, with the dilated duct *(DCT.)* behind, above the masseteric muscle (M. MASS.). **B,** sonographic image of a concrement (+. . .+, 7.2 mm in diameter) in the floor of the mouth congesting left Wharton's duct *(DUCT.)*. *GL. SM,* submandibular gland, *MM,* mylohyoid muscle.

and partly painful swelling is detected in the region of the affected salivary gland. In conventional radiography, 80% of the submandibular stones and 20% of the parotid stones are detectable (Fig 2). Because of their mineralogical components, 20% of the submandibular stones and 80% of the parotid stones are radiolucent.[13, 14]

The excellent axial resolution of high frequency ultrasound scanners

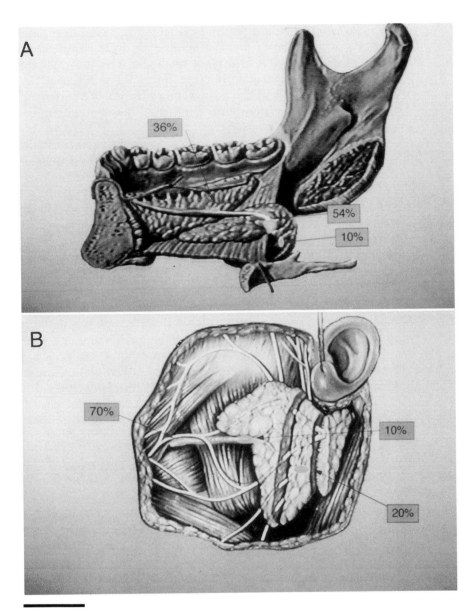

FIGURE 4.
A, frequencies of the different locations of the sialoliths in the submandibular gland. **B,** frequencies of the different locations of the sialoliths in the parotid gland.

allows concrements with diameters exceeding 1.5 mm to be detected in virtually all cases, independent of their mineralogical composition. Therefore, sonography should be the diagnostic imaging method of choice if sialolithiasis is suspected[15] (Fig 3,A and B). In inflammation-free intervals sialography may, in certain cases, provide additional information. With modern mini-endoscopes (external diameters of 0.6 to 2.0 mm) it is possible to examine the distal parts of the ducts and to verify the diagnosis by direct stone imaging. Scintigraphy of the salivary glands can give some general indications as to the secretory function of the afflicted gland.

It should be emphasized that the secretory function can regenerate completely after removal of the obstruction.[16, 17] In the application of modern minimally invasive treatment methods, it is essential not only to verify the diagnosis of sialolithiasis and to define the specific nature of the disorder, but to establish the exact localization of a concrement within the duct system important for a differential therapeutic approach which includes minimally invasive therapy.

Approximately 36% of all concrements in the submandibular duct are detectable in the vicinity of the ostium or in Wharton's duct as it passes through the floor of the mouth. In 54% of the cases the stones are located in the hilum and in 10% they are found in the intraglandular duct system (Fig 4,A). Seventy percent of the parotid stones are located in the distal part of Stensen's duct, 10% in the hilum, and 20% in the intraglandular duct system (Fig 4,B).

ESTABLISHED METHODS OF THERAPY (Table 1)

In the treatment of sialolithiasis no methods to dissolve concrements by medicaments have become available to date, nor has diet prophylaxis proven effective. This is in contrast to the treatment of stone diseases affecting the urogenital tract and especially the bile duct system; therefore, therapy of sialolithiasis has to be directed at complete stone removal. If stimulation of secretion, gland massage, or dilation of the orifice remain unsuccessful, the patient will have to undergo an operation.[18] If the concrement of the submandibular gland is lodged in the distal part of Wharton's duct near the orifice, the ductal orifice is enlarged by incision and the stone removed (Fig 5). In the case of more proximally positioned submandibular stones near the hilum, there is an imminent danger of injuring the lingual nerve when slitting the duct.[19]

Stenosis of Wharton's duct is rarely observed after performing duct incision. We reject an incision if sialolithiasis is detected in Stensen's duct, because of the danger of ductal strictures and stenosis resulting from scar formation.[20] Eight out of ten stenoses that occurred in the papillary region of the glandula parotis, which we observed during the last 4 years, were the result of incisions of the orifice of Stensen's duct that had been performed at other hospitals.

Up to now, surgical excision of the afflicted gland was required if removal of the concrement by careful probing and dilation or by incision

---

TABLE 1.
Established Therapies of Sialolithiasis

Established Methods of Therapy
    Sialagogues
    Duct dilation
    Duct slitting
    Gland extirpation
      (Chorda tympani neurectomy)

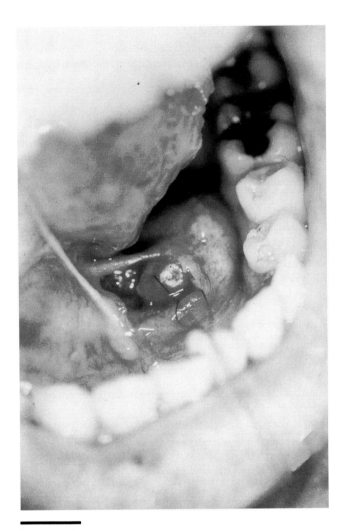

FIGURE 5.

Salivary stone coming out of left Wharton's duct after incision of the orifice.

of the duct was not successful. Complications that can arise during surgical removal of the submandibular gland, carried out using either general or local anaesthesia, include injuries of the mandibular branch of the facial nerve, of the lingual nerve, and of the hypoglossal nerve. These risks are well-described in the literature.[21, 22, 23]

Parotidectomy, which should be performed using general anaesthesia, bears the risk of causing irreversible injury to the facial nerve.[24] Frey's syndrome (gustatory sweating or auriculotemporal syndrome) is subjectively noticeable in 10% of the patients after parotidectomy and objectively detectable in nearly all patients.[25]

To spare patients suffering from a submandibular lithiasis the strain of undergoing submandibulectomy, Zalin and Cooney[26] recommended a tympanic neurectomy to reduce salivary secretion to a minimum by parasympathetic denervation of the submandibular gland. Following this transtympanally executed neurectomy a fairly rapid resolution of symptoms is noted, but this is accompanied by a partial loss of taste.[27] In addition, the concrement, as a possible source of consecutive infections, is left in the duct. Because of these disadvantages, tympanic neurectomy has not been able to assert itself as a therapeutic option.

NEW METHODS OF THERAPY

Efforts to establish minimally invasive methods in the treatment of sialo-lithiasis, i.e., to dispense with or to minimize surgical intervention, led to the introduction of intracorporeal, endoscopically controlled lithotripsy and extracorporeal, sonographically controlled lithotripsy as new treatment regimes in the management of sialolithiasis (Fig 6).

EXTRACORPOREAL SHOCKWAVE LITHOTRIPSY OF SALIVARY DUCT STONES

Extracorporeal shockwave lithotripsy (ESWL) was introduced in the treatment of kidney stones in 1980.[28] Within the last 13 years, 90% of all nephrotomies have been replaced by ESWL in the management of kidney stones.[29, 30] Extracorporeally, sonographically, and radiologically controlled lithotripsy also provides alternatives to cholecystectomy in treating noncalcified stones of the gallbladder. Furthermore, given certain indications, ESWL has also proved its effectiveness in the treatment of biliary duct and pancreatic duct stones.[31, 32]

In view of the continuing technical development of the first generation of lithotripters, it appeared possible to treat sialoliths by ESWL as well.[33] The small focal dimensions of the piezoelectric shockwave device (Piezolith 2500, R. Wolf Company, Knittlingen, Germany) appeared especially well adapted to applications in the head and neck region with its important and very sensitive peripheral and central nerve structures.

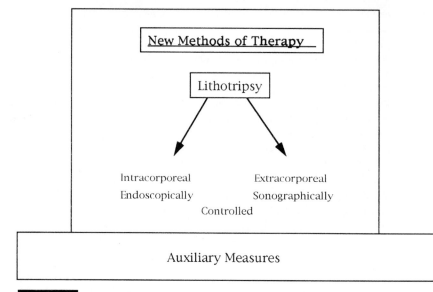

FIGURE 6.
New methods of therapy.

The feasibility of fragmenting sialoliths by piezoelectrically generated shockwaves was demonstrated in in vitro and animal experiments and other basic investigations.[34, 35] Moreover, animal experiments showed no structural and no severe tissue lesions in the head and neck region after exposure to piezoelectric shockwaves.[34]

Extracorporeal shockwaves are transduced into the body of the pa-

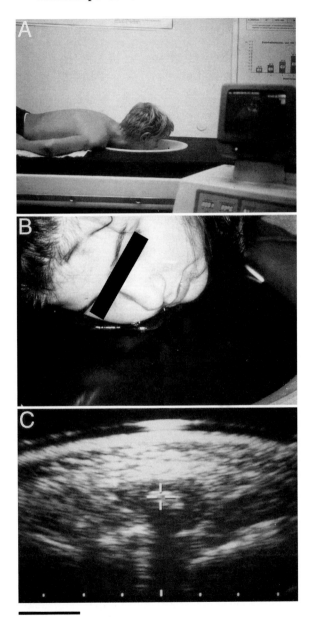

FIGURE 7.

A, twelve-year-old boy positioned above the extracorporeal shockwave generator during therapy of a sialolithiasis of the submandibular gland. **B,** 14-year-old girl with sialolithiasis of the parotid gland positioned above the shockwave generator during extracorporeal lithotripsy. **C,** calculus of the same young girl, sonographically localized and positioned in the focus of the lithotripter (+).

tient under sonographic control (Fig 7,A and B). Exact sonographic imaging and positioning of a salivary duct concrement into the focus zone of the lithotripter are decisive preconditions for implementing shockwave lithotripsy systems in the treatment of sialolithiasis in human patients (Fig 7,C). Clinical application of ESWL is possible without anaesthesia or sedoanalgesia, if these conditions are fulfilled. The first successful implementation of extracorporeal lithotripsy in human sialolithiasis was performed in 1989 by our group treating a patient afflicted by a parotid stone that measured 12 mm.[36] In a prospective study[37] we treated 60 patients suffering from sialolithiasis, giving consideration to the following criteria:

• The sialoliths had to cause clinical symptoms.
• Sonographic evidence had to be absolutely reliable.
• Removal of the stones by other measures such as duct incision was not possible.

An acute episode of sialadenitis or previously performed duct incisions are contraindications for lithotripsy because of the danger of scarred ductal strictures. Out of a total number of 60 patients, 41 suffered from submandibular calculi and 19 from parotid calculi. While complete stone fragmentation was achieved in all patients afflicted by parotid stones, in 7 of 41 patients suffering from submandibular stones, only partial fragmentation was shown by sonography after three ESWL sessions. The only side effects caused by ESWL were localized petechial bleedings and suggilations in the skin (13%), as well as temporary gland swellings (3%). During the average follow-up period of 12 months, all patients (100%) with parotid concrements and 85% of the patients with submandibular concrements remained free of symptoms. Complete elimination of stones was sonographically verified in 81% of the patients with parotid calculi (Fig 8), whereas stone fragments were still imaged in 60% of the patients exhibiting submandibular calculi. In summary, it can be conclusively stated that extracorporeal lithotripsy represents an effective minimally invasive therapy method for treating sialolithiasis that also ensures a high level of comfort for the patient. With the help of this new method, operations causing undesired side effects may be avoided. These experiences of our medical team are shared by Kater et al.[38]

INTRACORPOREAL SHOCKWAVE LITHOTRIPSY

Besides extracorporeal lithotripsy, the technique of intracorporeal shockwave lithotripsy (ISWL) is also currently available for treatment of salivary stones. With this method shockwaves are applied directly, under endoscopic control, to the surface of the stone lodged within the duct. An essential precondition for performing ISWL within the salivary ducts was the development of suitable mini-endoscopes with external probe diameters of 1.5 to 2.0 mm. In addition, a working channel of at least 0.5 mm for the laser probes and water irrigation has to be ensured (Fig 9).

In the field of ISWL different principles of shockwave generation

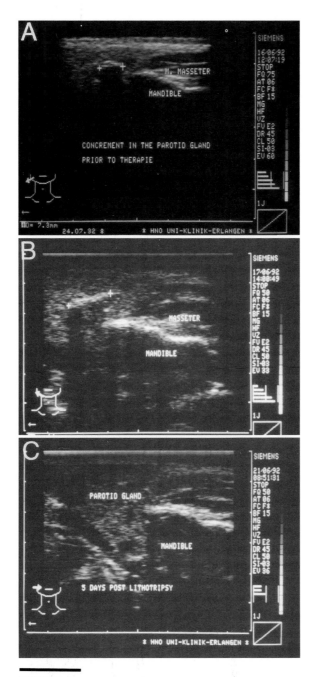

FIGURE 8.

A, sonographic image of a right parotid duct stone located in the hilum immediately before extracorporeal lithotripsy (+. . .+, 7.3 mm in diameter). **B,** the same concrement 24 hours after ESWL. Sonography shows a clearly enlarged stone signal (+. . .+, 14mm) as a sign of complete fragmentation. **C,** five days after therapy no concrement is detectable.

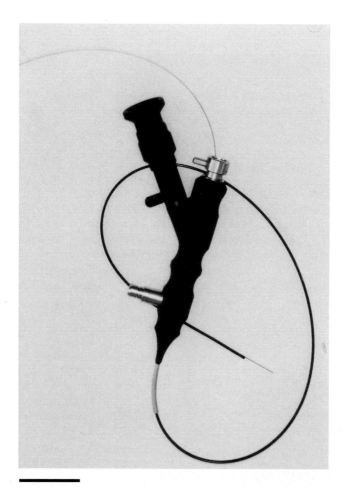

FIGURE 9.
Mini-endoscope (1.6 mm in diameter) with an inserted laser probe for ISWL (400 μm in diameter).

can be distinguished. Laser systems are being implemented on one hand, and on the other hand electrohydraulic shockwave generation systems, are also in use. In laser lithotripsy basically four different systems are available: the "Excimer-Laser," (Technolas Lasertechnologie, Germany) the "Neodymium-YAG-Laser," (LASAG-AG, Switzerland) the "Alexandrite-Laser," (Dornier Medizintechnik, Germany) and the so called "Rhodamine-6G-Dye-Laser" (595 nm, "Lithognost," Telemit-Company, Germany). Within the framework of detailed in vitro and animal experiments[39, 40] it was shown that the Nd-YAG-Laser (1064 nm) and the Alexandrite-Laser (755 nm) systems were not able to achieve fragmentation of calculi. With the Excimer-Laser (308 nm) it was indeed possible to achieve complete disintegration of salivary stones, but at the expense of a high risk of duct perforation if the tip of the probe comes into contact with the duct tissue. Tissue contact cannot always be avoided, especially in the narrow main salivary ducts with a maximum diameter of 1.2 to 1.8 mm. Although the Excimer-Laser is reliable in stone fragmentation, tissue lesions which might lead to consecutive scarred duct stenosis have to be anticipated. With the Rhodamine-6G-Dye-Laser (595 nm, "Lithognost," Telemit-Company, Germany) a system with an integrated stone/tissue detection system has become accessible. This laser is able to differentiate between tissue and stone material at the tip of the probe by optical analysis of fluorescent light which is emitted during laser-induced shockwave application. If tissue is detected in front of the probe, the laser pulse is terminated and shockwave emission is interrupted. Thus, this system can be applied without causing tissue lesions. After verification in vitro that salivary stones can be reliably disintegrated using the Rhodamine-6G-Dye-Laser, clinical application of this system for the treatment of sialolithiasis appears possible. Preconditions for the implementation of intracorporeal laser-induced lithotripsy are the following:

- A symptomatic disease
- The concrement cannot be extracted by duct dilation or incision
- Endoscopic visualization of the calculi

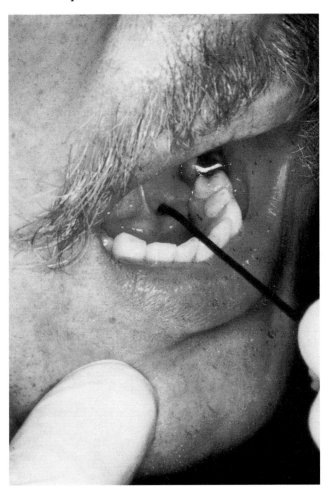

FIGURE 10.
Mini-endoscope introduced into Wharton's duct of a left submandibular gland for intracorporeal laser lithotripsy.

As the restricted dimensions of the distal ducts of the large salivary glands, especially near the orifices, tend to make incision and slitting of the duct necessary, the indication for intracorporeal laser lithotripsy is limited primarily to submandibular duct stones (Fig 10). As pointed out above, an incision of the orifice of Stensen's duct should be avoided. Like ESWL, ISWL can also be carried out using local anaesthesia. Complications of ISWL reported in the literature are intraglandular abscesses and acute episodes of sialadenitis.[41]

During the last two years various authors reported on their experiences with intracorporeal laser lithotripsy of salivary stones. The percent-

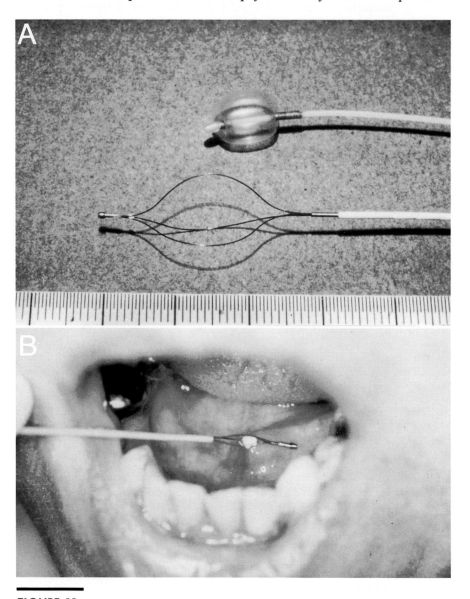

FIGURE 11.

A, three-wire dormia basket and balloon catheter ("auxiliary measures"). **B,** removal of a stone fragment after ESWL with the help of a dormia basket.

age of patients with submandibular stones that can become free of symptoms after treatment is as high as 88%.[41, 42] Up to now there have been no reports on stone clearance rates in patients who had received intracorporeal laser lithotripsy treatment.

Another method of shockwave generation and application besides laser lithotripsy is that of electrohydraulic intracorporeal lithotripsy. Whereas Königsberger et al[43] reported on very satisfactory success rates in electrohydraulic intracorporeal lithotripsy of salivary stones, our own research results clearly showed that the probability of tissue lesions and duct perforations is immense.[44] For this reason the clinical use of intracorporeal electrohydraulic lithotripsy should definitely not be recommended, particularly in view of the fact that better and less dangerous alternative methods such as ISWL and ESWL are available for therapy of sialolithiasis.

AUXILIARY MEASURES

Once the salivary stones have been fragmented by extracorporeally or intracorporeally generated shockwaves it is expected that the fragments will leave the ducts and the glands per vias naturales. The process of flushing out fragments can be facilitated by so-called auxiliary measures, which are applied by the patients or the physician. The patient should take sialagogues (i.e., sour drops) and regularly massage the affected gland to produce a continuous flow of saliva. Discharge of the concrements through the orifice can also be enforced by dilation of the duct using embolectomy balloons or by slitting of the duct. Stone extraction can be achieved by using small three-wire dormia baskets (probe diameters: 2.7 F), or balloon-catheters (probe diameters: 2 F; volume: 0.05 mL) (Fig 11,A and B).

SUMMARY

We use the following differential therapeutic scheme to manage salivary gland calculi depending, of course, on the afflicted gland and the sonographically determined stone location.

SUBMANDIBULAR GLAND (TABLE 2)

For stones located near the orifice in front of the papilla, extraction of calculi by duct incision with marsupialisation or manual mobilization of

TABLE 2.
Therapy of Submandibular Duct Stones

Localization of the Sialolith	Mode of Therapy
Vicinity of the orifice	Extraction, slitting
Distal parts of Wharton's duct	Slitting and marsupialisation
Hilum	Intracorporeal and extracorporeal lithotripsy
Intraglandular duct system	
Stone diameter < 12 mm	Extracorporeal lithotripsy
Stone diameter > 12 mm	Extirpation of the gland

TABLE 3.
Therapy of Parotid Duct Stones

Localization of the Sialolith	Mode of Therapy
Vicinity of the orifice	Extraction *without slitting*
Distal parts of Stensen's duct	Extracorporeal lithotripsy
Hilum	Extracorporeal lithotripsy
Intraglandular duct system	
All stone diameters	Extracorporeal lithotripsy

the stones is performed. If the concrement is located in the distal sections of Wharton's duct, slitting of the duct and marsupialisation will usually be the successful method of choice. Calculi of the hilum can be treated by extracorporeal or intracorporeal lithotripsy procedures. If the calculus is located in the intraglandular parts of the duct system, ESWL is the only possible option, because the available endoscopes are not small enough in diameter to be able to accede these sections of the duct system. If no success is reported after three treatment sessions within an overall period of one year (i.e., if the patient still exhibits symptoms) an extirpation of the submandibular gland has to be performed. Another indication for submandibulectomy is the size of the stone located in intraglandular regions: if the largest diameter of the stone reaches 12 mm in the sonographic image, chances of successful lithotripsy might be less than 20%.

PAROTID GLAND (TABLE 3)

In treating parotid gland stones, slitting of duct and incision of the orifice should be strictly avoided. Therefore, in our opinion, intracorporeal methods should not be implemented at the present time. Sometimes the removal of stones is possible by basket or balloon extractions. Stones located in the distal parts of Stensen's duct, in the hilum or in the intraglandular duct system are treated only by extracorporeal lithotripsy—independent of their sizes. Carrying out parotidectomy today to manage a sialolithiasis should be indicated only for isolated cases resistant to minimally invasive measures.

REFERENCES

1. Epker BN: Obstructive and inflammatory diseases of the major salivary glands. *J Oral Surg* 33:2, 1972.
2. Rauch S, Gorlin RJ: Diseases of the salivary glands, in Gorlin, RJ, Goldman, HM (eds), *Oral Pathology*. St. Louis, Mosby, 1970, p 962.
3. Perrotta RJ, Williams JR, Selfe RW: Simultaneous bilateral parotid and submandibular gland calculi. *Arch Otolaryngol* 104:469, 1978.
4. Anneroth G, Eneroth CM, Isacsson G: The relation of lipids to the mineral components in salivary calculi. *Oral Pathol* 6: 373, 1970.
5. Seifert G, Miehlke A, Haubrich J, et al: *Diseases of the Salivary Glands.* Stuttgart—New York, Thieme, 1986, p 91.

6. Harrill JA, King JS, Boyce WH, et al: Structure and compositions of salivary calculi. *Laryngoscope* 69: 481, 1959.
7. Epivatianos A, Harrison JD, Dimitriou T: Ultrastructural and histochemical observations on microcalculi in chronic submandibular sialoadenitis. *Oral Pathol* 16: 514, 1987.
8. Sakae T, Yamamoto H, Hirai G: Mode of occurrence of brushite and white-lockite in a sialolith. *Dent Res* 60: 842, 1981.
9. Yamamoto H, Sakae T, Takagi M, et al: Weddellite in submandibular gland calculus. *Dent Res* 62: 16, 1983.
10. Frame JW, Smith AJ: Large calculi of the submandibular salivary glands. *Oral Maxillofac Surg* 15: 769, 1986.
11. Donath K, Hirsch-Hofmann H-U, Seifert G: Zur Pathogenese der Parotislatro-phie nach experimenteller Gangunterbindung. Ultrastrukturelle Befunde am Drüsenparenchym der Rattenparotis. *Virchows Arch Abt A* 31:359, 1973.
12. Rettinger G, Stolte M, Bäumler C: Ausschaltung von Speicheldrüsen durch temporäre Okklusion des Gangsystems mit einer Aminosäurenlösung. Tier-experimentelle Studie zu einem neuen Therapieverfahren. *HNO* 29:294, 1981.
13. Stafne EC, Gibilisco JA: *Oral Roentgenographic Diagnosis*, 4th ed. Philadel-phia, WB Saunders Company, 1975.
14. Valvassori GE, Potter GD, Hanafee WN, et al: *Radiologie in der Hals-Nasen-Ohren-Heilkunde.* Stuttgart, Thieme-Verlag, 1984.
15. Foedra C, Kaarmann H, Iro H: Sonographie und Röntgennativaufnahme in der Speichelsteindiagnostik—experimentelle Untersuchungen. *HNO* 40: 25, 1992.
16. van den Akker P, Busemann-Sokole E: Submandibular gland function follow-ing transoral sialolithectomy. *Oral Surg* 56: 351 (1983).
17. Nishi M, Mimura T, Marutani K, et al: Evaluation of submandibular gland function by sialo-scinigraphy following sialolithectomy. *Oral Maxillofac Surg* 45: 567, 1987.
18. Seldin HW, Seldin SD, Rakower W: Conservative surgery for the removal of salivary calculi. *J Oral Surg* 6: 579, 1953.
19. Yoel J: *Pathology and Surgery of the Salivary Glands.* Springfield, Charles C. Thomas, Publisher, 1975, ch 22.
20. Seward GR: Anatomic surgery of salivary calculi. VII: Complications of sali-vary calculi. *Oral Surg* 26:137, 1968.
21. Kenefick JS: Some aspects of salivary gland disorders. *Br J Surg* 48: 435, 1961.
22. Lyall JB, Fleet J: Morbity study of submandibular gland excision. *Roy Coll Surg Engl* 68: 327, 1986.
23. Patey DH: Excision of submandibular gland, in Rob, C, Smith, R Wilson, JSP (eds.): *Operative Surgery: Head and Neck*, 3rd ed. London, Chapman and Hall, 1981, p 835.
24. Patey DH, Moffat W: A clinical and experimental study of functional paraly-sis of the facial nerve following conservative parotidectomy. *Br J Surg* 48: 435, 1961.
25. Hörmann K, Lemke T, Pirsig W: Komplikationslast und Rezidivhäufigkeit nach Enukleation, subtotaler sowie totaler Parotidektomie bei pleomorphen Adenomen. *Arch Otorhinolaryngol* 223: 200, 1979.
26. Zalin H, Cooney C: Chorda tympani neurectomy—a new approach to sub-mandibular salivary obstruction. *Br J Surg* 61: 391, 1974.
27. Chilla R, Brüner M, Arglebe C: Function of submaxillary gland following atro-genic damage to chorda tympani nerve. *Acta Otolaryngol* 87: 152, 1979.
28. Chaussy CH, Stähler G: Berührungsfreie Nierenstein-Zertrümmerung durch extrakorporal erzeugte, fokussierte Stoßwellen. *Beiträge zur Urologie Bd, 2,* 1980.

29. Marberger M, Türk C, Steinkogler I: Painless piezoelectric extracorporeal lithotripsy. *J Urol* 139: 695, 1988.
30. Zwergel U, Neisius D, Zwergel T, et al: Results and clinical management of extracorporeal piezoelectric lithotripsy (EPL) in 1321 consecutive treatments. *World J Urol* 5: 213, 1987.
31. Ell C, Kerzel W, Schneider HT, et al: Piezoelectric lithotripsy: Stone disintegration and follow-up results in patients with symptomatic gallbladder stones. *Gastroenterology* 99: 1439, 1990.
32. Sauerbruch T, Delius M, Paumgartner G, et al: Fragmentation of gallstones by extracorporeal shockwaves. *N Engl J Med* 314: 818, 1986.
33. Coleman AJ, Saunders JE: A survey of the acoustic output of commercial extracorporeal shock wave lithotripters. *Ultrasound Med Biol* 3: 213, 1989.
34. Iro H, Wessel B, Benzel W, et al: Gewebereaktionen unter Applikation von piezoelektrischen Stoßwellen zur Lithotripsie von Speichelsteinen. *Laryngo-Rhino-Otol* 69: 102, 1990.
35. Iro H, Nitsche N, Meier J, et al: Piezoelectric shockwave lithotripsy of salivary gland stones: An in vitro feasibility study. *Lith Stone Dis* 3: 211, 1991.
36. Iro H, Nitsche N, Schneider HT, et al: Extracorporeal shockwave lithotripsy of salivary gland stones. *Lancet* II: 115, 1989.
37. Iro H, Schneider HT, Födra C, et al: Shockwave lithotripsy of salivary duct stones. *Lancet* 339: 1333, 1992.
38. Kater W: Die Lithotripsie von Speichelsteinen als nicht invasive Behandlungsmethode. *Dtsch Ärztebl* 88: 1428, 1991.
39. Benzel W, Hofer M, Hosemann WG, et al: Laser-induced shock wave lithotripsy of salivary calculi with automatic feedback cessation in case of tissue contact: In vitro and animal experiments. *Eur Arch Otorhinolaryngol* 249: 437, 1992.
40. Iro H, Zenk J, Benzel W, et al: Experimentelle Untersuchungen zur Laser-Lithotripsie von Speichelsteinen. *Lasermedizin* 8:110, 1992.
41. Gundlach P, Scherer H, Hopf J, et al: Die endoskopisch kontrollierte Laser-lithotripsie von Speichelsteinen—in-vitro-Untersuchungen und erster klinischer Einsatz. *HNO* 38: 247, 1990.
42. Königsberger R, Feyh J, Goetz A, et al: Die endoskopisch kontrollierte Laser-lithotripsie zur Behandlung der Sialolithiasis. *Laryngo-Rhino-Otol* 69: 322, 1990.
43. Königsberger R, Feyh J, Götz A, et al: Endoscopically-controlled electrohydraulic intracorporeal shock wave lithotripsy of salivary stones. *Can J Otolaryngol* 22:12, 1993.
44. Zenk J, Benzel W, Hosemann WG, et al: Experimental research on electrohydraulic lithotripsy of sialolithiasis. *Eur Arch Otorhinolaryngol* 249: 436, 1992.

Reconstruction of Laryngotracheal Stenosis in the Adult

J. Paul Willging, M.D.

Assistant Professor, Otolaryngology, Department of Pediatric Otolaryngology, Children's Hospital Medical Center, Cincinnati, Ohio

Robin T. Cotton, M.D.

Professor, Otolaryngology, Department of Pediatric Otolaryngology, Children's Hospital Medical Center, Cincinnati, Ohio

ETIOLOGY

Laryngeal stenosis in the adult patient is most commonly related to trauma. The inciting event may be an indwelling endotracheal tube that causes pressure necrosis of the underlying mucosa, resulting in chondritis of the cricoid cartilage. Healing leads to an accumulation of scar tissue that is responsible for obstructing the airway.[1] Other types of trauma may result from external blunt forces that have an impact upon the laryngeal framework, such as an individual striking the steering wheel in a motor vehicle accident. Inhalation of heated and toxic gases in house fires may lead to severe laryngotracheal injuries from thermal and chemical injuries. Caustic ingestion, frequently intentional in the adult population, may lead to severe laryngeal stenosis at multiple levels depending on the nature and volume of the material ingested.

Laryngeal stenosis is not always a sequela of trauma. Stenosis may also develop in the adult as a consequence of the spectrum of collagen vascular disease. Wegener's granulomatosis may involve the larynx with necrotizing granulomatous lesions and vasculitis.[2] Sarcoidosis may occasionally involve the larynx and lead to destruction of the laryngeal framework. Relapsing polychondritis may attack any cartilage of the body including the laryngotracheal airway. The gradual destruction of cartilage leads to stenosis. Laryngeal amyloidosis is an idiopathic disease process whereby a diffuse protein and polysaccharide complex is deposited in the laryngeal mucosa causing obstruction. Amyloidosis has a predilection for the anterior subglottic area.[3] True idiopathic subglottic stenosis is rare. It typically affects females in their twenties and thirties with no underlying etiology for their laryngeal obstruction.

Infectious causes of laryngeal stenosis are rare in the postantibiotic era but have been reported in cases of tuberculosis,[4] secondary or tertiary syphilis, and leprosy (Hansen's disease).

Advances in Otolaryngology—Head and Neck Surgery®, vol. 9
© 1995, Mosby–Year Book, Inc.

PRESENTATION

Patients with laryngotracheal stenosis usually present with air hunger. Exercise intolerance in the mild cases may be confused with exercise-induced asthma. More severe stenosis will present with obvious stridor on exertion and occasionally at rest. Stenosis of the subglottic and glottic airway will produce biphasic stridor. Stenosis of the supraglottic airway will typically present with inspiratory stridor only. Stenosis of the thoracic trachea will lead to expiratory stridor. With inspiration, the surrounding negative pressure in the pleural spaces tends to open the trachea, while expiration causes compression of the trachea, worsening the underlying narrow segment. Pain is rarely present with stenosis. Alterations in the quality of the voice are common. Feeding difficulties may occasionally be present in the adult population as a consequence of laryngeal stenosis. If the glottis is incompetent as the result of a vocal cord paralysis in a lateral position, symptoms of aspiration may be present.

EVALUATION

After a thorough history that specifically explored all areas of potential laryngeal trauma is obtained, a routine examination of the head and neck is performed. Visualization of the larynx and hypopharynx must be achieved to rule out a laryngeal or hypopharyngeal neoplasm. The position and function of the vocal cords as well as the structural appearance of the supraglottic larynx must be documented. It is essential to have an adequate evaluation. Flexible nasopharyngoscopy should be performed in the office in those cases in which the indirect examination is suboptimal. Airway films (posterior-anterior and lateral [PA/LAT] chest radiography with PA/LAT neck) should be obtained to define any defects of the airway below the level of the cords.

Direct laryngoscopy and bronchoscopy are the mainstay for diagnosis of airway pathology. Great care must be given to the evaluation of each anatomic unit of the airway—supraglottic, glottis, subglottic, and trachea—so that an accurate determination of the extent of the stenosis can be documented. A biopsy specimen should be obtained as indicated by the appearance of the lesion. It is important to minimize trauma to the larynx during the endoscopic evaluation, as edema may obstruct a marginal airway, leading to an uncontrolled situation where the airway must be secured.

During the preoperative evaluation, the safety of the patient's airway needs to be addressed. If on viewing the larynx a very small aperture is identified or a significant obstruction of the airway is identified radiographically, tracheotomy should be performed under local anesthesia. A slowly progressive stenosing lesion in an adult may have a diameter of only 4 mm with minimal symptoms present in the patient at rest. Never be lulled into complacency when confronted with a patient presenting with a possible airway obstruction. In the morbidly obese patient in whom a tracheotomy under local anesthesia would be difficult, or in the case of a mid-tracheal stenosis where concern arises about being able to pass the tracheotomy cannula through the obstructing lesion, femoral cardiopulmonary bypass may offer additional safety in the establishment of the airway.[5] With the patient awake, the groin can be anesthetized and the femoral vessels isolated. The vessels can be cannulated and connected to the cardiopulmonary bypass machine. Induction of anesthesia can then take place and the patient can undergo intubation, tracheotomy, or the passage of a bronchoscope through the stenotic lesion to establish a safe airway. Should difficulty occur in the establishment of the airway, the bypass circuit could be opened and oxygenation maintained until the airway is secured. With prior preparation of the bypass equipment, cardiopulmonary bypass can be established within seconds of opening the clamps. We have utilized this technique on a morbidly obese female with a mid-tracheal stenosis of 3 mm diameter and 1.5 cm length. Having the option of utilizing the bypass equipment minimized the anxiety experienced by otolaryngologists and anesthesiologists alike.

Computed tomography and magnetic resonance imaging are rarely of value in cases of stenosis. The stenotic area can be visualized and the length of the stenosis and residual lumen determined with these techniques; however, this is the same information that is obtained at bronchoscopy. The imaging studies will not replace endoscopic evaluation of the airway as they are unable to differentiate between immature and mature stenoses, and soft and dilatable stenoses from firm, incompressible lesions.

STAGING OF STENOSIS

Multiple staging systems exist for subglottic stenosis. There is no optimal system. The ideal system would be easy to implement among multiple institutions, have little risk of improper classification, be objective, and have relevance with regard to the outcome of the surgical repair. The system developed at the Children's Hospital Medical Center in Cincinnati, Ohio, is based upon the degree of subglottic narrowing.[6] This system has four subjective grades. Grade I stenosis is a mild impairment of the airway, the degree of narrowing being no more than 70% of the subglottic airway. Grade II stenosis is an obstruction between 70% to 90% of the total subglottic lumen. Grade III stenosis is severe, with greater than 90% of the lumen obstructed. As long as a channel exists through the stenosis the lesion is considered grade III. Grade IV lesions are indicated by complete obstruction of the laryngeal airway. The prognosis for decannulation is dependent upon the stage of the stenosis at the time of the reconstruction. The number of operations required to achieve decannulation is also generally dependent upon the surgical stage of the stenosis. Grade IV lesions always require multiple reconstructions. Grade I and II lesions are almost always successfully decannulated after a single procedure.

Sizing of the airway is useful. The magnification achieved with the Storz-Hopkins endoscopes makes determination of the actual diameter of the airway difficult. By passing a cuffless endotracheal tube of known size into the airway, the diameter of the airway can be measured. The appropriate endotracheal tube will pass easily into the airway, and when connected to the anesthetic circuit will allow a leak of gases around the tube into the hypopharynx at a pressure less than 30 cm H_2O. By recording both the endotracheal tube size and the leak pressure, a given airway can be followed sequentially and lumenal expansion verified. It is important to pass the endotracheal tube the same distance below the vocal cords each time to standardize the measurement.

ANCILLARY STUDIES

Gastroesophageal reflux may complicate the postoperative healing of a laryngeal reconstruction. Generally, the adult patient can give a history consistent with this problem. With a positive history of gastroesophageal reflux, a gastric emptying scan is obtained to quantify gastric emptying time and also visualize gastroesophageal reflux. Delayed emptying of the stomach is treated with metaclopromide. Twenty-four-hour pH probes are obtained to define the clinical significance of the gastroesophageal reflux. Two probes are used, one near the gastroesophageal junction, the other at the mid-esophageal level. H_2 blockers, either ranitidine or omeprazole, are administered to control mild to moderate reflux of the acidic gastric secretions. Severe cases of reflux require a fundoplication prior to airway reconstruction.

Pulmonary function tests are reliable in adults. They will define the obstructive characteristics of the lesion. Although not useful in the initial evaluation of a stenosis, they offer objective follow-up data on the airway that may obviate the need for repeated endoscopy under anesthesia once the reconstruction has healed and all granulation tissue has resolved.

Videostroboscopy, with formal voice evaluation by a speech pathologist, is a valuable study to define the functional effect of the stenosis on voice. Although voice is not the primary priority in airway reconstruction, the maintenance of maximal vocal function is important. Compensation techniques utilized by the patient to overcome glottic incompetence (false cord phonation, arytenoid displacement anteriorly into the glottis, reverse phonation) may be identified, which will direct the speech therapist in the postoperative sessions.

SURGICAL TREATMENT

Every case of laryngotracheal stenosis must be individualized. A standard treatment to fit all patients is not available. The degree of stenosis, the location of the stenosis, and the extension of the stenosis to adjacent areas will have a significant impact on the success of reconstruction. The general medical condition of the patient also needs to be considered. Specifically, the pulmonary status of the patient must be adequate to support the patient postoperatively. Airway reconstruction is a stressful procedure to the pulmonary system. Secretions are increased for a period of time in response to the surgical trauma to the airway and in response to indwelling stents. Aspiration may be a problem until protective reflexes return to protect a compromised airway from oropharyngeal secretions. A patient with marginal pulmonary reserve may require supplemental oxygen or even ventilator support postoperatively, which stresses the repair site and increases the risk of postoperative complications. Patients with a marginal medical status are best treated conservatively, postponing the reconstruction until their condition improves.

An immature stenosis should not be reconstructed. Active fibrosis and inflammation should be avoided as the final degree of stenosis is unknown. The underlying process of fibrosis may extend beyond the bounds of the identifiable stenosis, which could lead to an inadequate repair. Conversely, immature stenoses may respond to conservative management with steroids and antireflux measures making operative intervention unnecessary.

FIVE STEPS OF AIRWAY RECONSTRUCTION

The reconstruction of the stenosis can be divided into five distinct stages.[7] Stage I is complete evaluation of the airway. This is the most important preliminary aspect of reconstruction. An inaccurate assessment will lead to an inadequate or overly aggressive attempt to repair the airway. It is critical that the anatomic and functional status of the larynx be evaluated at all levels. Areas proximal and distal to the stenosis need to be examined for contributions to the obstruction of the airway. For example, significant redundancy of the oropharyngeal airway or a posteriorly displaced tongue base may not permit decannulation of an improved yet marginal airway. Distal pulmonary disease may contribute in a similar fashion to the prevention of decannulation.

Stage II involves the expansion of the subglottic lumen with presentation of laryngeal function. The precise method involved will vary with the pathology.

Stage III deals with the stabilization of the expanded laryngeal framework. This may be fulfilled by use of an endotracheal tube as a short-term stent or a teflon or silicone stent for prolonged periods of support. The duration of stenting is dependent upon the inherent instability of the repair.

Stage IV is the time required for healing of the operative site. The surgeon has least control over this stage of the reconstruction. This stage may range from a few days to 6 months.

Stage V is the end point of the reconstruction, decannulation of the patient after proper healing has been documented, with the establishment of an adequate airway.

ENDOSCOPIC REPAIR

Endoscopic management of laryngotracheal stenosis is successful in cases of mild airway stenosis. Many grade I lesions can be managed endoscopically, but it is unusual for more advanced lesions to be successfully resolved by this treatment approach. Endoscopic techniques are commonly applied to the postoperative care of patients having open surgical reconstruction to maintain maximal lumen size and minimize the development of partially obstructing lesions.

Endoscopic management of stenosis has a success rate between 60% and 80%.[8] Careful selection of patients is required to maximize the success of the procedure. Endoscopic failures are associated with circumferential scarring, stenosis extending more than 1 cm in the vertical dimension, arytenoid fixation secondary to fibrosis of the interarytenoid area, and a history of a previous severe bacterial infection associated with tracheotomy that may result in substantial loss of skeletal support of the airway.[8] Cases which have failed previous endoscopic treatment carry an increased risk of failure with repeated endoscopic techniques.

Endoscopic treatment options include cryotherapy, microcautery, dilation, laser treatments, and submucosal resection of the stenosis with formation of micro-trapdoor flaps. Cryotherapy[9] is rarely used, as the depth of tissue injury is difficult to control. Significant loss of cartilaginous structural support is possible with injury to the underlying perichondrium. Microcauterization[10] remains a viable technique in the postoperative period where exuberant granulation tissue can be removed. The Bugby electrocautery device passed through the side port of a bronchoscope, at low power settings, offers the ability to debulk the subglottic or

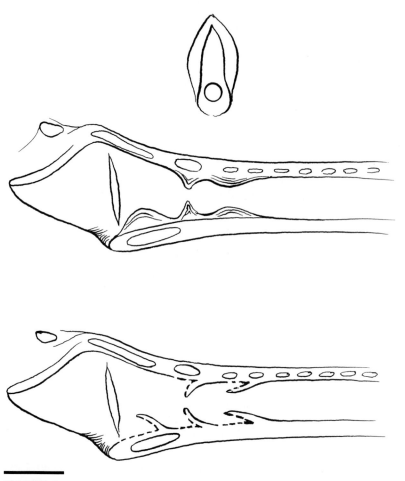

FIGURE 1.
A, irregular circumferential stenosis of the subglottis and cervical trachea. **B,** inferiorly based mucosal flaps are created and the fibrotic component of the stenosis removed. The flaps are then returned to their anatomic position.

tracheal airway while maintaining hemostasis. Electrocautery as a primary treatment modality for stenosis has limited usefulness.

Dilation[11] as a primary treatment modality has limited success in the maintenance of an open airway. Combined with the excision of excess granulation tissue and systemic antibiotics and steroids, it is useful as an adjuvant method of maintaining a lumen prior to open reconstruction techniques. As the ability to successfully decannulate after a single reconstructive procedure is related to the grade of stenosis, prevention of the development of a grade IV lesion will improve surgical outcome.

The CO_2, argon, and KTP lasers are the most commonly utilized endoscopic tools due to their precise and predictable tissue characteristics.[12, 13] Tissue destruction is proportional to the energy delivered to the tissue. The energy density and duration of exposure are critical parameters that must be controlled to limit the zone of tissue injury. The improperly applied laser can make a stenosis worse.[14, 15] The laser is most appropriately applied to early stenoses with granulation tissue and thin circumferential webs.[16] The laser can be combined with dilation techniques to minimize the overall trauma and maximize the results.[17] The laser has also been used to submucosally resect the area of stenosis and maintain inferiorly based mucosal flaps, which are then repositioned over the resection site to provide coverage of the denuded area (Fig 1).[18] The success of all endoscopic techniques depends upon reepithelialization of the defect before granulation tissue maturation and scar tissue formation occurs.[19]

The advantages of endoscopic treatment approaches to laryngotracheal stenosis include the low morbidity rates of the procedures, minimal damage to the surrounding tissues, and the ability to avoid tracheotomy in those patients presenting without a cannula.[20] Failure of endoscopic techniques will not preclude the application of other reconstructive techniques to improve the airway.[21]

OPEN RECONSTRUCTIVE TECHNIQUES

Grade I lesions rarely need open surgical intervention and usually are handled well by endoscopic techniques. Grade II lesions may be managed by either endoscopic or open procedures depending on the surgeon's experience with reconstructive techniques. In general, lesions classified as grade III or IV will require open procedures to establish an airway adequate to permit decannulation. There are multiple techniques available to reconstruct a severely compromised larynx. It must be remembered that a successful outcome depends as much on the preoperative assessment of the stenosis as on the surgical reconstruction. Failure to appreciate the extent of the lesion will lead to an inadequate repair and unsuccessful reconstruction.

Not all patients are candidates for open reconstructive techniques. Contraindications include

1. Contraindication for general anesthesia
2. A situation where a patient will be tracheotomy dependent despite an adequate airway, for example, a patient suffering the effects of a

stroke that makes him or her unable to handle oral secretions, putting him or her at risk for chronic aspiration and recurrent pneumonias

3. A patient with severe gastroesophageal reflux who is at risk for complications developing in the airway as a result of this chronic irritation.

These patients may be candidates for surgical reconstruction after correction with an anti-reflux procedure.

Open laryngotracheoplasty is a combination of techniques chosen specifically for an individual lesion. These techniques can be classified broadly as splits, augmentations, and resections. Stenting is an adjunctive measure that is used for a variable length of time depending upon the instability of the larynx after surgical reconstruction. The materials used for stenting as well as the position of the stent and duration of stenting are tailored to the individual reconstructive procedure.

SPLITS

The anterior cricoid split is performed in the neonate or young child in whom extubation has failed on several occasions.[22, 23] Distraction of segments beyond 3 mm results in soft tissue fibrosis that will prolapse into the airway, thus obstructing the newly created lumen. In adults, the use of the anterior cricoid split as the sole reconstructive method has limited applicability. Most stenoses will require lumenal expansion much greater than 3 mm. The adult larynx has achieved its final size, thus no expansion with normal developmental growth can be expected. Lumenal expansion at the end of the operation must be adequate to maintain the patient's airway.

In addition to the anterior laryngofissure, however, the posterior cricoid plate may be divided in the midline, exposing the median raphe of the cricopharyngeus. Lateral division of the cricoid cartilage is also possible to gain maximal expansion of the laryngeal framework (Fig 2).[24] The lateral cuts are made at the 3 o'clock and 9 o'clock positions, taking care not to incise the outer perichondrium which protects the recurrent laryngeal nerves from injury.[25] Long-term stenting is required in these multiple split procedures to permit fibrosis between the divided segments of the cricoid cartilage. Frequently, distraction alone is not successful in allowing decannulation. Generally, this technique is required in grade IV lesions to establish a rudimentary lumen which may then be augmented as a separate reconstructive procedure.

AUGMENTATION GRAFTS

Augmentation of the laryngotracheal complex is required when the distraction of the laryngeal framework is greater than 3 mm. Autologous tissue interposed between the divided cartilage reestablishes the structural integrity of the larynx. The larynx may be augmented anteriorly as well as posteriorly. Tissue available for augmentation includes costal cartilage, thyroid cartilage,[26] auricular cartilage,[27] hyoid bone, epiglottic cartilage, myocutaneous flaps, myo-osseous flaps, and myoperiosteal flaps.

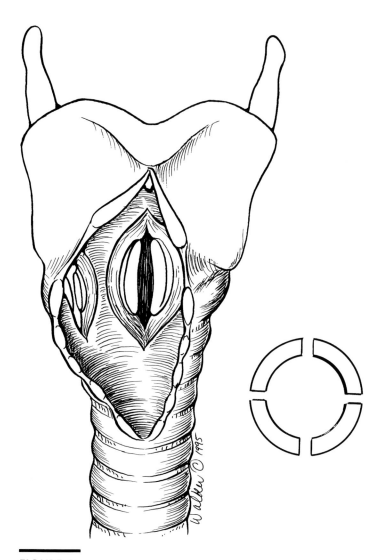

FIGURE 2.

The cricoid may be divided in the midline through the anterior cricoid arch and the posterior cricoid plate for routine expansion. Lateral division on the cricoid allows further expansion ability and can be accomplished without interruption of the growth centers.

Costal Cartilage Graft.—Costal cartilage grafts offer a wide variety of flexibility in the reconstruction of the airway. The cartilaginous portion of the rib is harvested, leaving the perichondrium attached only to the lateral surface, and the perichondrium is dissected off the cartilage on the remaining three sides of the graft. The perichondrium is placed intralumenally. The graft revascularizes through a process of embouchment, with the vascular supply coming from the overlying strap muscles for anterior grafts or the cricopharyngeus for posterior grafts. The perichondrium resists infection and provides a collagen framework for rapid epithelialization.

The anterior graft is shaped as an ellipse. Wide flanges are preserved lateral to the inset portion of the graft to prevent prolapse of the graft into the airway. The graft is secured with mattress sutures of 4-0 polypropylene monafilament, taking care to keep all sutures extralumenal. It is vital to make a single pass through the cartilage graft with the needle as necrosis of the cartilage along the suture tract occurs (Fig 3).[28]

Posterior grafts need to fit flush between the divided posterior cricoid lamina. A graft that is excessively thick will compromise swallowing as well as the airway. The posterior division of the cricoid must be at right angles to the plane of the cartilage. A beveled incision prohibits maximal contact between graft and cricoid cartilage and predisposes the graft to projecting into the lumen.[28] All posterior laryngeal divisions require stenting despite the presence of graft to maintain the distraction. Com-

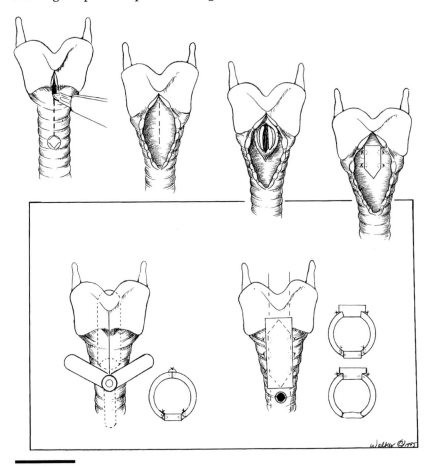

FIGURE 3.

Expansion grafting can be performed in several combinations. Dividing the thyroid cartilage, cricoid arch, and upper cervical tracheal rings provides access to the stenotic airway lumen. The posterior cricoid plate may be divided in the midline and an autogenous costalcartilage graft secured for adequate distraction of the segments. An anterior graft can simultaneously be used to further expand the lumen. Either grafting technique can be used as the sole mode of reconstruction dependent upon the nature of the stenosis. Laryngeal stents are generally used to stabilize the laryngeal framework.

bined anterior and posterior division of the larynx induces marked instability in the laryngeal framework that must be addressed to prevent shearing forces from interfering with adequate integration of the graft material.

HYOID GRAFT.—The laryngeal skeleton of the patient older than 40 years of age has undergone significant calcification. Calcification can also be seen in younger patients with laryngeal fractures. Because of the diminished metabolic activity of bone, pedicle grafts may be considered in these instances to maximize blood supply and graft tissue viability. The hyoid bone interposition may be used as both a pedicled or free graft.[29, 30] The curvature of the hyoid bone closely matches the profile of the cricoid arch. The sternohyoid muscle is left attached to the central portion of the hyoid bone. The muscle is dissected free and the graft interposed into the laryngeal framework (Fig 4). There is no donor site morbidity due to resection of the anterior hyoid bone. There is no additional incision required to harvest the graft.[31] This technique may also be used to reconstruct high cervical trachea defects. Pedicle grafts can only be used to augment anterior defects.

EPIGLOTTIS.—Epiglottic reconstruction for laryngeal stenosis has been reported as a technique with good results.[32] The petiole of the epiglottis is sectioned and the epiglottic cartilage retracted inferiorly between the cartilage edges of the anterior laryngofissure (Fig 5). The blood supply of the

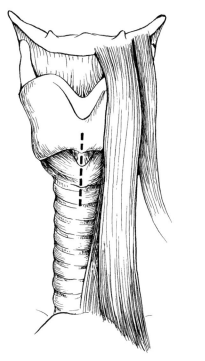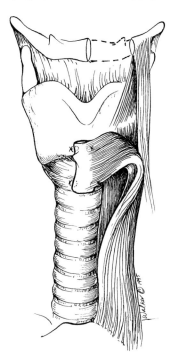

FIGURE 4.

The central portion of the hyoid bone is isolated with preservation of the muscular attachments of the sternohyoid muscle. The pedicled bone is transposed into an anterior defect to maintain distraction.

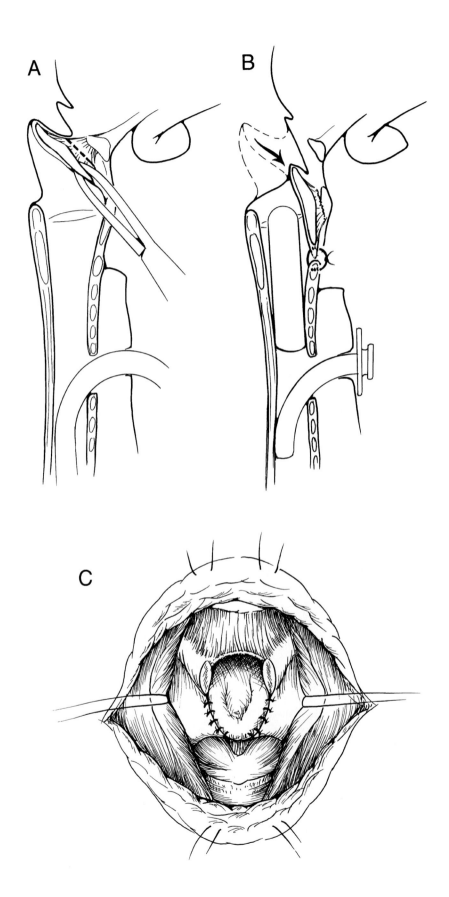

flap is maintained by preserving the mucosal connection at the lingual epiglottic junction.[33] Splaying of the anterior commissure with poor vocal function frequently requires secondary procedures to improve voice. Occasionally, aspiration may complicate the reconstruction if glottic incompetence was present because of impaired vocal function, and the protective retroflexion movement of the epiglottis is abolished by the pull-down procedure.

CLAVICULAR MYO-OSSEUS FLAPS.—The sternocleidomastoid myoperiosteal flap was described for the reconstruction of the subglottic airway. This flap consists of the clavicular perichondrium pedicled to the sternocleidomastoid muscle.[34] The periosteum provides an airtight, tension-free closure with vascularity provided by the transposed muscle (Fig 6). Bone formation resulting from periosteal activity provides a rigid subglottic framework.[35] The clavicle can be partially resected medially, the cancellous bone removed from the central portion of the clavicle to create a concavity, and this rigid support used to reconstruct laryngotracheal defects.[36] This myoosseus flap is also based on the sternocleidomastoid muscle. One-half or less of the circumference of the clavicle is utilized depending on the defect to be reconstructed. A buccal mucosal graft lines the concave surface of the clavicular graft. Free perichondrium and periosteum have also been used to reconstruct moderate defects.[37] As long as infection was prevented, the grafts produced a firm substrate that was able to support and maintain the subglottic lumen.[38]

MYOCUTANEOUS FLAP.—The sternohyoid myocutaneous flap offers a single-stage reconstruction that lines the laryngeal surface of the repair and provides structural support because of the tension inherent in the muscular system.[39] It is suggested that during inspiration the intact muscle contracts and tends to open the airway in a dynamic fashion.[40] The bipedicled muscle flap is rotated 180° so that the overlying skin is placed intralumenally. Adjacent neck skin is undermined to close the donor defect.

MICROVASCULAR GRAFTS.—Advances in microvascular surgery have permitted distant tissue transfer to the airway. Jejunum has been transplanted for tracheal defects[41] and free iliac crest grafts have reconstructed the subglottis.[42] The complexity of these surgical procedures and the potential for devastating complications should the vascular anastomosis fail have prevented widespread adoption of these techniques.

EXTERNALIZATION OF THE LARYNX

In cases of severe stenosis or where multiple reconstructive efforts have failed, the creation of a trough after resection of the stenotic area allows

---

FIGURE 5.

A, petiole of the epiglottis is detached from the thyroid cartilage and freed from the pre-epiglottic fat. **B,** epiglottis is pulled inferiorly to reconstruct a laryngeal defect. A laryngeal stent supports the reconstruction. **C,** anterior epiglottic augmentation graft to the larynx sutured in place.

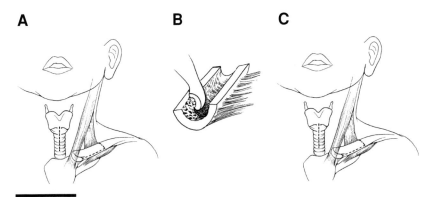

FIGURE 6.

A, the medial aspect of the clavicle is resected, leaving the medial and lateral heads of the sternocleidomastoid muscle attached. Up to half of the circumference of the clavicle may be taken. **B,** removal of the cancellous bone from the clavicular graft. A buccal mucosal graft is used to line the concavity. **C,** reconstruction of a laryngotracheal defect, with a stent providing support to the buccal graft lining the clavicle.

epithelialization of the interlumenal larynx.[43] The patients are maintained on a T-tube during the reconstruction. In a staged procedure, mesh is implanted subcutaneously adjacent to the trough. Final closure of the trough is accomplished by reconstructing the anterior wall with the mesh reinforced skin, and rotating local flaps to close the donor defect. The disadvantage to this procedure is the multiple stages required to accomplish the reconstruction and the possibility of introducing a hair-bearing flap into the larynx. In some patients, however, improper epithelialization of the subglottic airway is the primary reason for repeated failure and this technique offers improved visualization of the healing process and the opportunity to alter the process.

RESECTION

With end-to-end anastomosis, tracheal lesions may be isolated, resected, and the proximal and distal tracheal segments mobilized with primary anastomosis. Neck flexion and hyoid release are frequently all that are required to achieve a tension-free anastomosis. The patient may be extubated on the operating table or the following day.

Subglottic stenosis that does not extend superiorly to involve the glottis is potentially amenable to a partial cricoid resection.[44] We prefer to have 1 cm of normal airway below the vocal cords to allow ample space for the resection and subsequent anastomosis. After isolating the subglottic segment, a subperichondrial resection is performed to remove the ste-

FIGURE 7.

A, stenotic segment of cricoid and upper cervical trachea to be resected. **B,** resection of the inferior cricoial cartilage, leaving the superior aspect of the posterior cricoid plate and arytenoids. Subperichondrial dissection protects the recurrent laryngeal nerves. **C,** anastomosis of the cervical trachea to the thyroid cartilage and posterior cricoid plate remnant.

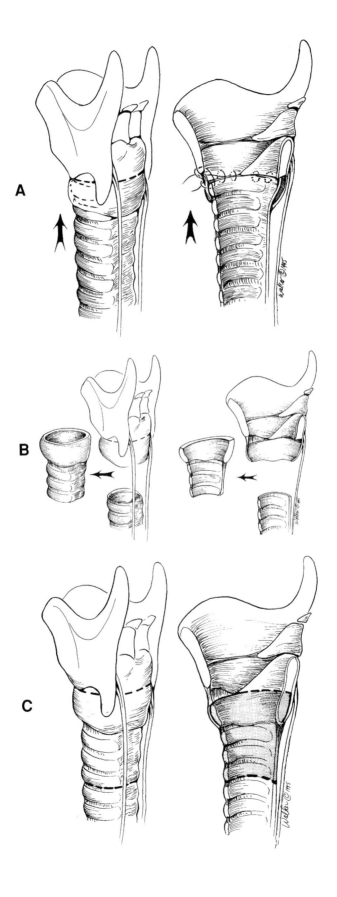

A

B

C

nosis and surrounding cricoid cartilage.[45] Primary end-to-end anastomosis is performed, taking care laterally not to extend beyond the perichondrium with the suture, which may injure the recurrent laryngeal nerves
(Fig 7). The patient needs to be intubated for a week or maintained with
a tracheotomy as significant edema of the glottis and subglottic airway
follows this procedure.

Advantages of the surgical resection of a laryngotracheal stenosis include the provision of a stable anastomosis with good healing potential,
as it is a single-stage procedure, as well as the maintenance of good mu-
cociliary function as respiratory epithelium is preserved. The number of
patients who would be satisfactory for this procedure is low because of
the prevalence of stenosis extending into multiple areas of the larynx.

SKIN GRAFTING

In major reconstruction, large areas of raw tissue may be exposed intralumenally. In these cases, some type of covering is required to minimize
granulation tissue formation. Split-thickness skin grafts as well as mucosal grafts taken from the oral cavity or nasal septum are utilized to reline
the subglottic airway. Skin grafting is rarely required with current reconstructive techniques.

STENTING

Laryngeal stents are often required in laryngotracheal reconstruction. The
primary function of the stent is to provide stability to the newly reconstructed airway. Not all forms of reconstruction require stenting. When
the airway is destabilized by multiple cricoid divisions, stenting is recommended so as to stabilize the larynx during the act of swallowing, head
turning, and ambulation. The stent will minimize shearing forces between
opposing laryngeal structures, thus maximizing healing.

As the function of stents varies from providing structural support for
mucosal and cartilage grafts to maintaining structural integrity of the larynx and forcing distraction of cartilaginous segments in the larynx with
multiple divisions, the duration of stenting will vary. Periods of 3 months
to 6 months are required when the larynx has been divided and the dis-
tracted segments need to be fixed by fibrosis to maintain the distraction.
Cartilage grafting generally requires 4 weeks to 8 weeks to allow adequate
intrinsic support to develop between the graft and the native laryngeal
cartilage. Stenting of mucosal and skin grafts requires only 3 days to 5
days.

The ideal stent should not induce any inflammatory response. It
should conform to the contours of the larynx, provide structural support
to the laryngeal framework without causing mucosal injury, remain stable
within the lumen to avoid shearing forces, and be easily removable from
the airway. The ideal stent would be resistant to bacterial colonization.
There is no ideal stent material.

There is a wide range of material that has served as a laryngeal stent.
Common stents include the rolled silastic sheeting,[46] preformed silastic
stents,[47-49] polyvinyl chloride endotracheal tubes,[50] teflon tubes,[51] and

the foam finger cot.[52] The actual stent that is chosen is generally one with which the surgeon has the most experience, experiences the least complications, and fulfills the theoretic functions of a stent. Stenting is an adjuvant to surgical reconstruction and improper stenting may lead to unsuccessful outcome.

SUMMARY

Laryngotracheal stenosis is a complex problem for which multiple divergent and radically different reconstructive options are available. The precise method of reconstruction chosen for a given lesion must be based on sound judgement to maximize the chances for a successful outcome and minimize the potential for making the stenosis worse. Laryngotracheal reconstruction is not necessarily within the realm of all otolaryngologists. Experience is required to manage these complex abnormalities of the airway.

REFERENCES

1. Quiney RE, Gould SJ: Subglottic stenosis: A clinicopathologic study. *Clin Otolaryngol* 10:315–327, 1985.
2. Hoare TJ, Jayne D, Evans PR, et al: Wegener's granulomatosis, subglottic stenosis and anti-neutrophil cytoplasm antibodies. *J Laryngol Otol* 103:1187–1191, 1989.
3. Heiner ER: Primary amyloidosis of the larynx. *Arch Otolaryngol Head Neck Surg* 87:413–415, 1968.
4. Herzog JA, Donovan DT: Complete subglottic stenosis secondary to tuberculosis. *Otolaryngol Head Neck Surg* 93:666–669, 1985.
5. Phillips SJ, Ballentine B, Slonire D, et al: Percutaneous initiation of cardiopulmonary bypass. *Ann Thorac Surg* 36:223–225, 1983.
6. Cotton RT, Gray SD, Miller RP: Update of the Cincinnati experience in pediatric laryngotracheal reconstruction. *Laryngoscope* 99:1111–1116, 1989.
7. Cotton RT, Myer CM, O'Connor DM: Innovations in pediatric laryngotracheal reconstruction. *J Pediatr Surg* 27:196–200, 1992.
8. Simpson GT, Strong MS, Healy GB, et al: Predictive factors of success or failure in the endoscopic management of laryngeal and tracheal stenosis. *Ann Otol Rhinol Laryngol* 91:384–388, 1982.
9. Rodgers BM, Talbert JL: Clinical applications of endotracheal cryotherapy. *J Pediatric Surg* 13:662–668, 1978.
10. Kirchner FR, Toledo PS: Microcauterization in otolaryngology. *Arch Otolaryngol Head Neck Surg* 99:198–202, 1974.
11. Campbell BH, Dennison BF, Durking GE, et al: Early and late dilation for acquired subglottic stenosis. *Otolaryngol Head Neck Surg* 95:566–573, 1986.
12. Holinger LD: Treatment of severe subglottic stenosis without tracheotomy. *Ann Otol Rhinol Laryngol* 91:407–412, 1982.
13. Healy GB: An experimental model for the endoscopic correction of subglottic stenosis with clinical applications. *Laryngoscope* 92:1103–1115, 1982.
14. Cotton RT, Tewfik TL: Laryngeal stenosis following carbon dioxide laser in subglottic hemangioma. Report of three cases. *Ann Otol Rhinol Laryngol* 94:494–497, 1985.
15. Duncavage JA, Ossoff RH, Toohill RW: Carbon dioxide laser management of laryngeal stenosis. *Ann Otol Rhinol Laryngol* 94:565–569, 1985.

16. Schmidt FW, Piazzo LS, Chipman TJ, et al: CO_2 laser management of laryngeal stenosis. *Otolaryngol Head Neck Surg* 95:485–490, 1986.
17. Shapshay SM, Beamis JF, Hybels RL, et al: Endoscopic treatment of subglottic and tracheal stenosis by radial incision and dilation. *Ann Otol Rhinol Laryngol* 96:661–664, 1987.
18. Dedo HH, Sooy CD: Endoscopic laser repair of posterior glottic, subglottic and tracheal stenosis by division on micro-trapdoor flap. *Laryngoscope* 94:445–450, 1984.
19. Hall RR: The healing of tissues incised by carbon dioxide laser. *Br J Surg* 58:222–225, 1971.
20. Holinger LD: Treatment of severe subglottic stenosis without tracheotomy—a preliminary report. *Ann Otol Rhinol Laryngol* 91:407–412, 1982.
21. Friedman EM, Healy GB, McGill TJI: Carbon dioxide laser management of subglottic and tracheal stenosis. Review. *Otolaryngol Clin North Am* 16:871–877, 1983.
22. Cotton RT, Myer CM, Bratcher GO, et al: Anterior cricoid split, 1977–1984. *Arch Otolaryngol Head Neck Surg* 114:1300–1302, 1988.
23. Cotton RT, Seid AB: Management of the extubation problem in the premature child. Anterior cricoid split as an alternative to tracheotomy. *Ann Otol Rhinol Laryngol* 89:508–511, 1980.
24. Drake AF, Contencin P, Narcy R, et al: Lateral cricoid cuts as an adjunctive measure to enlarge the stenotic subglottic airway: An anatomic study. *Int J Otorhinolaryngol* 18:129–137, 1989.
25. Cotton RT, Mortelliti AJ, Myer CM: Four-quadrant cricoid cartilage division in laryngotracheal reconstruction. *Arch Otolaryngol Head Neck Surg* 118:1023–1027, 1992.
26. Fearon B, Cinneamond M: Surgical correction of subglottic stenosis of larynx: Clinical results of Fearon-cotton operation. *J Otolaryngol* 5:457–478, 1976.
27. Morgenstein K: Composite auricular graft in laryngeal reconstruction. *Laryngoscope* 82:844–847, 1972.
28. Cotton RT: The problem of pediatric laryngotracheal stenosis: A clinical and experimental study on the efficacy of autogenous cartilaginous grafts placed between the vertically divided halves of the posterior lamina of the cricoid cartilage. *Laryngoscope* 101 (suppl 12) 56:1–34, 1991.
29. Alonso WA, Druck NS, Ogura JH: Clinical experience in hyoid arch transposition. *Laryngoscope* 86:617–624, 1976.
30. Wong ML, Finnegan DA, Kashima HK, et al: Vascularized hyoid interposition for surgical and upper tracheal stenosis. *Ann Otol Rhinol Laryngol* 87:491–497, 1978.
31. Freeland AP: The long-term results of hyoid-sternohyoid grafts in the correction of subglottic stenosis. *J Laryngol Otol* 100:665–674, 1986.
32. Olson NR: Laryngeal suspension and epiglottic flap in laryngopharyngeal trauma. *Ann Otol Rhinol Laryngol* 85:533–537, 1976.
33. Kennedy TL: Epiglottic reconstruction of laryngeal stenosis secondary to cricothyroidectomy. *Laryngoscope* 90:1130–1136, 1980.
34. Friedman M, Toriumi DM, Owens R, et al: Experience with the sternocleidomastoid myoperiosteal flap for reconstruction of subglottic and tracheal defects: Modification of technique and report of long-term results. *Laryngoscope* 98:1003–1111, 1988.
35. Friedman M, Garybauskas VT, Toriumi DM, et al: Reconstruction of the subglottic larynx with a myoperiosteal flap: Clinic and experimental study. *Head Neck* 8:286–295, 1986.
36. Schuller DE, Parris RT: Reconstruction of the larynx and trachea. *Arch Otolaryngol Head Neck Surg* 114:278–286, 1988.

37. Rice DH, Coleman M: Repair of subglottic stenosis with a free perichondrium graft. *Arch Otolaryngol Head Neck Surg* 108:25–27, 1982.
38. Kon M, Vanden Hoof A: Cartilage tube formation by perichondrium: A new concept for tracheal reconstruction. *Plast Reconstr Surg* 72:791–797, 1983.
39. Eliachar I, Marcovich A, Shai Y: Rotary door flap in laryngotracheal reconstruction. *Arch Otolaryngol Head Neck Surg* 110:580–585, 1984.
40. Eliachar I, Roberts JK, Welker KB, et al: Advantages of the rotary door flap in laryngotracheal reconstruction: Is skeletal support necessary? *Ann Otol Rhinol Laryngol* 98:37–40, 1989.
41. Jones RE, Morgan RF, Marcella KL, et al: Tracheal reconstruction with autogenous jejunal microsurgical transfer. *Ann Thorac Surg* 41:636–638, 1986.
42. Kambic V, Godina M, Zupevc A: Epithelialized microvascular iliac crest flap for reconstruction of subglottic and upper tracheal stenosis: A preliminary report. *Am J Otolaryngol* 7:157–162, 1986.
43. Biller HF, Lawson W, Weisberg V: Staged repair of extensive tracheal and laryngotracheal stenosis. *Ann Otol Rhinol Laryngol* 95:586–589, 1986.
44. Pearson FG, Cooper JD, Nelems JM, et al: Primary tracheal anastomosis after resection of the cricoid cartilage with preservation of recurrent laryngeal nerves. *J Thorac Cardiovasc Surg* 70:806–816, 1975.
45. Monnier P, Savary M, Chapuis G: Partial cricoid resection with primary tracheal anastomosis for subglottic stenosis in infants and children. *Laryngoscope* 103:1273–1283, 1993.
46. Evans JNG, Todd GB: Laryngotracheoplasty. *J Laryngol Otol* 88:589–597, 1974.
47. Montgomery WW: T-tube tracheal stent. *Arch Otolaryngol Head Neck Surg* 82:320–321, 1965.
48. Eliacher I, Nguyen D: Laryngotracheal stent for internal support and control of aspiration without loss of phonation. *Otolaryngol Head Neck Surg* 103:837–840, 1990.
49. Maran AG, Geissler PR: A new material for laryngeal prosthesis. *J Laryngol Otol* 84:1147–1151, 1970.
50. Passy V, Kulber H, Ermshar CB: The K.E.B. laryngeal-tracheal stent. *Laryngoscope* 82:271–275, 1972.
51. Zalzal GH: Use of stents in laryngotracheal reconstruction in children. Indications, technical consideration and complications. *Laryngoscope* 98:849–854, 1988.
52. Olsen NR: Skin grafting of the larynx. *Otolaryngol Head Neck Surg* 104:503–507, 1991.

Congenital Perilymphatic Fistula

Peter C. Weber, M.D.
Assistant Professor, Director, Division of Neurology/Otology, Director, Center for Hearing and Balance Disorders, Department of Otolaryngology, Medical University of South Carolina, Charleston, South Carolina

Barry E. Hirsch, M.D.
Associate Professor, Department of Otolaryngology, University of Pittsburgh Eye and Ear Institute, Pittsburgh, Pennsylvania

P erilymphatic fistula (PLF) is defined as a condition that consists of an abnormal communication between the inner and the middle ear. Unfortunately, diagnosis of PLF is controversial. This controversy is in part related to the myriad of nonspecific signs and symptoms associated with PLF and with the surgeon's subjective diagnosis at the time of exploratory tympanotomy. These signs and symptoms include tinnitus; progressive, fluctuating, or (rarely) sudden sensorineural hearing loss, which may or may not be associated with vertigo; and vertigo or disequilibrium, which may be present without hearing loss.[1–11]

Unfortunately, exploratory tympanotomy, currently the only way of actually making the diagnosis of an active PLF, is also fraught with controversy.[12–14] Fluids other than perilymph may be seen in the middle ear at the time of exploration, including local anesthetic, serous fluid, and/or blood. There are various intraoperative procedures and maneuvers designed to enhance the visualization of a PLF such as jugular vein compression, Valsalva's maneuver, Trendelenburg positioning, or ossicular chain manipulation. Despite these efforts, an active PLF may not be confirmed.

Disagreement still remains regarding the existence, incidence and treatment of PLF. It should be noted that most would agree that congenital PLFs indeed exist as do traumatic or iatrogenic fistulas.[15–16] What is really in question is whether or not the "spontaneous" PLF is indeed a valid disease entity.[17] This chapter will not try to delineate whether or not the diagnosis of a spontaneous PLF is valid, but rather will center on the advances in the diagnosis of perilymphatic fistulas. We will do this by looking at recent papers that describe correlations between PLF and magnetic resonance imaging results, computed tomography (CT) scan results, congenital middle ear abnormalities, electrocochleography, fluorescein testing, posturography, endoscopic examination, and beta-2 transferrin testing. We will also be looking at the results of exploratory tympanotomies on children suspected of having a PLF.

Advances in Otolaryngology—Head and Neck Surgery®, vol. 9
© 1995, Mosby–Year Book, Inc.

MIDDLE EAR ABNORMALITIES

Nenzelius was the first to describe a temporal bone malformation as a predisposing condition for a congenital PLF, deafness, and recurrent meningitis.[18] Since this first description, other early reported cases of congenital PLF have been described.[19-22] Subsequent to those early reports, other surgeons have described congenital middle ear abnormalities in association with PLF.[6, 15, 16] Although it is well known that inner ear abnormalities such as an enlarged vestibular aqueduct and a Mondini type deformity have a high association with PLFs and with sensorineural hearing loss, the correlation between middle ear abnormalities and PLF has not been as well defined. Recent evidence has shown that this correlation does exist.[6, 15, 16] A recent report by Weber and associates demonstrated an 80% correlation between a positive PLF and a middle ear abnormality.[15] In their retrospective review of 94 patients (117 ears), 60 patients (80 ears) were thought to have a PLF at the time of surgery. Forty-eight patients, or 80%, also had a middle ear abnormality at the time of exploration (Fig 1). Although this correlation exists, the presence of a middle ear abnormality does not imply that a PLF is present. Of the 34 patients who were not identified as having a PLF at the time of surgery, 12 (35%) also had a middle ear abnormality.

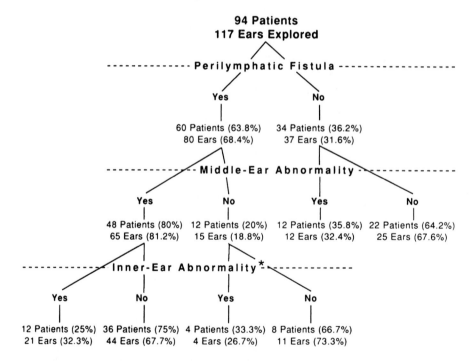

*Note: No patient had inner-ear abnormality on CT who did not have PLF observed.

FIGURE 1.

The incidence of perilymphatic fistula and congenital middle ear and inner ear abnormalities in 94 children, 1980 to 1989. (From Weber P, Bluestone C, Perez B, et al: *Laryngoscope* 103:160–164, 1993. Used by permission.)

Weber and co-workers also noted that CT confirmed inner ear abnormalities were found in 25% of patients that were identified as having a PLF.[15] Interestingly, all patients who had an inner ear abnormality on CT scan had a PLF observed.

The most common middle ear anomalies found in this study were that of the stapes superstructure.[15] The stapes superstructure was abnormal in approximately 60% of cases. Figure 2 demonstrates the most common stapes abnormalities. The second most common type of middle ear malformations associated with PLF involved the round window. This was seen in approximately 31% of the patients. The incus was deformed in approximately 17% of cases. This study demonstrated that the oval window was the most common site of a PLF, observed in 60% of ears, while the round window was involved in 22.5% of the cases, and both windows were the site of PLF in 17.5% of patients. Perilymphatic fistulas were also noted to be bilateral in 20 patients (33%).

The CT scan provides a method of determining temporal bone anatomy and development of the otic capsule and middle ear. Unfortunately, it has always been difficult to make a diagnosis of a middle ear abnormality by CT. A recent study by Weisman and associates has shown that with 1mm fine-cut high-resolution CT scans that the stapes superstructure can be well visualized and abnormalities can be documented accurately.[23] These high resolution CT scans however, can not detect an abnormally facing round window or an abnormal curvature of the incus. It is also very difficult to ascertain a type 3 stapes malformation from a CT scan (see Fig 2). Thus, there are limitations of CT imaging, namely that it does not provide consistent identification of the middle ear round window or ossicular chain abnormalities. However, a CT scan is still recommended in the evaluation of a PLF since it will identify inner ear abnormalities, which although not as common as middle ear abnormalities, have a high correlation with PLFs in those patients who are symptomatic.

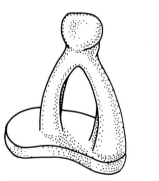 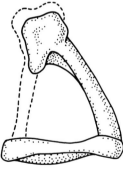 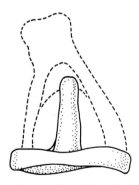

Ant. crus in middle of footplate   Columellar Type I   Columellar Type II

FIGURE 2.

The three types of stapes superstructure malformations. (From Weber P, Bluestone C, Perez B, et al: *Laryngoscope* 103:160–164, 1993. Used by permission.)

MAGNETIC RESONANCE IMAGING

Interestingly, magnetic resonance imaging (MRI) may also prove to be useful in the detection of a PLF. Although an MRI scan does not demonstrate bony abnormalities and, thus, cannot predict a middle ear or inner ear abnormality, the test may be useful in identifying a leak when used with Gadolinium, an intravenous contrast agent. Since cochlear perilymph is thought to be an ultrafiltrate of cerebral spinal fluid, Gadolinium, a nonionic paramagnetic contrast agent, may someday be used to help identify these leaks. Morris and co-workers injected Gadolinium intrathecally into six healthy adult cats in which they had created a PLF in the round window.[24] They demonstrated pooling of the Gadolinium in the middle ear and mastoid air cells. Unfortunately, the study was limited to six cats and there was no control group without fistulas. Thus, it is difficult to ascertain whether the Gadolinium indeed came from the cerebral spinal fluid, or whether it was absorbed into the blood stream and because of the recent surgery was found in the middle ear and mastoid from the blood. This study does bring up the possibility that in the future, MRI with Gadolinium may be a very useful test in a preoperative diagnosis of a PLF.

ELECTROCOCHLEOGRAPHY

Interest regarding the use of electrocochleography (ECoG) as a useful preoperative diagnostic test for PLF has been renewed. Gulya and associates demonstrated no clinical usefulness for ECoG in the diagnosis of a PLF in an experimental study using a guinea pig model.[25] In contrast, Arenberg and co-workers demonstrated the usefulness of the ECoG if a patent fistula was maintained in the guinea pig model, and in patients with an active PLF.[26] Arenberg made the point that in addition to creating a fistula in the round window or oval window, perilymph actually must leak out and be active in order for there to be an abnormality in the ECoG. Gibson monitored ECoG changes in patients undergoing stapedectomy or round window cochleostomy.[27] In his recent study assessing outpatient ECoG criteria in predicting a PLF, he demonstrated no ECoG changes until perilymph was actually removed. He looked at ECoG recordings from 206 ears suspected of having a PLF. Forty-six of the 206 patients underwent exploration that showed a positive identification of a PLF in 38 ECoGs. Evaluation of the electrocochleography results showed a high correlation between strongly positive ECoG and the presence of a PLF, and a weak ECoG with the absence of a PLF. Furthermore, in 116 patients with negative ECoG findings, 32 underwent exploration, and 10 (31%) were found to have a PLF, thus indicating that electrocochleography can not be used to exclude a PLF. Gibson concluded that reduced perilymph volume was the cause for a strongly positive ECoG but the reduced perilymph volume diminished the likelihood of being able to identify an active PLF at the time of the surgery. Furthermore, ears having a readily visible, active PLF may have a normal ECoG since the actual volume of perilymph should be close to normal. Nevertheless, for patients suspected of having a PLF, Gibson recommended exploration despite negative preoperative ECoG data. Two other recent studies have also revealed that ECoG changes may be demonstrated in both vestibular endolymphatic hydrops (no cochlear signs or symptoms) and cochlear endolymphatic hydrops (no vestibular signs or symptoms).[28, 29] Unfortunately, these studies point out that abnormal ECoG results are found in both endolymphatic hydrops and PLF. Thus, ECoG testing is not specific to the diagnosis of PLF.

FLUORESCEIN

Fluorescein is a synthetic dye with a low molecular weight that has fluorescent properties when excited by light. Fluorescein absorbs light in the blue end of the spectrum and is visible in the mixed light of the green/yellow spectrum. It has been used by ophthalmologists for many years in the detection of various ocular disorders, and in the past was used in otology research to trace the flow of labyrinthine fluids. Syms and co-workers reported on the intravenous injection of fluorescein in order to detect PLFs both in humans and in dogs.[30] He proposed that fluorescein crossed the blood-brain barrier, diffused into the cerebral spinal fluid, and then into perilymph. Other investigators have refuted this theory by demonstrating that fluorescein, injected intravenously, is taken up by the soft tissues and mucosa of the middle ear and remains visible for up to three and one-half hours.[31, 32] These studies also convincingly demonstrated that when a controlled PLF was achieved in the study animals and complete hemostasis was obtained using a laser, no detection of fluorescein could be documented. These two studies demonstrated that what was thought to be PLF identification by Syms may have been leakage of fluorescein from blood vessels.

Research has also been done on the use of intrathecal injection of fluorescein for the detection of PLFs in animals and although there is a quick leakage of fluorescein from a PLF with intrathecal injection, the increased chance of seizure activity associated with intrathecal injection of fluorescein would contraindicate this use in humans. In summary, it appears that intravenous fluorescein is not clearly useful in diagnosing a PLF.

PLATFORM POSTUROGRAPHY

Shepard and associates, investigating the use of posturography with varied positive and negative pneumatic pressure to the tympanic membrane, suggested that this method may be a useful preoperative diagnostic test for PLF.[33] In this prospective study using six different protocols for platform posturography testing, they demonstrated a sensitivity ranging from 53% to 100% and specificity ranging from 56% to 89%. The problem in using this or any other preoperative test still stems from the lack of a final objective test determining whether or not a PLF actually exists at the time of exploratory tympanotomy. Therefore, these authors felt that due to the variability of their selection criteria and the inability to make an accurate diagnosis by surgical observation, clear conclusions regarding the accuracy of preoperative platform pressure test could not be achieved. Interestingly, their study also demonstrated that vestibular rehabilitation may be helpful in certain groups of patients with PLF, thus obviating the need for surgical exploration. The one group of patients who did not do well with vestibular rehabilitation were those patients who had a traumatic PLF.

FISTULA TEST

Historically, nystagmus observed with positive or negative pressure during pneumatic otoscopy (Hennebert's sign) was believed to be a sign of a PLF. Unfortunately, less than 50% of patients with a PLF demonstrate a positive fistula test and 30% of patients with hydrops may have a positive fistula test.[34] Wall and Casselbrandt report a 92% correlation with electronystagmogram (ENG)-electro-oculographic response measurement with the fistula test in an animal model.[35, 36] These results do not appear as promising in adult humans.[34]

MIDDLE EAR ENDOSCOPY

An exciting new opportunity to make the diagnosis of PLF is afforded by middle ear endoscopy. Recent advances in endoscope technology have made available 1 mm flexible endoscopes and small rigid telescopes with a diameter of 1.7 mm to evaluate the middle ear. In an awake patient these endoscopes can be passed through a small myringotomy to examine the oval or round window niche for possible PLF and to identify middle ear abnormalities. Currently, endoscopes of 0.5 mm diameter are being evaluated. Poe and co-workers recently reported their experience with middle ear endoscopy for PLF both in the feline model and in human subjects.[37] Their excellent endoscopic examination of the middle ear and observation of PLF in the feline model was the basis for future investigation. Twenty patients with possible PLF were endoscopically examined. No active PLFs were noted, although four had a positive fistula test shown by Valsalva's maneuver. Blood patches were placed on seven patients with good resolution of the fistula test on follow-up examination. No patients had discernible hearing loss following endoscopic examination. An advantage of endoscopic examination is that no injectable anesthetic is necessary and, thus, this eliminates any transudate or lidocaine in the middle ear, which may obscure a possible diagnosis of a PLF. Poe and associates recommend the use of a rigid telescope for superior resolution rather than a fiberoptic endoscope. Although this is an exciting field for the evaluation of PLFs, it should be recognized that this technique is mainly for use in adult patients, since children would have difficulty remaining still without general anesthesia.

PROTEINS

It has been known for some time that the protein component of perilymph is distinctly different from that of serum and cerebral spinal fluid. Schweitzer and colleagues, and Woodson and associates analyzed the amino acid components of perilymph in both guinea pig and human aspirates.[38, 39] In their study analyzing 19 free amino acid concentrations by chromatography, there were distinct differences in these samples. However, no distinct patterns could be elicited to exactly make the diagnosis of perilymph versus serum or cerebral spinal fluid. These two papers are indeed promising, and suggest that in the future this may be a viable way of making an objective diagnosis of PLF. Further identification of perilymph proteins was described by Paugh and co-workers, who again studied differences between perilymph, serum, and cerebral spinal fluid.[40] Their paper used a two-dimensional gel electrophoresis separating the proteins by an isoelectric point. A small number of perilymph proteins not found in plasma were identified in both the guinea pig and human specimens. This finding demonstrates that perilymph does have unique proteins which may permit the development of a sensitive marker to aid in the diagnosis of PLF. Silverstein published a report using a rapid protein test for perilymphatic fistula.[41] His paper test, which was a real-time test, showed the presence of protein with a light green or dark green color change depending on the protein concentration. Silverstein suggested that perilymph has a protein content of 524 mg%, whereas in acoustic neuromas or cerebral spinal fluid, the protein content is markedly increased at 2,260 mg%. The problem with this method for diagnosing a PLF is the effect that serum or blood contamination may have on the analysis.

β-2 TRANSFERRIN

β-2 transferrin, a variant of β-1 serum transferrin, was first described in the early 1960s as a unique protein or transferrin specific for cerebral spinal fluid.[42, 43] There are two theories for the origin of β-2 transferrin. One describes cleavage of a sialic acid from the β-1 transferrin through a neuramidase in the brain parenchyma. The other suggests β-2 transferrin is produced entirely by dark cells of the brain tissue.[44] Since its first description, authors have advocated the use of β-2 transferrin as a diagnostic means for detecting cerebral spinal fluid leaks.[45–49] β-2 transferrin has also been isolated from vitreous humor[50] and more recently from perilymph.[51–53] Two recent studies suggest that β-2 transferrin should be used to diagnose a PLF.[54, 55] An early report failed to demonstrate β-2 transferrin in perilymph during acoustic neuroma surgery, but unfortunately no methodology for the determination of β-2 transferrin was reported in this article.[56] Because β-2 transferrin is only identified in cerebral spinal fluid, perilymph, and vitreous humor, and normally can not be detected in serum or local anesthetics, it is believed that β-2 transferrin would be a useful test to objectively determine whether a PLF exists.

A recent prospective study involving 10 children operated on for PLF and 10 controls demonstrated that β-2 transferrin was negative in all 10 control patients.[54] Nine of the 10 patients operated on for a PLF were thought to have a perilymphatic fistula at the time of exploratory tympanotomy. Six of the nine tested positive for β-2 transferrin. These results indicated that no false-positive results occurred in the control group and that the one child who was explored surgically for a possible PLF and found not to have one also tested negative for β-2 transferrin. Interestingly, of the nine patients diagnosed with a PLF at the time of surgery, seven had middle ear abnormalities. Of these seven patients, six tested positive for β-2 transferrin, thus, demonstrating a strong correlation between PLF and abnormal middle ear anatomy.

Based upon this pilot study a subsequent prospective study evaluated 43 children with suspected PLF over a three-year period.[55] There were 23 positive and 20 negative PLFs identified at the time of exploration (Fig 3). Of the 20 patients who were thought to be negative for a PLF, 18 also tested negative for β-2 transferrin. Of interest are the two patients who tested positive for β-2 transferrin despite having a negative exploration at the time of surgery. Both of these patients had a congenital middle ear abnormality. This may be interpreted as a false-positive test or that an intermittent fistula was present that was not readily identifiable at the time of exploration. This finding further supports the theory that PLFs are associated with middle ear anomalies (Fig 4). Of the 23 patients considered to have a PLF at the time of surgery, six (26%) tested positive for β-2 transferrin. All six of these patients had middle ear abnormalities. There were 16 control patients in this study and all tested negative for β-2 transferrin as would be expected.

Although β-2 transferrin is a very promising objective test in the confirmation of PLFs, there are problems with the test. First, the western blot assay for the test takes approximately 3 hours to complete and, thus, it is not a real-time test which can be used during the actual surgery. Second, the actual sensitivity and specificity of this test is not known. Because samples are taken with Gelfoam (Upjohn, Kalamazoo, Mich) from the oval and round window and may dessicate in a test tube and need to

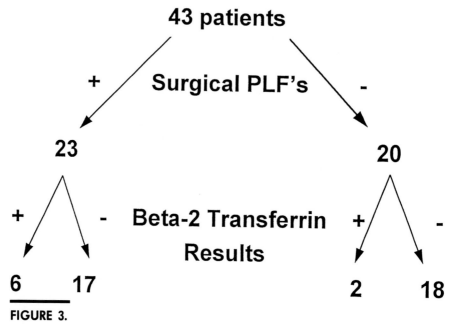

FIGURE 3.

The correlation of β-2 transferrin and middle-ear abnormalities in congenital perilymphatic fistula. (From Weber P, Bluestone C, Kenna M, et al: *Am J Otology,* in press. Used by permission.)

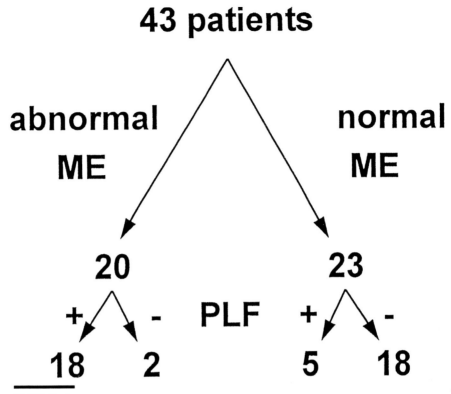

FIGURE 4.
Correlation of β-2 transferrin and middle ear abnormalities in congenital peri-lymphatic fistula. (From Weber P, Bluestone C, Kenna M, et al: *Am J Otology*, in press. Used by permission.)

be reconstituted, the dilutional effect may increase the number of false-negative results. Further testing for the best method and material for sample collection needs to be defined. The testing of control samples of perilymph and cerebral spinal fluid is currently in progress so the true sensitivity and specificity of this analysis can be determined. It should be noted that patients with severe liver failure have abnormal levels of serum proteins. On rare occasions, blood from these patients may test positive for β-2 transferrin.[57]

TREATMENT

The treatment of suspected PLF at the time of exploration remains a controversial issue. Hughes completed a survey of otologists that illustrates the difference in management philosophies.[12] Some otologists believe that all ears should be packed at the oval and round window regardless of the intraoperative findings. Other otologists believe that if an active leak is not identified the ear should not be packed. Two of the concerns of packing every ear despite no evidence of a fistula are the fear of subsequent development of hearing loss or obscuring future explorations. Iatrogenic hearing loss was not a problem in a study performed at the University of Iowa[6] nor in a retrospective chart review of 94 children (117 ears) operated on for a possible congenital PLF at the University of Pittsburgh.[54] In the latter study a total of 80 ears (60 patients) had a PLF identified, while 37 ears (35 patients) did not have a PLF identified. Of the 80 ears positive for a PLF, 8 actually demonstrated an improvement in their hearing greater than 10 dB while 2 demonstrated a decrease in their hearing greater than 10 dB, and 63 had no appreciable change. Seven patients were unavailable for follow-up examination. Of the 37 ears that were negative for a PLF, 34 had no appreciable change in hearing while 2 ears continued to have hearing loss (>20 dB) despite packing and 1 was lost to follow-up. Stabilizing hearing was determined to be a success since the progression of hearing loss was abated. It should be noted that all ears were packed in this study regardless of a positive or negative PLF.

The second area of treatment that needs to be addressed are those patients with vestibular complaints. Previous studies have demonstrated that patients with vestibular complaints are helped by exploration and packing for a suspected PLF. In the study by Weber and co-workers,[58] of the 60 children with a PLF, 24 had vestibular complaints preoperatively. Seventeen of these 24 had improvement in their symptoms, 4 had no change, 1 patient felt worse, and 2 were unavailable for follow-up examination.

Recurrences are always a complication that may be associated with PLFs. In the study by Weber and associates their reexploration rate was approximately 10%.[58] Of these, a PLF was only found in half of the ears reexplored. To diminish the recurrence rate or the need for reexploration, Black and co-workers recommended using autologous fibrin glue with the use of the laser to ensure an adequate seal. This method works well for these patients, although other reports advocate using temporalis muscle or fascia without the laser, which allows for equal results.[6, 54]

CONCLUSION

The diagnosis and management of PLF continues to be controversial. Many of the proposed and established preoperative tests cannot be accurately verified when the "gold standard" for diagnosing a PLF is a subjective interpretation. The advent of β-2 transferrin analysis provides the potential ability to objectively make the diagnosis of a PLF. Unfortunately, problems still do exist with this test that need to be addressed in future investigations. When identified, surgery for perilymphatic fistulas is not only safe but also effective in the vast majority of patients and should be offered if the diagnosis of a PLF is of concern.

REFERENCES

1. Stroud MH, Calcaterra TG: Spontaneous perilymph fistulas. *Laryngoscope* 80:479–487, 1970.
2. Singleton G, Weider D: Panel discussion: Perilymphatic fistula. *Am J Otolaryngol* 8:355–363, 1987.
3. Shelton C, Simmons FB: Perilymph fistula: The Stanford experience. *Ann Otol Rhinol Laryngol* 97:105–108, 1988.
4. Weider DJ, Johnson GD: Perilymphatic fistula: A New Hampshire experience. *Am J Otolaryngol* 9:184–196, 1988.

5. Pappas DG, Schneiderman TS: Perilymphatic fistula in pediatric patients with a preexisting sensorineural loss. *Am J Otol* 10:499–501, 1989.
6. Seltzer S, McCabe BF: Perilymph fistula: The Iowa experience. *Laryngoscope* 94:37–49, 1986.
7. Reilly JS: Congenital perilymphatic fistula: A prospective study in infants and children. *Laryngoscope* 99:393–397, 1989.
8. Supance JS, Bluestone CD: Perilymph fistulas in infants and children. *Otolaryngol Head Neck Surg* 91:663–671, 1983.
9. Althaus SR: Perilymph fistulas. *Laryngoscope* 91:538–562, 1981.
10. Grundfast KM, Bluestone CD: Sudden or fluctuating hearing loss and vertigo in children due to perilymph fistula. *Ann Otol Rhinol Laryngol* 87:761–771, 1978.
11. Bluestone CD: Otitis media and congenital perilymphatic fistula as a cause of sensorineural hearing loss in children. *Pediatr Infect Dis J* 7:S141–145, 1988.
12. Hughes GB, Sismanis A, House JW: Is there consensus in perilymph fistula management? *Otolaryngol Head Neck Surg* 102:111–117, 1990.
13. Rizer FM, House JW: Perilymph fistulas: The House Ear Clinic experience. *Otolaryngol Head Neck Surg* 104:239–243, 1991.
14. House JW, Morris MS, Kramer SJ, et al: Perilymphatic fistula: Surgical experience in the United States. *Otolaryngol Head Neck Surg* 105:51–61, 1991.
15. Weber PC, Bluestone CD, Perez BA: Congenital perilymphatic fistula and associated middle ear abnormalities. *Laryngoscope* 103:160–164, 1993.
16. Weber PC, Kelly RH, Bluestone CD, et al: Beta-2 transferrin confirms perilymphatic fistula in children. *Otolaryngol Head Neck Surg* 110:381–386, 1994.
17. Shea JJ: The myth of spontaneous perilymph fistula. *Otolaryngol Head Neck Surg* 107:613, 1992.
18. Nenzelius C: On spontaneous cerebrospinal otorhea due to congenital malformations. *Acta Otolaryngol (Stockh)* 39:314–328, 1951.
19. Ban B, Wensall J: Cerebro-spinal otorrhea with meningitis in congenital deafness. *Arch Otolaryngol Head Neck Surg* 81:26–28, 1965.
20. Crook JP: Congenital fistula in the stapedial footplate. *South Med J* 60:1168, 1967.
21. Rice WJ, Waggoren LG: Congenital cerebrospinal fluid otorrhea via defect in the stapes footplate. *Laryngoscope* 77:341–349, 1967.
22. McCabe BF: The incidence, site, treatment and fate of labyrinthine fistula. *Clin Otolaryngol* 3:239–242, 1948.
23. Weisman J, Weber PC, Bluestone CD: Computed tomography in assessing middle-ear abnormalities associated with congenital perilymphatic fistula. *Otolaryngol Head Neck Surg* (in press).
24. Morris MS, Kil J, Carvlin MJ: Magnetic resonance imaging of perilymphatic fistula. *Laryngoscope* 103:729–734, 1993.
25. Guyla AJ, Boling LS, Mastroianni MAP: EcoG and perilymphatic fistula: An experimental study in the guinea pig. *Otolaryngol Head Neck Surg* 102:132–139, 1990.
26. Arenberg IK, Ackley RS, Ferraro J, et al: EcoG results in perilymphatic fistula: Clinical and experimental studies. *Otolaryngol Head Neck Surg* 99:435–443, 1988.
27. Gibson WPR: Electrocochleography in the diagnosis of perilymphatic fistula: Intraoperative observations and assessment of a new diagnostic office procedure. *Am J Otolaryngol* 13:146–151, 1992.
28. Comphill KCM, Savage MM, Harker LA: Electrocochleography in the presence and absence of perilymphatic fistula. *Ann Otol Rhinol Laryngol* 101:403–407, 1992.

29. Donhoffer JI, Arenberg IK: Diagnoses of vestibular Meniere's disease with electrocochleography. *Am J Otolaryngol* 14:161–164, 1993.

30. Syms CA, Atkins JS, Murphy TP: The use of fluorescein for intraoperative confirmation of perilymph fistula—a preliminary report, in Arenberg IK (ed): *Proceedings of the third international symposium and workshops on the surgery of the inner ear*. New York, Kugler & Ghedini Publications, 1992, pp 383–385.

31. Bojrab DI, Bhansali SA: Fluorescein use in the detection of perilymphatic fistula: A study in cats. *Otolaryngol Head Neck Surg* 108:548–555, 1993.

32. Poe DS, Gadre AK, Rebeiz EE, et al: Intravenous fluorescein for detection of perilymphatic fistulas. *Am J Otol* 13:529–534, 1992.

33. Shephard NT, Telian SA, Riparko JK, et al: Platform pressure test in identification of perilymphatic fistula. *Am J Otol* 13:49–54, 1992.

34. Calhoun KH, Strenk CL: Perilymph fistula. *Arch Otolaryngol Head Neck Surg* 118:693–694, 1992.

35. Wall C, Casselbrandt ML: System identification of perilymphatic fistula in an animal model. *Am J Otol* 13:443–448, 1992.

36. Hammerschlag PE: Management of vestibular disorders current opinion. *Otolaryngol Head Neck Surg* 108:39–45, 1993.

37. Poe DS, Rebeiz EE, Pankratov MM: Evaluation of perilymphatic fistulas by middle ear endoscopy. *Am J Otol* 13:529–533, 1992.

38. Schweitzer VG, Woodson BT, Mawhinney TD, et al: Free amino acid analysis of guinea pig perilymph: A possible clinical assay for the PLF enigma? *Otolaryngol Head Neck Surg* 103:981–985, 1990.

39. Woodson BT, Fujita S, Mawhinney TD, et al: Perilymphatic fistula: Analysis of free amino acids in middle ear microspirates. *Otolaryngol Head Neck Surg* 104:796–802, 1991.

40. Paugh DR, Telian SA, Disher MJ: Identification of perilymph proteins by two-dimensional gel electrophoresis. *Otolaryngol Head Neck Surg* 104:517–525, 1991.

41. Silverstein H: Rapid protein test for perilymph fistula. *Otolaryngol Head Neck Surg* 105:422–426, 1991.

42. Pette D, Stupp I: Die B-Fraktion in liquor cerebrospinalis. *Klin Wschr* 38:109–110, 1960.

43. Parker W, Bearn A: Studies on the transferrin of adult serum cord serum and cerebrospinal fluid. *Exp Med* 115:83–105, 1962.

44. Reisinger PW, Hochstrasser K: The diagnosis of CSF fistulae on the basis of detection of beta-2 transferrin by polyacrylamide gel electrophoresis and immunoblotting. *J Clin Chem Clin Biochem* 27:169–172, 1989.

45. Meurman OH, Irjala K, Suonpaa J, et al: A new method for the identification of cerebrospinal fluid leakage. *Acta Otolaryngol (Stockh)* 87:366–369, 1979.

46. Oberscher G: Cerebrospinal fluid otorrhea—new trends in diagnosis. *Am J Otol* 9:102–108, 1988.

47. Oberscher G, Arrer E: Erste Klinische erfahrangen nit Beta-2 transferrin bei oto und rhinoliquorrhoe. *HNO* 34:151–155, 1986.

48. Oberscher G: A modern concept of cerebrospinal fluid diagnosis in oto and rhinorrhea. *Rhinology* 26:89–103, 1988.

49. Irjala K, Suonpaa J, Laurent B: Identification of CSF leakage by immunofixation. *Arch Otolaryngol Head Neck Surg* 105:447–448, 1979.

50. Tripathi RC, Millard CD, Tripathi BJ, et al: A fraction of transferrin is present in human aqueous humor and is not unique to cerebrospinal fluid. *Exp Eye Res* 50:541–547, 1990.

51. Naiberg JB, Flemming E, Patterson M, et al: The perilymphatic fistula—the end of an enigma. *J Otolaryngol* 19:260–263, 1990.

52. Bassiouny M, Hirsch BE, Kelly RH, et al: Beta-2 transferrin application in otology. *Am J Otol* (accepted for publication).
53. Arrer E, Oberscher G, Gibitz HJ: Protein distribution in the human perilymph. *Acta Otolaryngol (Stockh)* 106:117–123, 1988.
54. Weber PC, Kelly RH, Bluestone CD, et al: Beta-2 transferrin confirms perilymphatic fistula in children. *Otolaryngol Head Neck Surg* 110:381–386, 1994.
55. Weber PC, Bluestone CD, Kenna MA, et al: Correlation of beta-2 transferrin and middle ear abnormalities in congenital perilymphatic fistula. *Am J Otol* (in press), 1994.
56. Thomsen J, Saxtrup O, Tos M: Quantitated determination of proteins in perilymph in patients with acoustic neuromas. *ORL J Otorhinolaryngol Relat Spec* 44:61–65, 1982.
57. Skedros DG, Carso SP, Hirsch BE, et al: Sources of error in use of beta-2 transferrin analysis for diagnosing perilymphatic and cerebral spinal fluid leaks. *Otolaryngol Head Neck Surg* 109:861–864, 1993.
58. Weber PC, Bluestone CD, Perez BP: Outcome of hearing and vertigo following surgery for congenital perilymphatic fistula in children. *Ann Otol Rhinol Laryngol* (submitted).

The Extended Subperiosteal Coronal Face-Lift: An Improved Approach in Facial Rejuvenation Surgery

Howard A. Tobin, M.D.
Medical Director, Facial Plastic and Cosmetic Surgical Center, Abilene, Texas

George T. Goffas, M.D., D.D.S.
Private Practice, Facial Plastic and Maxillofacial Surgery, Birmingham, Michigan

C ervicofacial rhytidectomy, or face-lift surgery, continues to evolve and remains a popular cosmetic procedure. Originally consisting of skin excision, later techniques emphasized first undermining and then plication or dissection and repositioning of deeper fascial layers to improve results. More recently, surgeons have utilized the deepest tissue layer, periosteum, to advance face-lifting techniques. This "third generation face-lift," known as the extended subperiosteal coronal lift (ESCL), offers an improved approach in facial rejuvenation surgery of the middle and upper third of the face.

Although traditional face-lift techniques are effective in the lower face and neck, they become less effective in the middle and upper face and minimally improve the forehead and brow region. Attempting to overcome these limitations, surgeons have extended the scope of traditional techniques by combining procedures such as coronal brow lifting with lower face-lifts. Others have expanded the traditional approaches with modifications, such as the composite face-lift proposed by Hamra,[1,2] with variable results.

Advancing craniofacial principles, Tessier[3] first proposed the concept of extending the coronal lift by developing a subperiosteal plane of dissection from the forehead onto the zygoma and maxilla. Psillakis et al.[4] adopted the technique and described a four-year experience involving 105 patients. Operating through a bicoronal incision, his technique included subperiosteal dissection of the upper orbit, glabella, zygoma and anterior zygomatic arch, as well as the upper maxilla. Although his results were encouraging, a 7% incidence of temporary paralysis of the frontal branch of the facial nerve convinced him to limit dissection to the middle third of the zygomatic arch. Psillakis believed that lateral dissection placed the nerve at greater jeopardy since it passes closely over the arch in the mid-zygomatic region. Nevertheless, 3 of the 85 patients that underwent the

Advances in Otolaryngology—Head and Neck Surgery®, vol. 9
© 1995, Mosby–Year Book, Inc.

more limited dissection still experienced temporary forehead weakness.

While the surgical technique will be described in detail below, the principles of the operation are reviewed here. Surgery is carried out under general anesthesia, supplemented with infiltration of lidocaine and adrenaline. The operation is begun with intraoral subperiosteal dissection of the maxilla, anterior zygoma, lateral nasal bones, and includes the anterior masseteric space. This effectively mobilizes the muscles of facial expression in the midface and perioral region (Fig 1). Although the operation is referred to as "subperiosteal," it is actually performed in four distinct planes (Fig 2). These planes are

1. Subperiosteal
2. Subgaleal
3. Subtemporal
4. Submasseteric

Initially, the forehead is approached in the subgaleal plane, similar to standard coronal lifting techniques. Once the brow is approached, the dissection is deepened from the subgaleal plane to a subperiosteal level. However, as the incision is continued laterally, the temporalis muscle is encountered. At this point, a plane of dissection is developed beneath the superficial layers of the temporal fascia—giving rise to the subtemporal plane. From this upper approach, elevation over the zygoma and maxilla continues, returning to a subperiosteal plane.

The fourth plane of dissection is developed inferior to the zygomatic arch in a plane just deep to the masseteric fascia. This represents the sub-

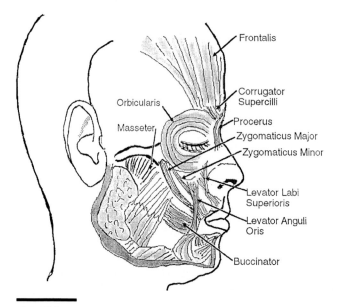

FIGURE 1.

The extended subperiosteal coronal face-lift (ESCL) is carried out in a plane that is deep to the muscles of facial expression, as indicated. This plane of dissection is immediately superficial to the masseter muscle but is actually carried out in a plane that is beneath the masseteric fascia. This plane is chosen to avoid injury to the overlying buccal branch of the facial nerve and parotid duct.

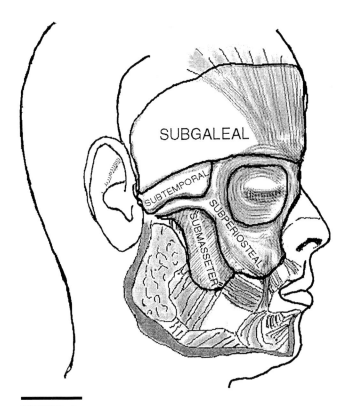

FIGURE 2.

Although the operation is described as "subperiosteal" it is carried out in several planes. This illustration depicts the planes of dissection in the various areas of the face. While several levels are used, they are all connected to create a single, deep, musculofascial flap containing the subcutaneous tissue, muscles of facial expression, and branches of the facial nerve and parotid gland. This strong flap has generous attachments to the overlying skin, acting as a vehicle for "lifting" the facial skin.

masseteric plane. As discussed later, this plane is developed beneath the most superficial fibers of the masseter muscle to provide protection for the buccal branch of the facial nerve and Stenson's duct.

Ramirez et al.[5] made two contributions that improved both the safety and effectiveness of the ESCL procedure. First, he described a plane of dissection beneath the superficial temporal fascia, overlying the temporalis muscle, extending inferiorly to the zygomatic arch. Ramirez felt this was a safer approach to the zygomatic arch because dissection in the subperiosteal plane along the lateral surface of the arch ensured that the frontal branch of the facial nerve was superficial to the plane of dissection, therefore, decreasing vulnerability to injury. Also, working beneath this fascial plane provides a strong flap to help anchor and vertically support the deeper tissues that are dissected free.

Ramirez further described a "back cut" made perpendicular to the zygomatic arch from deep to superficial.[6] This incision was made after completion of the submassateric deep plane elevation, and was designed to free up the flap attachments to the lateral zygoma, temporal bone, ear cartilage, and temporomandibular joint.

We have developed an improvement in the technique whereby the "back cut" is replaced by an initial preauricular incision with dissection carried down to the capsule of temporomandibular joint and the zygomaticotemporal suture line. This technique enables the surgeon to safely dissect the lateral zygomatic arch, since it is approached in a subperiosteal plane, assuring avoidance of the temporal branch of the facial nerve. Additionally, this facilitates mobilization of the entire deep plane, resulting in less traction on the nerve during subsequent dissection of the zygoma and masseteric muscle.

SURGICAL TECHNIQUE

Patients are instructed to wash their hair the night before and the morning of surgery. General endotracheal anesthesia is utilized, along with perioperative administration of corticosteroids and intravenous antibiotics. We prefer cephalosporins, because the operation involves incision through the oral mucosa. Dexamethasone acetate (Decadron LA), 8 mg intramuscularly, and dexamethasone sodium phosphate (Decadron), 4 mg intravenously, are used to reduce postoperative edema. An initial prep is performed with isopropyl alcohol, saturating the hair as well as the skin. The hair is then thoroughly rinsed with sterile water to avoid any flame hazard from use of the electrosurgical unit.

Modified tumescent infiltration is used for hemostasis and to facilitate dissection. A solution of 50 mL of 2% lidocaine, 2.5 mL of 1:1000 epinephrine, and 250 mL of normal saline is freshly prepared for each patient. Using a Klein electric roller pump and a 22 gauge needle, this mixture is infiltrated throughout the soft tissues of the forehead, face, and neck. Tumescent infiltration eliminates much of the bleeding that might otherwise be associated with the dissection.

Surgery is carried out using a headlight, supplemented with 3.5 power magnification utilizing Zeiss loops. While much of the operation can be carried out under direct lighting without magnification, the use of the loops and headlight is invaluable when working in the deeper areas. It also allows much more precise dissection and hemostasis.

The initial approach is through an incision made in the canine fossa with an electrosurgical knife. This soft tissue is electrosurgically dissected to the periosteum, after which an elevator is introduced in a subperiosteal plane, to further lift the periosteum away from the anterior surface of the maxilla. We carry out this part of the dissection primarily by feel, occasionally peeking through the small incision with the assistance of an Aufrecht retractor.

Dissection is continued medially over the nasal bones, superiorly to the inferior orbital rim, avoiding the infraorbital nerve, and laterally to the anterior surface of the zygoma and over the zygomatic arch (Fig 3). With experience, this dissection can be performed blindly through a very small vertical incision, although it is acceptable to use a larger incision to allow dissection under direct visualization.

Once the soft tissue and periosteum have been elevated off bone, a sharp elevator is used to sever some of the soft tissue overlying the masseter muscle. Operating intraorally, the elevation is then advanced to the

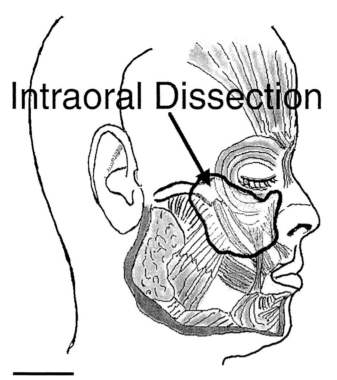

FIGURE 3.

Initial dissection is carried out through a small vertical canine fossa incision. Dissection is subperiosteal except over the masseter muscle.

zygomatic arch and swept inferiorly in a beveled manner, cutting muscle fibers and detaching the masseteric fascia. At this level, care must be exercised to prevent the dissection from becoming too superficial, as one is dissecting just beneath Stenson's duct and the buccal branch of the facial nerve.

It is not necessary to obtain complete detachment of the masseter at this stage, since that will be completed later through the coronal approach. If the mucosal incisions remain small, there is no need to close them. However, if they are torn, or surgically extended for access, they are closed with buried 4-0 chromic catgut suture. It is best to delay closure until completion of the entire operation to allow for drainage and inspection of the wound.

After the intraoral dissection, a bicoronal flap is outlined. This incision will extend inferiorly in a preauricular fashion and terminate just below the tragus. Two possible surgical approaches can be used, depending on the location of the anterior hairline (Fig 4). In patients with a high, prominent forehead, an incision is made centrally at the hairline. This incision is made in a "zig-zag" pattern and beveled anteriorly to preserve the bulbs of the hair follicles, allowing hair to grow through the scar upon healing. In the temporal scalp, the incision extends superiorly then curves downward to join the preauricular incision.

Incisions are similar for patients with a low hairline except for the coronal incision which extends directly across the head, at least 6 cm be-

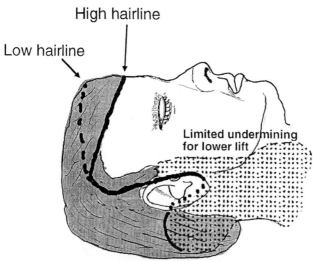

Subperiosteal lift <u>with</u> facelift

FIGURE 4.
When the hairline is high, an anterior incision is selected, as shown. With a relatively low hairline, a bicoronal incision is utilized. When combined with lower face-lifting, a standard face-lift incision is used. If only a subperiosteal lift is being carried out, the incision ends inferiorly behind the ear for better camouflage. Undermining in the face is limited because of the extensive subperiosteal and submasseteric dissection in that region.

hind the hairline. This results in better scar camouflage and less numbness, although it does elevate the hairline somewhat. Also, it is important to place the bicoronal incision far enough posteriorly to ensure that the resulting scar remains behind the hairline when the excess scalp is excised. Similar to the anterior incision, the lateral extension of this incision is carried forward to the preauricular region.

After the initial incision is made, dissection is performed using an electrosurgical knife with an ultra-fine needle tip and a low-power cutting current. Small bleeding vessels are cauterized as encountered. This dissection is performed anterior to the ear and extends along the tragal cartilage posterior to the parotid gland, until the zygoma and capsule of the temporomandibular joint are encountered. This plane of dissection is similar to that used in parotidectomy and temporomandibular joint surgery, and will be familiar to those experienced in these types of surgery.

Numerous small vessels may be encountered, including the superficial temporal artery and veins. However, this plane of dissection is safe, with no risk of damage to motor nerves or other vital structures. Once the posterior body of the zygoma has been identified, an elevator is used to lift the periosteum from the posterior half of the bone. At that point, the dissection shifts to the forehead.

The forehead incisions are made sharply and beveled at an extreme angle. We prefer using a broken razor blade as it is somewhat sharper than a conventional scalpel. After the initial incision, dissection is continued with the electrosurgical needle tip and a low-power pure cutting current. Once the plane of dissection is away from the hair follicles, a low-power blended current and a thin spatula-type tip is selected for improved hemostasis. Dissection progresses to the subgaleal plane. This is an avascular plane which can be elevated quickly and safely (Fig 5).

Combined sharp and blunt subgaleal dissection continues to approximately 2 cm above the superior orbital rim. At this level, the periosteum is incised and dissection continues subperiosteally over the frontal bone. Laterally, the incision is carried across the temporalis fascia (Figs 5 and 6) and curved inferiorly where it meets the previous incision, in the fascia overlying the zygoma, made during the initial preauricular dissection. Periosteal elevation continues effortlessly over the frontal bone and laterally to the frontozygomatic suture line, where sharp periosteal elevation is necessary to free up the dense condensation of fibrous attachments to the suture line.

Dissection over the frontal bone is continued inferiorly until the supraorbital neurovascular bundle is encountered at the level of the superior orbital rim. Since the dissection is subperiosteal, the foramina are easily identified thereby minimizing the risk of injury to the neurovascular structures themselves (see Fig 6).

Attention is then directed to the incision that is made in the superficial layer of the temporalis fascia. Although commonly described in

Subgaleal Dissection

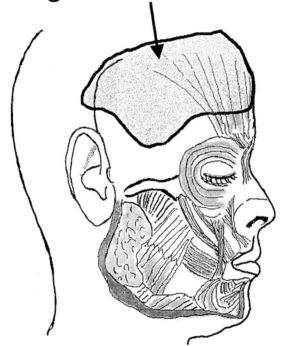

FIGURE 5.

Initial dissection from the coronal approach is carried out in a subgaleal plane until the temporalis fascia and brow are encountered. The plane is then deepened to a subperiosteal plane anteriorly, and a subtemporal plane laterally.

Upper Subperiosteal Dissection

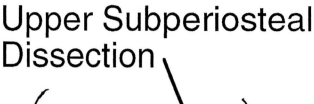

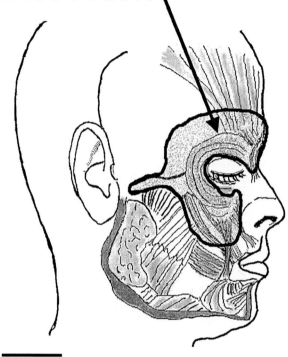

FIGURE 6.

Additional subperiosteal dissection is carried out from above, completely exposing the zygomatic arch and ultimately joining the dissection over the maxilla that was initiated through the canine fossa incision.

anatomy texts as a single layer, this fascial layer actually develops into a more complex structure as it descends towards the zygomatic arch (Fig 7). The fascia splits into an outer and inner layer that envelops the temporal fat pad and zygomatic arch.

In developing a plane of dissection beneath the outermost layer of fascia, there is no risk of injury to the temporal branch of the facial nerve, as this plane will safely guide the surgeon to the zygomatic arch. It is this (outer) superficial layer that attaches to the arch, while the (inner) deeper layer passes beneath the arch along with the temporalis muscle. This is a key part of the dissection because the temporal branch of the facial nerve traverses the zygomatic arch in close proximity to the bone. As long as the surgeon dissects beneath this superficial layer of the temporal fascia, the nerve is safe from direct injury and remains superficial to the plane of dissection (Fig 8).

One must avoid dissecting beneath the deep layer of the temporalis fascia since it will lead you deep to the zygomatic arch. This approach is commonly used by maxillofacial surgeons in the anatomic reduction of zygomatic arch fractures. It is also important to keep the plane of dissection above the temporal fat. If one goes deep to the fat, it will be carried

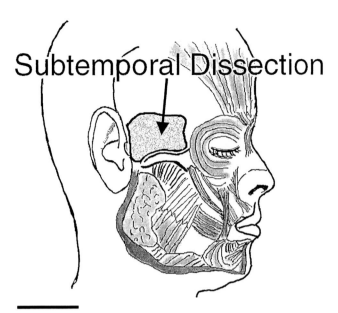

FIGURE 7.
Subtemporal dissection is carried out between the two layers of the temporalis fascia, usually deep to the fatty tissue that is between these layers. This plane brings the surgeon to the zygomatic arch where the plane again becomes subperiosteal.

upward as the flap is retracted, and can lead to a hollowing of the fossa above the zygoma.

Once this plane is established, the zygomatic arch can be completely freed by combining the access gained through

1. The initial canine fossa dissection
2. The preauricular dissection
3. The dissection beneath the superficial layer of the temporalis fascia

Once the entire arch is exposed, dissection continues forward toward the body of the zygoma. Again, great care must be taken because of close proximity to the temporal branch of the facial nerve. In addition to direct trauma, nerve injury can also occur with overzealous traction, and, in fact, this is probably the main cause of the weakness seen following this operation.

Dissection is continued in the subperiosteal plane toward the orbit, along the anterior surface of the zygoma and maxilla, where it fully joins the previous intraoral dissection. Care must be taken to identify and preserve the infraorbital nerve.

The depth to which dissection is performed within the orbit is variable. Extensive dissection will allow greater elevation of the lateral canthal periosteum, as will incising the periosteum within the orbit. Although it is debatable whether a lateral canthal "tendon" truly exists, one can completely release the lateral canthal fascia to considerably elevate the corner of the eye when the final subperiosteal flap is vertically anchored (Fig 9). We have never been able to discern a tendinous structure, either in the anatomy laboratory or during actual operations.

Some authors[7] have recommended fixation sutures to secure the lat-

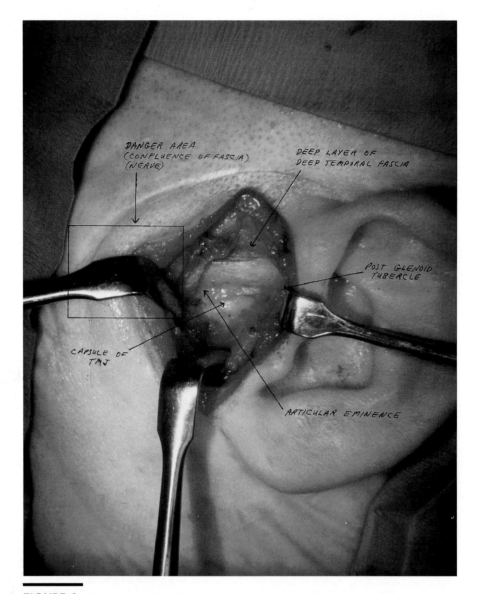

FIGURE 8.

The operative anatomy of posterior zygomatic arch dissection. This permits safe and complete dissection of the zygoma in a subperiosteal plane. (Photograph courtesy of T. William Evans, M.D.)

eral canthal "tendon" in its new position. We have not found this necessary nor desirable. One of the striking improvements from this operation is the significant elevation of the lateral aspect of the eye. In fact, one must be careful not to overcorrect this region, for it is easy to exaggerate the elevation of the lateral corner of the eye—a problem that can be very slow to resolve.

The next step in the operation involves mobilizing the soft tissues of the cheek, jowl, and nasolabial fold. This is performed by dissection over the masseter muscle (Fig 10). The buccal branch of the facial nerve and

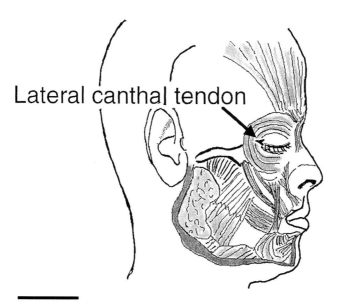

Lateral canthal tendon

FIGURE 9.

The lateral canthal ligament can be completely detached from the orbit when carrying out the extended subperiosteal lift. This allows for considerable elevation of the lateral orbit which is generally long lasting even without fixation to bone.

the parotid duct cross over the muscle, just superficial to the masseteric fascia. Therefore, to avoid injury to these structures, it is essential that the plane of dissection be deep to this fascia. Since the masseteric fascia is so thin, it is safest to dissect just beneath the superficial-most fibers of the masseter muscle. This is best performed utilizing a sharpened elevator. The dissection extends downward to about the level of the alveolar ridge of the mandible, and proceeds forward to meet the previously made intraoral dissection.

Attention is now directed to the glabellar region (Fig 11). Periosteal dissection is carried out over the nasal dorsum and continued laterally over the nasal bones to free up the insertions of the corrugator supercilii and procerus muscles. Although the levator labii superioris and the levator anguli oris do not have periosteal attachments, they are nonetheless mobilized by this maneuver. Finally, the undersurface of the flap is addressed. This may include resecting or avulsing the procerus or corrugator muscles. Additionally, transverse forehead rhytids can be corrected by a crisscross division, or gridding of the galea and frontalis muscle.

Our approach to the frontalis tends to be conservative, unless the forehead lines are severe, or the patient is particularly troubled by them. If we transect the frontalis, we only go through the muscle fibers, and keep the dissection limited to the middle third of the forehead.

With the dissection now complete, the musculofascial flap which has been mobilized is advanced in a superior direction. It is usually possible to overlap the edges of the temporalis fascia at least two or three centimeters. Occasionally, the flap seems immobile, regardless of the surgeon's efforts to free it. This is especially true in patients who have had previous face-lift surgery. Several mattress sutures of 3-0 silk are used to an-

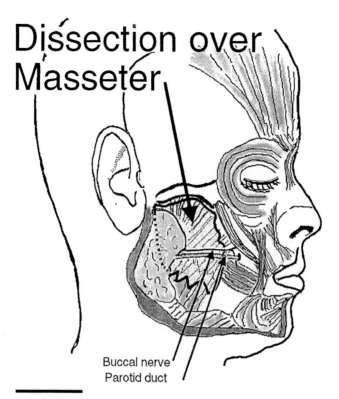

Dissection over Masseter

Buccal nerve
Parotid duct

FIGURE 10.

It is important to elevate the tissue over the masseter muscle for adequate mobilization. This plane lies beneath the masseteric fascia and often encompasses the outermost fibers of the masseter muscle. This plane of dissection avoids injury to the buccal nerve and the parotid duct.

chor the flap to the deep temporal fascia. The skin flap is then advanced in a superior and lateral direction and the excess is trimmed and beveled to match the original incision.

We avoid tension on the skin flap, because the pull is primarily in the deeper plane. Staples are used to close the incision in hair-bearing regions, while subcutaneous chromic and running 6-0 plain catgut sutures are used to close the remainder of the incisions.

If a lower face-lift is planned, it is performed in a relatively routine manner. Subcutaneous dissection over the cheek should be very limited, since detachment of skin from the preparotid fascia would reduce the effectiveness of the deeper subperiosteal lift. Treatment of the neck can be accomplished with standard superficial musculo-aponeurotic system or platysmal techniques.

More recently, in cases where we plan both upper and lower lift, we have been carrying out the lower lift first. The dissection is somewhat easier, because the tissues have not yet been tightened by elevation of the fascial flap.

Another change that seems promising is to completely avoid the incision in front of the ear. The incision for the upper lift can be made either behind the helix or in front of it, curving inferiorly to the upper tra-

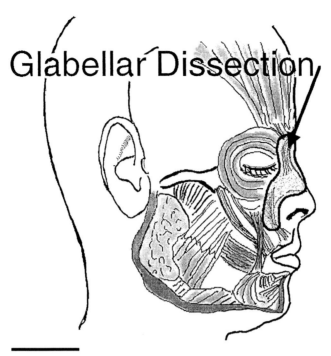

FIGURE 11.

Glabellar dissection is carried out in a subperiosteal plane, elevating the procerus muscle as well as the levator labii superioris. Care is taken to avoid injury to the infraorbital nerve and the lacrimal sac. This dissection also joins the dissection carried out through the canine fossa approach.

gus. The incision for the lower lift can be limited to behind the ear. We have used this approach in approximately six patients. There is a bunching of skin in front of the ear that tends to resolve, although in one case it required revision. The avoidance of a preauricular scar would seem to make this a worthwhile addition, even if a minor secondary revision is required. Of course, this approach should be limited to patients without major skin redundancy.

RESULTS

The technique described above represents an evolution based on the descriptions and results of others. The senior author has been performing the ESCL since 1989, with progressive extention of dissection. Initially, patients had what would be considered a traditional coronal lift with extended dissection over the zygoma and maxilla. Subsequent changes in technique involved subperiosteal dissection of the forehead, dissection through the canine fossa, and elevation of the masseteric fascia. The most recent changes have been incorporation of the initial preauricular approach to the posterior zygoma; performance of the lower lift first, when also performing a lower lift; and avoidance of the preauricular incision in selected cases. This technique has been used with little change since the end of 1992.

For a period of time, we adopted the technique described by Ramirez.[6]

This involved approaching the zygomatic arch entirely from above, dissecting beneath the temporalis fascia. He then recommended a "back cut" to sever the fibrous attachments of the temporomandibular joint and the perichondrium of the ear and temporal bone. In 1992, 23 patients underwent ESCL by using this technique. With the exception of four patients, the majority had lower face-lifting as well.

Except for neuropraxia of the temporal division of the frontal nerve, complications have been uncommon. Forehead weakness has occurred in approximately 5% of patients, although nearly all eventually recovered function. We are aware of one patient who retained forehead weakness past two years, and two who have remained weak for approximately 1 year. Recovery from neuroproxia has varied from 1 week to 12 months. We have not found any significant decrease in the incidence of nerve weakness by adopting the approach to the zygomatic arch as described by Ramirez.[8]

One patient had profound weakness of the buccal branch of the facial nerve; however, this improved within 3 weeks. Another patient experienced mild weakness of the buccal nerve that completely resolved after several weeks. Some patients have described discomfort while chewing for several weeks postoperatively. This was probably related to the masseteric dissection. There have been no hematomas of the coronal portion of the lift, although there have been two minor hematomas of the lower neck. We have not seen any instances of forehead weakness with the modification to the approach from in front of the ear, as discussed.

Although variable, there can be significant swelling postoperative. This generally resolves in approximately 3 weeks, but patients are cautioned to allow at least 6 weeks for full recovery. One patient had considerable facial edema that persisted for 8 weeks. This may have been related to failure of the canine fossa incisions to heal promptly.

Exaggerated elevation of the lateral canthus is often present for the first few weeks but usually resolves in 4 to 8 weeks. Surprisingly, trismus has not been a major problem, especially when one considers the extensive masseteric dissection. There have been no instances of skin necrosis, even in several patients who were heavy smokers.

Although long-term follow-up is not available, the results seem promising. This technique offers more improvement in the upper and middle face compared to traditional techniques. While conventional coronal lifting elevates the brow, the extended operation provides a stronger and longer lasting result. In the malar region, a "natural" augmentation occurs secondary to elevation of ptotic tissue over the malar eminence.

Even with this, it is not uncommon to include a small malar implant, which can easily be inserted through the surgical approach under direct visualization. We place the implants from above and secure them directly with one or two titanium bone screws. We prefer the anatomical design of malar implant.

The ESCL produces an elevation of the lateral canthal region of the eye, the cheek, and oral commisure. Indeed, no other technique produces such an elegant elevation of the lateral canthus. Additionally, the oral commisures are elevated producing a more youthful, smiling appearance at rest.

Ramirez[8] stated that the operation was an improvement over traditional techniques in eliminating the nasolabial fold. However, we have not observed significant improvement in this region and frequently resort to fillers when needed. We do not feel that this operation is the answer to the elusive problem of the nasolabial fold, although frequently there is considerable improvement. The most striking advantage is the balanced look that results from this operation. The entire face is rejuvenated—unlike the "segmental" results obtained from traditional techniques.

DISCUSSION

Unlike traditional face-lift techniques, which use lifting face in a posterior direction, the ESCL primarily uses a strong vertical lift. This directly counteracts the ptotic effects of facial aging that tend to be vertically oriented. Also, this technique differs from others, in that the primary force is exerted on deeper connective tissues as well as the facial muscles. These structures remain attached to the overlying skin and are repositioned enbloc.

Furnas[9] described retaining ligaments in the cheek and mandible that he believed bound the skin to the periosteum. Furthermore, he suggested severing these ligaments to allow for maximum lift during rhtytidectomy. Assuming his theory is correct, it would appear that lifting the periosteum, without detaching these ligaments, would result in a stronger and more permanent correction.

Since Mitz and Peyronie[10] originally described the "superficial musculo-aponeurotic system" (SMAS) in 1976, there has been great emphasis on this layer when discussing face-lifting. Surgeons often think of the SMAS as a true fibrous sheet that can be "pulled" to exert force on distant facial structures. Jost et al.[11] is probably more correct in recognizing that the SMAS may actually be a fibrous extension of the platysma over the jaw and parotid gland. Clinically, its strength varies from individual to individual. In some cases, muscle fibers can be seen in the tissue overlying the parotid, while in others, it represents only a thin gossamer layer.

Newer concepts of facial rejuvenation recognize the importance of a balanced approach to the entire face. This is opposed to traditional face-lifting techniques which emphasize the lower face and neck. Because the eyes and malar eminence are a focus of attention, early signs of aging in these areas are readily noted by observers. Traditional face-lift techniques are relatively ineffective and frequently ignore these important regions. Malar augmentation enjoys popularity because it helps correct this deficiency.[12] These implants also "lift" soft tissue which has dropped beneath the malar eminence. With the ESCL, this region is directly rejuvenated through soft tissue elevation, reducing the need for synthetic implants. In cases of true malar hypoplasia, augmentation can be performed under direct visualization using titanium screws for precise implant fixation.

While the results of the ESCL are superior, the recovery is longer and there is greater risk of injury to the frontal branch of the facial nerve. This is counterbalanced by the fact that there is less risk of flap necrosis—

even in heavy smokers. Although the subperiosteal plane is relatively avascular, numerous small veins are encountered and dissection of the masseter muscle can result in significant bleeding. This can obscure the operative field, making dissection more difficult while increasing postoperative edema. We have found that by combining tumescent infiltra-

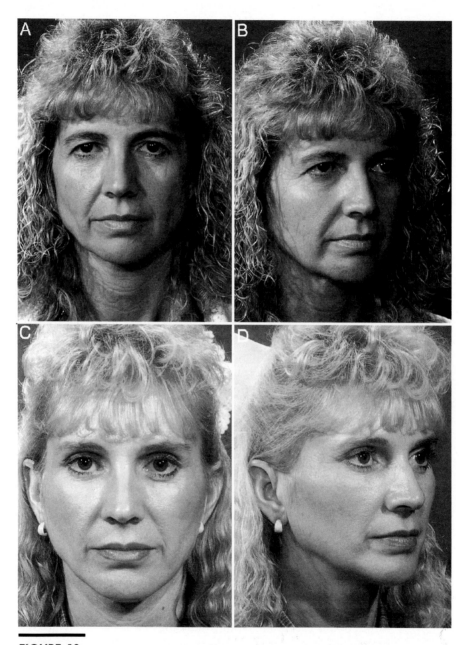

FIGURE 12.

43-year-old patient who underwent subperiosteal lift and neck lift with upper and lower transconjunctival blepharoplasty. Appearance before **(A and B)** and 6 months after **(C and D)** surgery. Notice the recontouring of the cheek, softening of the nasolabial fold, and marked improvement of the eyes.

tion with electrosurgical dissection bleeding is minimal, resulting in a dry operative field. The use of surgical loops and headlight illumination is also helpful.

The lengthened postoperative recovery period must be considered. We advise patients to anticipate 3 weeks before they look fairly normal,

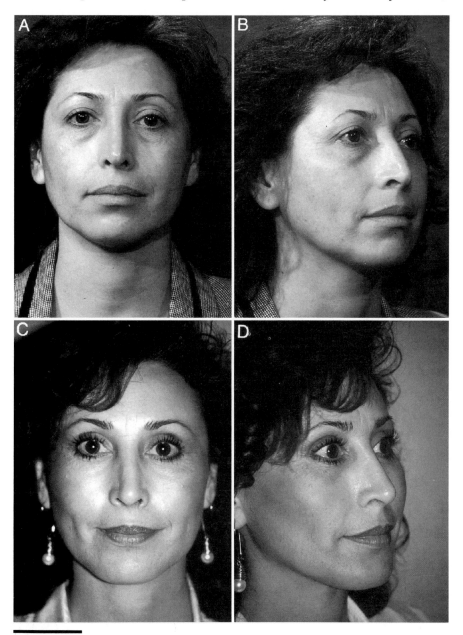

FIGURE 13.

42-year-old patient who underwent subperiosteal lift, upper and lower transconjunctival blepharoplasty, malar/chin augmentation, and tip rhinoplasty. Appearance before **(A** and **B)** and 6 months after **(C** and **D)** surgery. No lower face/neck lift performed. Notice the elevation of the lateral area of the orbit, and rejuvenation of the cheek and jowl region.

and 6 weeks until they feel normal. Faivre[13] reported a modification of the ESCL in which he limits the temporal incision. While elevating over the zygoma and maxilla, he does not dissect beneath the masseter. This approach reduces postoperative edema, and may have merit in younger patients with less ptosis of the cheek and jowl region.

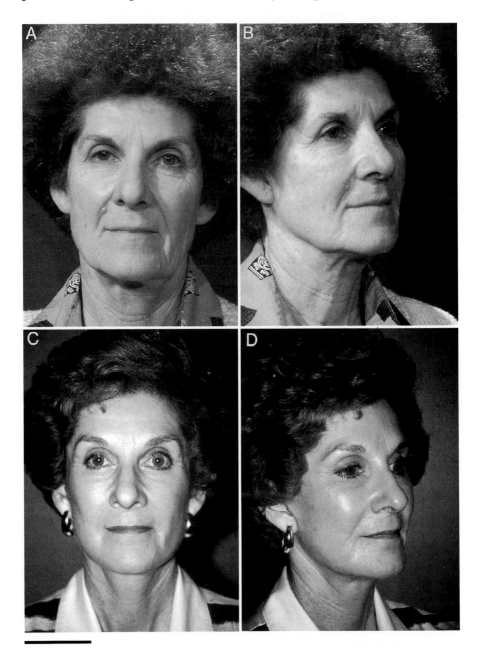

FIGURE 14.

67-year-old patient before **(A** and **B)** and 9 months after **(C** and **D)** subperiosteal lift, lower lift, upper and lower blepharoplasty, perioral chemical peel, and mole excision of right cheek. Note rejuvenation of the eyes, elevation of the eyebrows, and marked improvement of the nasolabial fold.

The greatest concern with this technique involves the risk of facial nerve injury. This generally involves the frontal branch, although the buccal nerve is also vulnerable. The cause of frontal weakness is not completely understood. While the plane of the dissection is certainly in close proximity to the nerve as it crosses over the zygomatic arch, direct injury

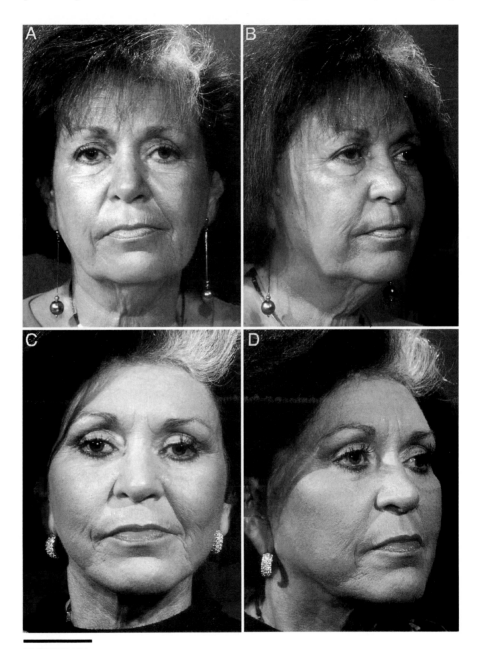

FIGURE 15.
55-year-old patient before (**A** and **B**) and 9 months after (**C** and **D**) subperiosteal lift, lower lift, upper and lower blepharoplasty, and malar/chin augmentation. Notice elegant elevation of lateral canthal region, improvement of the frown wrinkles, and softening of the nasolabial fold.

is unlikely since nearly all patients have recovered. It remains possible that weakness results from either tension placed on the nerve during flap advancement, or from nerve traction during zygomatic arch exposure.

With our new modifications, there is less need for vigorous retraction because the zygomatic arch is safely dissected from a posterior and

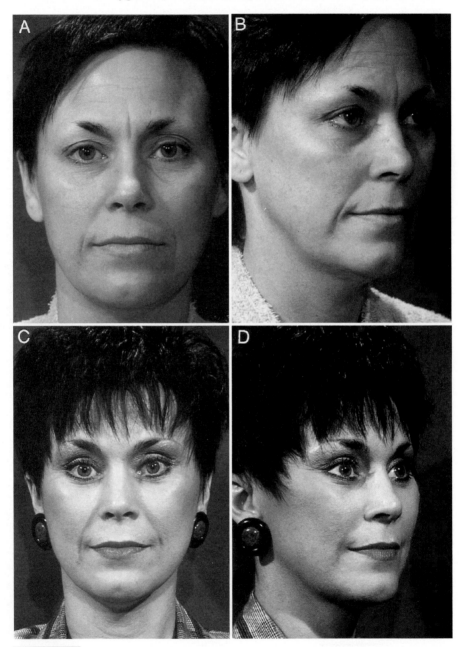

FIGURE 16.
A–D, 44-year-old patient who underwent subperiosteal lift, upper and lower transconjunctival blepharoplasty, and lower lid chemical peel. No lower face/neck lift performed. Note rejuvenation of the eyes and upper face, along with remodeling of the jowl region and improvement of mandibular contour.

superior approach. There have not been any instances of frontal nerve weakness since we adopted this approach. Another significant advantage is the fact that it completely mobilizes the deep flap compared to the "back cut" which was previously used. By dissecting the deep tissues away from the ear cartilage, temporomandibular joint, and posterior parotid gland, we have gained substantial mobilization of the entire face. This permits enhanced rejuvenation of the cheek, jowl, and oral commissure (Figs 12–16) Improvement is also seen in the nasolabial fold although we still believe the ESCL falls short of ideally correcting this difficult region.

With experience, operating time for the ESCL is not much greater than that required for traditional coronal lifting. Because dissection of the lower face is more limited, total operating time is comparable to traditional face-lifting techniques. The overall results are superior and naturally balanced, making this the procedure of choice for an increasing number of patients. Therefore, it remains an option that deserves the consideration of surgeons and patients contemplating facial rejuvenation surgery.

REFERENCES

1. Hamra ST: *Composite rhytidectomy*. St. Louis, Quality Medical Publishing, 1993.
2. Hamra ST: Composite rhytidectomy. *Plast Reconstr Surg* 90: 1–13, 1990.
3. Tessier P: Facelifting and frontal rhytidectomy, in JF Ely (ed), *Transactions of the 7th International Congress of Plastic and Reconstructive Surgery*, Rio De Janiero, 1980, pp 393–396.
4. Psillakis JM, Rumley TO, Camargos A, et al.: Subperiosteal approach as an improved concept for correction of the aging face. *Plast Reconstr Surg* 82: 383–392, 1988.
5. Ramirez O, Maillard GF, Musolas A, et al.: The extended subperiosteal facelift: A definitive soft-tissue remodeling for facial rejuvenation surgery. *Plast Reconstr Surg* 88: 227–236, 1991.
6. Ramirez O: Personal communication. 1st annual workshop on facial rejuvenation: The subperiosteal and deep plane techniques. Baltimore, Md, April 1992.
7. Hinderer UT, Urriolagoitia F, Vildosola R, et al.: The blepharoperiorbitoplasty: Anatomical basis. *Ann Plast Surg* 18: 437–453, 1987.
8. Ramirez O: The subperiosteal rhytidectomy: The third-generation face-lift. *Ann Plast Surg* 28: 218–232, 1992.
9. Furnas DW: Retaining ligaments of the cheek. *Plast Reconstr Surg* 83: 11–16, 1989.
10. Mitz V, Peyronie M: The superficial musculo-aponeurotic system (SMAS) in the parotid and cheek area. *Plast Reconstr Surg* 58: 80–88, 1976.
11. Jost G, Wassef M, Lever Y, et al.: Subfascial lifting. *Aesthetic Plast Surg* 11: 163–170, 1987.
12. Tobin H: Malar augmentation as an adjunct to facial cosmetic surgery. *Am J Cosm Surg* 3: 13–16, 1986.
13. Faivre J: Deep temporal facelift: Its indications in surgery for aging of the upper third of the face. *Am J Cosm Surg* 8: 155–165, 1991.

Advances in Coding Strategies for Cochlear Implants*

Blake S. Wilson

Director, Center for Auditory Prosthesis Research, Research Triangle Institute, Research Triangle Park, North Carolina; Adjunct Associate Professor, Division of Otolaryngology—Head & Neck Surgery, Duke University Medical Center, Durham, North Carolina

Dewey T. Lawson, Ph.D.

Senior Scientist, Center for Auditory Prosthesis Research, Research Triangle Institute, Research Triangle Park, North Carolina; Adjunct Assistant Professor, Division of Otolaryngology—Head & Neck Surgery, Duke University Medical Center, Durham, North Carolina

Mariangeli Zerbi, M.S.

Research Engineer, Center for Auditory Prosthesis Research, Research Triangle Institute, Research Triangle Park, North Carolina

---

N ew strategies for representing acoustic information have produced large improvements in speech recognition for cochlear implant users. In this chapter we present basic considerations in the design of processing strategies for implants and then describe two particularly effective strategies, the *continuous interleaved sampling* (CIS) approach now used with several implant systems and the *spectral peak* (SPEAK) approach now used with the Nucleus device. In a final section we suggest several possibilities for further improvements in processor performance.

DESIGN CONSIDERATIONS

Essential elements of implant systems are shown in Figure 1. A microphone senses pressure variations in a sound field and converts them into electrical variations. The electrical signal from the microphone is processed to produce stimuli for an implanted electrode or array of electrodes. The stimuli are sent to the electrode(s) through a transcutaneous link (top panel) or through a percutaneous connector (bottom panel). A typical transcutaneous link includes encoding of the stimulus information for electromagnetic transmission from an external transmitting coil to an implanted receiving coil. Carrier frequencies for such electromag-

*Work in our laboratory was supported by NIH projects N01-DC-2-2401, N01-DC-9-2401, and P01-DC-0-0036.

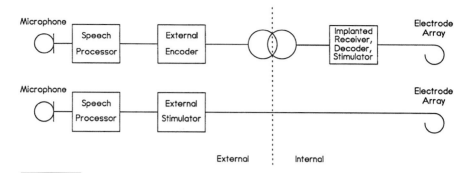

FIGURE 1.

Components of prosthesis systems. A system with a transcutaneous transmission link is illustrated in the top panel, and a system with a percutaneous connector in the bottom panel. (From Wilson BS: Signal processing, in Tyler RS (ed): *Cochlear Implants: Audiological Foundations.* San Diego, Calif, Singular Publishing Group, 1993, pp 35–85. Used by permission.)

netic transmission usually are several MHz or higher. The signal received at the implanted coil is decoded to specify stimuli for the electrodes.

ELECTRODES

The range of choices in the design for each of these elements, along with possible sources of variation among patients, is indicated in Figure 2. Electrodes may be placed on the medial wall or round window of the cochlea ("extracochlear"), in the scala tympani ("intracochlear"), within the modiolus, or on the surface of the cochlear nucleus. Among these, extracochlear placements are least invasive and those on the surface of the cochlear nucleus most invasive.

The most common placement by far is within the scala tympani. This placement positions electrodes close to surviving ganglion cells and peripheral processes of the auditory nerve, which are spread along the length of the cochlea in an orderly, tonotopic arrangement. Multiple electrodes can be used to mimic, in a crude way, the "place" representation of frequencies in the normal cochlea. In particular, the presence of high frequency sounds in the environment can be conveyed by stimulating electrodes toward the basal end of the cochlea, whereas lower frequencies can be indicated by stimulating electrodes closer to the apical end of the cochlea.

The quality of the place representation presumably depends on the number and spacing of perceptually independent sites of stimulation. Loss of excitable neurons in particular areas would be expected to degrade or distort the representation. In an extreme case, for example, survival of neurons might be limited to only one small region of the cochlea. Any of the electrodes in a multielectrode array then could only stimulate the same set of neurons. The patient would not be able to distinguish stimuli delivered through the different electrodes. In this case, one electrode might be as good as one hundred.

At the other extreme, excellent survival of neurons may support an effective representation of frequencies by place of stimulation. Indeed,

Electrodes

- extracochlear

  intracochlear

  modiolar

  cochlear nucleus

- number and spacing of contacts

- orientation with respect to excitable tissue

Processing Strategy

- number of channels

- number of electrodes

- analog

  pulsatile

- waveform representation

  feature extraction

Patient

- peripheral nerve survival

  surgical placement of electrodes

  function of central auditory pathways

  cognitive and language skills

Transmission Link

- percutaneous

  transcutaneous

FIGURE 2.

Principal design options and considerations for cochlear prostheses. (Adapted from Wilson BS: Signal processing, in Tyler RS (ed): *Cochlear Implants: Audiological Foundations.* San Diego, Calif, Singular Publishing Group, 1993, pp 35–85. Used by permission.)

many patients with multichannel implants can discriminate among electrodes on the basis of differences in pitch or timbre.[1]

TRANSMISSION LINK

Another distinction among implant designs is the method used for transmitting stimuli from an external processor to the implanted electrodes. A principal advantage of a percutaneous connector is signal transparency; that is, the specification of the stimuli is in no way constrained by the limitations imposed by any practical design for a transcutaneous transmission system. An advantage of a transcutaneous system is that the skin is closed over the implanted components, which may reduce the risk of infection.

PATIENT

Great variability in outcomes among patients is a common finding in studies of implant performance. While any of several implant devices can support relatively high levels of speech recognition for some patients, other patients have poor outcomes with each of those same devices. Obviously, characteristics of individual patients can exert a strong influence on performance. Factors contributing to this variability may include differences among patients in the survival of neural elements in the implanted co-chlea, surgical placement of the electrodes, integrity of the central auditory pathways, and cognitive and language skills.

PROCESSING STRATEGY

A final difference among implant designs is in the strategy used for transforming speech inputs into stimuli for the electrodes. As indicated in Figure 2, processing strategies can be classified according to number of channels, number of electrodes, whether analog or pulsatile stimulation is used, and whether particular features of the speech inputs are explicitly detected and then encoded in the patterns of stimulation.

The remainder of this chapter will be concerned mainly with the effects of various differences among processor designs. Emphasis is given to within-subject comparisons, in which effects of processor variables may be separated from effects of patient variables and electrode design.[2] The comparisons include CIS with a *compressed analog* (CA) strategy and SPEAK with a *multipeak* (MPEAK) strategy. These comparisons illustrate issues in the design of speech processors for cochlear implants and show what is possible with the CIS and SPEAK processors. Descriptions of the many other approaches to design that have been proposed or used throughout the history of cochlear implants are presented in a number of excellent reviews on the subject.[3-10]

CONTINUOUS INTERLEAVED SAMPLING STRATEGY

Recent studies in our laboratory have included comparisons of CA and CIS processors.[11, 12] Both processors use multiple channels of stimulation, and both represent waveforms or envelopes of speech inputs. No specific features of the inputs, such as the fundamental or formant frequencies for voiced speech sounds, are extracted or explicitly represented. Compressed analog processors use continuous analog signals as stimuli, whereas CIS processors use pulses.

DESIGNS OF COMPRESSED ANALOG AND CONTINUOUS INTERLEAVED SAMPLING PROCESSORS

The designs of the two processors are illustrated in Figures 3 through 5. In CA processors, a microphone input, varying over the wide dynamic range of speech and other environmental sounds, is compressed or restricted to the narrow dynamic range of electrically evoked hearing[13-15] with an automatic gain control (AGC). The AGC output is filtered into four contiguous frequency bands for presentation to each of four electrodes. As shown in Figure 4, information about speech sounds is contained in the relative amplitudes of the stimuli for each of the four electrodes. In addition, temporal details in the waveforms for individual electrodes reflect details of the speech input.

A concern associated with the CA approach is that much of the information that is presented may not be perceived by implant patients. For example, most patients cannot perceive frequency changes in stimulus waveforms for frequencies above about 300 Hz.[1] Thus, many of the tem-

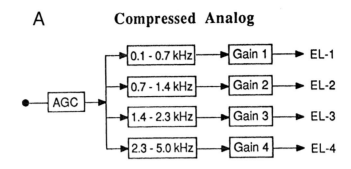

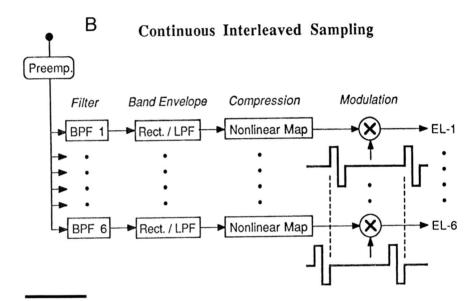

FIGURE 3.

Block diagrams of major processing steps in CA and CIS strategies. **A,** a CA strategy uses a broadband automatic gain control *(AGC),* followed by four channels of bandpass filtering. The outputs of the bandpass filters can be adjusted by independent gain controls. The outputs of gain stages are connected to four intracochlear electrodes *(EL-1 to EL-4).* **B,** a CIS strategy uses a preemphasis filter *(Preemp.)* to attenuate strong low frequency components in speech that otherwise might mask important high frequency components (high frequency emphasis is accomplished in CA processors through adjustment of the channel gain controls). The preemphasis filter is followed by multiple channels of processing, usually five or six for CIS processors used in conjunction with the Ineraid implant. Each channel includes stages of bandpass filtering *(BPF),* envelope detection, compression, and modulation. The envelope detector consists of a rectifier *(Rect.)* followed by a lowpass filter *(LPF).* Carrier waveforms for two of the modulators are shown immediately below the two corresponding multiplier blocks. (From Wilson BS, Finley CC, Lawson DT, et al: *Nature* 352:236–238, 1991. Used by permission.)

poral details present in CA stimuli are not likely to be perceived by the typical patient.

In addition, the simultaneous presentation of stimuli across electrodes may produce significant interactions among channels through vector summation of the electric fields from each electrode.[16] The resulting degradation of channel independence would be expected to reduce the salience of channel-related cues. The neural response to stimuli from one

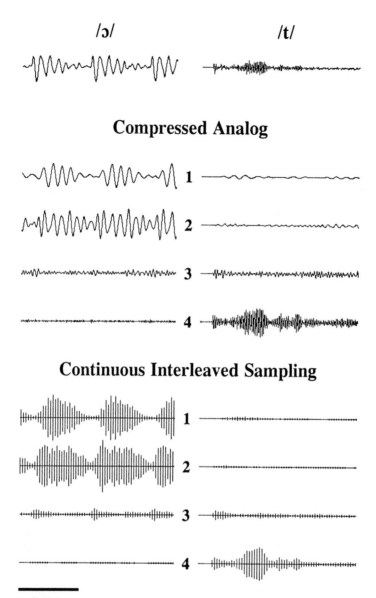

FIGURE 4.

Waveforms produced by simplified implementation of CA and CIS strategies. The top panel shows preemphasized (6 dB/octave attenuation below 1.2 kHz) speech inputs. Inputs corresponding to a voiced speech sound ("aw") and an unvoiced speech sound ("t") are shown in the left and right columns, respectively. The duration of each trace is 25.4 ms. The remaining panels show stimulus waveforms for CA and CIS processors. The waveforms are numbered by channel, with channel one delivering its output to the apicalmost electrode. To facilitate comparisons between strategies, only four channels of CIS stimulation are illustrated here. In general, five or six channels have been used for that strategy. The pulse amplitudes reflect the envelope of the bandpass output for each channel. In actual implementations the range of pulse amplitudes is compressed using a logarithmic or power-law transformation of the envelope signal. (From Wilson BS, Finley CC, Lawson DT, et al: *Nature* 352:236–238, 1991. Used by permission.)

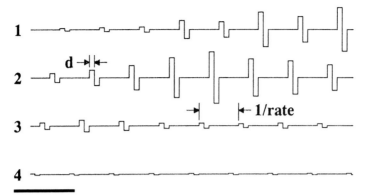

FIGURE 5.

Expanded display of CIS waveforms. Pulse duration per phase (d) and the period between pulses on each channel (1/rate) are indicated. The sequence of stimulated channels is 4-3-2-1. The total duration of each trace is 3.3 ms. (From Wilson BS, Finley CC, Lawson DT, et al: *Nature* 352:236–238, 1991. Used by permission.)

electrode may be greatly distorted, or even counteracted, by coincident stimuli from other electrodes.

The problem of channel interactions is addressed in the CIS approach through the use of interleaved nonsimultaneous stimuli (see Figs 3 and 5). Trains of biphasic pulses are delivered to each electrode with temporal offsets that eliminate any overlap across channels. No more than one channel is stimulated at any instant. The amplitudes of the pulses are derived from the envelopes of bandpass filter outputs (see Fig 3). The envelope signals are produced by rectification and lowpass filtering. A logarithmic or power-law transformation is used to convert the magnitudes of the envelope signals into pulse amplitudes, so that envelope signals at or near zero will produce pulse amplitudes corresponding to auditory thresholds while envelope signals at high levels will produce pulse amplitudes corresponding to "most comfortable loudness" (MCL) percepts. A logarithmic mapping approximates a normal relationship between loudness and sound input levels across the dynamic range of electrically evoked hearing.[17, 18]

An important feature of CIS is relatively high rates of stimulation on each electrode channel (see Fig 4). Continuous interleaved sampling processors generally use rates of 500 pulses/sec or higher for each channel, so that rapid variations in speech can be tracked by variations in pulse amplitudes.

WITHIN-SUBJECT COMPARISONS

We have compared the performance of CA and CIS processors in tests with 11 users of the Ineraid cochlear prosthesis. Seven of the subjects were selected for their high levels of performance with the Ineraid CA processor (Smith and Nephew Richards, Bartlett, Tenn) and four were subsequently selected for relatively poor performance with that processor. The "high performance" subjects were representative of the best results, in terms of speech recognition scores, obtained as of 1991 with any commercially available implant system.[11] All of the subjects had at least 1 year of daily experience with the clinical system at the time of our tests, and most had multiple years of such experience. Each subject's performance with the CA processor was compared to that with the best CIS version identified in the first several days of a one-week fitting and evaluation period. The standard four channels of stimulation were used for the clinical CA processors,[19] whereas five or six channels were used for the CIS processors, to take advantage of additional implanted electrodes and reduced interactions among channels.

The comparison tests included identification of 16 consonants (/b, d, f, g, dʒ, k, l, m, n, p, s, ʂ, t, θ, v, z/) in an /a/-consonant-/a/ context ("aba," "ada," etc.)[20] and the open-set tests of the Minimal Auditory Capabilities (MAC) battery.[21] All tests were conducted with hearing alone, and all tests used single presentations of recorded material without feedback as to correct or incorrect responses. Results for the consonant tests were expressed as percent information transfer for various articulatory and acoustic features of consonants,[22] and results for the open-set tests as the percentage of correct responses.

Results for the consonant tests are presented in Figure 6. The top panel shows scores for the "high performance" group of seven subjects (high CA group), and the bottom panel shows scores for the "low performance" group of four subjects (low CA group). Both sets of subjects show gains for all consonant features. Especially large gains are found for nasality and frication for both sets, and large gains also are found in the low CA group for voicing and envelope features. The extent of increases for these latter features may have been limited by ceiling effects for the high CA group. Note that the overall pattern of improvement is similar for the two groups of subjects.

Results from the open-set tests are presented in Figure 7. The tests included recognition of 25 two-syllable words (spondees), 100 key words in the Central Institute for the Deaf (CID) sentences of everyday speech, the final words in each of 50 sentences from the Speech Perception in Noise (SPIN) test (presented in our studies without noise), and 50 one-syllable words from Northwestern University Auditory Test 6 (NU-6). In Figure 7, lines connect CA scores with CIS scores for each of the subjects. Scores for the "high performance" subjects are indicated by the endpoints of the thinner lines near the top of each panel, and scores for the "low performance" subjects are indicated by the endpoints of the thicker lines closer to the bottom of each panel.

As is evident from the figure, scores for all 11 subjects are improved with the use of a CIS processor. The average scores across subjects increased from 57% to 80% correct on the spondee test ($P < 0.002$), from 62% to 84% correct on the CID test ($P < 0.005$), from 34% to 65% correct on the SPIN test ($P < 0.001$), and from 30% to 47% correct on the NU-6 test ($P < 0.0005$).

Perhaps the most encouraging of these results are the improvements for the four low-performance subjects. One subject, for instance, achieved scores on each test with the CIS processor that would, with the clinical CA processor, have qualified him for membership in the high performance

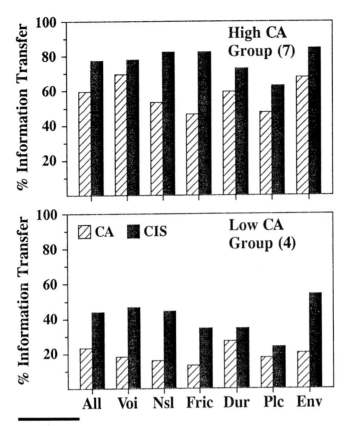

FIGURE 6.

Percent information transfer scores for CA and CIS processors. The top panel shows scores derived from the sum of stimulus/response matrices for seven subjects with high levels of performance with the clinical CA processor, and the bottom panel shows scores derived from the summed matrix for four subjects with low levels of performance with that processor. Consonant features include overall information transfer *(All)*, voicing *(Voi)*, nasality *(Nsl)*, frication *(Fric)*, duration *(Dur)*, place of articulation *(Plc)*, and envelope cues *(Env)*. At least 10 presentations of each of 16 consonants by a recorded male speaker, and 10 presentations of each consonant by a recorded female speaker, were used in the tests with each processor and subject. (From Wilson BS, Lawson DT, Zerbi M, et al: *Am J Otol*, in press. Used by permission.)

group. Another subject's scores on the spondee test increased from 0% to 56% correct, on the CID test from 1% to 55% correct, on the SPIN test from 0% to 26% correct, and on the NU-6 test from 0% to 14% correct.

The consistency and magnitude of improvements with CIS are especially impressive when one considers the large disparity in experience with the two types of processor. At the time of our tests each subject had 1 year to 5 years of daily experience with the CA processor, but only several hours over a few days with CIS. In previous studies involving within-subjects comparisons, such differences in experience have strongly favored the processor with the greatest duration of use.[23, 24] This suggests the possibility that even higher scores could be obtained with additional experience in using CIS processors.

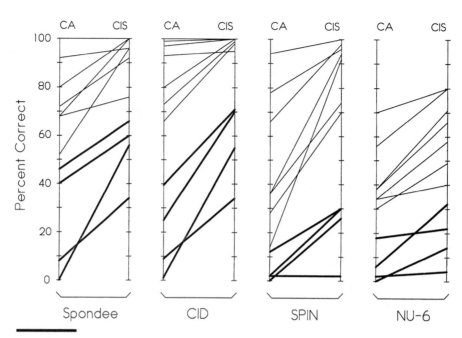

FIGURE 7.
Speech recognition scores for CA and CIS processors. A line connects the CA and CIS scores for each subject. Light lines correspond to the seven subjects selected for their excellent performance with the clinical CA processor, whereas the heavier lines correspond to the four subjects selected for relatively poor performance. (From Wilson BS, Lawson DT, Zerbi M, et al: *Am J Otol,* in press. Used by permission.)

EFFECTS OF NOISE INTERFERENCE

An additional aspect of CIS performance is illustrated in Figure 8. Here we show performances of CIS and CA processors with speech inputs degraded by the addition of noise. No special provisions for noise reduction were used with either processor. Consonant identification first was measured under quiet conditions, and then progressively greater amounts of multitalker speech babble were added to the primary speech signal. Signal-to-noise ratios (SNRs) included 15 dB, 10 dB, 5 dB, and 0 dB, with 0 dB corresponding to the babble signal amplitude exceeding the maximum consonant waveform amplitude about once per second on average. The tests were conducted with one of the two subjects who achieved the highest NU-6 score in Figure 7. A 24 consonant test was used instead of a 16 consonant test, to increase test sensitivity for this subject, who was scoring at or near 100% correct on the 16 consonant test with a variety of CIS processors.

Although the presence of noise reduces the performance of both processors, relatively high percent correct scores are maintained down to a SNR of 5 dB. The scores for the CIS processor are higher than those for the CA processor at all SNRs. This is especially encouraging inasmuch as the CA processor in the Ineraid device has been identified as the most resistant to the deleterious effects of noise interference among several tested implant systems.[10, 25]

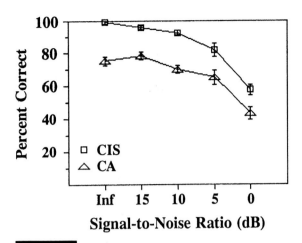

FIGURE 8.

Performance of CA and CIS processors as a function of signal-to-noise ratio (SNR). Percent correct scores from tests of consonant identification with Ineraid subject SR2 are shown. The SNR of *"Inf"* refers to presentation of the primary speech signal without any accompanying noise. Five presentations of each of 24 consonants by a recorded male speaker were used in the tests for each processor at each SNR. The presentations were arranged in block randomized order, providing a percent correct score after each set of randomized presentations of all 24 consonants. The *square symbols* show averages of these scores (from five randomized sets) for the CIS processor, and the *triangles* show the averages for the CA processor. Standard errors of the mean are indicated by the *vertical bars*. (From Wilson BS, Lawson DT, Zerbi M, et al: Recent developments with the CIS strategies, in Hochmair-Desoyer IJ, Hochmair ES (eds): *Advances in Cochlear Implants.* Vienna, Manz, 1994, pp 103–112. Used by permission.)

Similar results have been obtained with this and other subjects using the SPIN sentences, presented at the standard 8 dB SNR. All subjects studied to date have demonstrated a higher level of performance with CIS than with CA processors.

One possible factor underlying the relatively high levels of CIS performance is a good representation of envelope cues. In particular, covariation in envelope information across channels may help maintain high levels of speech recognition in noise.[26] Such across-channel information may allow a listener to follow the correlated cues of the primary speech signal, while rejecting the uncorrelated variations produced by the noise.

GENEVA STUDY

Our comparisons of CA and CIS processors have been replicated and extended in recent studies conducted by the cochlear implant team in Geneva, Switzerland.[27, 28] Fifteen users of the Ineraid device participated in the Geneva study. Unlike our study, subjects were not selected for either high or low levels of performance with the clinical CA processor. Also, six different native languages were represented among the subjects: French, German, Italian, Spanish, Albanian, and Swahili. Fourteen of the subjects had more than 2 years of daily experience with the CA processor at the time of the tests, and the remaining subject had 3 months of such experience. In contrast to our study, a standard set of parameters was used for all but a few subjects. Most subjects were fit with a five-channel CIS processor, which presented 50 μsec/phase pulses at the rate of 2,000/sec on each channel. Fitting time for these standardized CIS processors approximated 1 hour. As in our studies, the subjects had only 2 or 3 hours of aggregated experience with CIS prior to testing.

Results from consonant tests conducted in our laboratory and in the Geneva laboratory are presented in Figure 9. Our tests included 16 consonants, presented by both male and female speakers, whereas the Geneva tests included 14 consonants, presented by a different male speaker. Means and standard deviations of scores for overall information transfer are shown for both laboratories. Note the similarities in standard deviations and in the difference between CA and CIS results for the two laboratories. Absolute scores are somewhat lower for the Geneva laboratory for both CA and CIS processors, presumably because our subject population was biased toward high levels of performance, with seven subjects in a "high CA" group and four subjects in a "low CA" group. Performances among subjects in the Geneva study had a broad and more uniform distribution of performance levels with the clinical CA processor. Paired-t

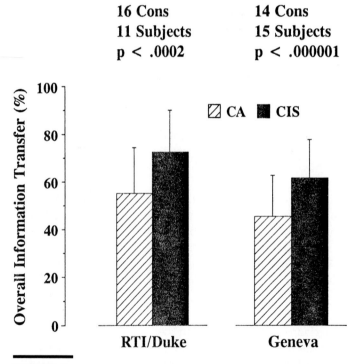

FIGURE 9.

Means and standard deviations of speech test scores from studies conducted in our laboratory (*RTI/Duke*) and in Geneva, Switzerland (*Geneva*), comparing the CA and CIS processors. Tests of consonant identification were administered in both laboratories. Sixteen consonants, presented by both male and female speakers, were used in the RTI/Duke tests, whereas 14 consonants, presented by a different male speaker, were used in the Geneva tests. Scores for percent overall information transfer are shown. (From Wilson BS, Lawson DT, Zerbi M, et al: *Am J Otol,* in press. Used by permission.)

comparisons of the subject scores for the two processors show highly significant differences for both laboratories ($P < 0.0002$ for our laboratory and $P < 0.000001$ for the Geneva laboratory).

The Geneva results replicate ours by demonstrating a large and highly significant difference between CA and CIS processors. The Geneva results extend ours by showing that such a difference is maintained with a standardized fitting and across six different native languages.

PARAMETRIC STUDIES WITH CIS PROCESSORS

In recent studies[12, 29, 30] we have evaluated effects produced by changes in parameters for CIS processors. We have compared performances with processors using (a) different numbers of channels, (b) nonsimultaneous versus simultaneous stimulation across channels, (c) different pulse durations and rates, and (d) different update orders for the channels within each cycle of nonsimultaneous stimulation. Findings to date indicate that each of these manipulations can affect performance and that the best choices for some parameters can vary from patient to patient. The findings may be summarized by the following:

- In studies with one subject, increases in the number of CIS channels in steps of one, from one channel to six, produced significant increases in percent correct scores on the 24 consonant test at each step, for both male and female speakers. Studies with other subjects also have demonstrated improvements in performance with the addition of CIS channels.
- Use of simultaneous stimulation produced large decrements in consonant identification for three tested subjects. This result was consistent with the idea that simultaneous stimulation might produce strong interactions among channels and thereby degrade the representation of channel-related cues.
- Effects of changes in pulse durations and rates have been studied with several subjects. Results for a subject in the "low CA" group indicated a maximum of performance on the 16 consonant test with a pulse rate of 833/sec and a pulse duration of 33 μsec/phase. Use of a higher (2,525/sec) or lower (500/sec or 417/sec) rate produced a decrement in performance. Also, use of pulses with greater durations (at rates below 2,525/sec, where such pulses can be used in a six channel processor without overlaps across channels) produced scores about the same as or lower (sometimes substantially lower) than those obtained with 33 μsec/phase pulses. Results for other subjects, in the "high CA" group, indicated small but significant increases in performance on either the 16 or 24 consonant test as the pulse rate was increased from 833/sec to 1,365/sec, and from 1,365/sec to 2,525/sec, using 33 μsec/phase pulses.
- In standard implementations of CIS processors a "staggered" order of channel updates has been used. This order imposed the maximum possible spatial separation between sequentially stimulated channels for each stimulus cycle (e.g., for a six channel processor an order of six-three-five-two-four-one has been used, where electrode one is the apicalmost electrode and electrode six is the basalmost electrode). In tests

conducted near the beginning of our studies with CIS processors we compared the staggered order with a base-to-apex order. A base-to-apex order mimics the direction of the traveling wave of mechanical displacements along the basilar membrane found in normal hearing. We therefore anticipated a possible advantage to the base-to-apex order. The results, however, showed that the staggered order was as good as, or substantially better than, the base-to-apex order for the studied subjects. As a control, we decided in recent studies with three subjects to compare the staggered order with an apex-to-base order. We expected that the apex-to-base order might produce a decrement in performance, inasmuch as it placed sequentially stimulated channels adjacent to each other, as in the base-to-apex order and was opposite to the direction of the traveling wave found in normal hearing. To our surprise, the apex-to-base order was clearly superior for two of the three subjects. Large increases in information transfer for the place of articulation feature were seen for both subjects. In addition, the apex-to-base order produced large gains in the transmission of voicing, duration, and envelope information for one subject. Both subjects performing better with it expressed a strong preference for the apex-to-base order, and said that processors using that order sounded more natural, more intelligible, and lower in overall pitch than otherwise identical processors using the staggered update order. In contrast, results for the third subject did not demonstrate a clear difference in performance with the two orders.

IMPORTANCE OF PROCESSOR FITTING

Findings presented in the previous section indicate that choices of pulse rate, pulse duration, and channel update order can have large effects on the performance of CIS processors. Such effects are illustrated further in Figure 10, which shows a history of improvements for one subject over the course of three successive visits to our laboratory. The subject used his Ineraid CA clinical device daily before and between visits to our laboratory.

In the first visit, this subject was fitted with a CIS processor using relatively long pulses (167 μsec/phase), a relatively low pulse rate (500/sec), and a staggered order of channel updates. As shown in the figure, application of this processor produced a quite large improvement over the clinical CA processor used in his daily life. The score for consonant identification improved from 25% to 56% correct. The scores for the open set tests also improved, as indicated here for the CID sentence and NU-6 word tests. These increases in performance were obtained with no more than several hours of aggregated experience with CIS processors, compared with more than 1 year of daily experience with the CA processor.

Seventeen months later the subject returned to the laboratory for a second visit, this time to evaluate effects of manipulations of pulse duration and pulse rate. The best combination of tested durations and rates for this subject was 33 μsec/phase pulses presented at 833/sec. We decided at the end of the visit to evaluate fully a CIS processor using these parameters. We also repeated the consonant test for the CA processor, to evaluate the possibilities that his performance with that processor had

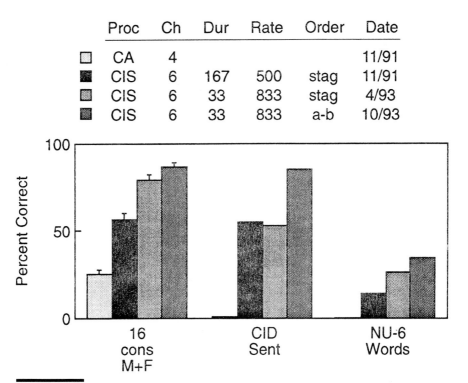

	Proc	Ch	Dur	Rate	Order	Date
☐	CA	4				11/91
■	CIS	6	167	500	stag	11/91
▨	CIS	6	33	833	stag	4/93
▨	CIS	6	33	833	a-b	10/93

FIGURE 10.

Improvements in speech processor performance for Ineraid subject SR10. The table above the bar chart specifies different processors. The leftmost column *(Proc)* indicates the general strategy, CA or CIS. The remaining columns indicate, from left to right, the number of channels *(Ch)* in CA or CIS processors, the duration per phase *(Dur)* of pulses used in CIS processors, the rate of pulses on a single channel in CIS processors *(Rate)*, the order of channel updates used in CIS processors *(Order;* the order is either staggered *[stag]* or apex-to-base *[a-b]),* and the date of testing. The error bars show standard errors of the mean for the consonant test.

improved through additional daily experience, or that his performance on the consonant test had improved through additional practice and familiarity with the test.

The subject again obtained a score of 25% correct for the consonant test (combined male and female speakers) with the CA processor. Scores for the CIS processor were generally better than those obtained during the first visit, with a CIS processor using a much longer pulse duration and a lower pulse rate. The score for the consonant test improved from 56% to 79% correct; the score for the CID test stayed about the same, from 55% to 53% correct; and the score for the NU-6 test almost doubled, from 14% to 26% correct.

Six months later, during a third visit to our laboratory by this same subject, we compared CIS processors with different update orders, and found that an apex-to-base order produced an improvement over the staggered order. Based on this finding, we again decided at the end of the visit to evaluate a CIS processor with an apex-to-base update order in greater detail, and to repeat the consonant test for the CA processor.

The subject's performance on the consonant test with the CA processor improved, from 25% to 37% correct. Most of the improvement was for the female speaker. The improvement may have reflected better use of cues provided by the CA processor through additional experience, or increased familiarity with the female version of the consonant test (which had been used more intensively than before during this third visit).

Performance with the apex-to-base CIS processor was substantially better than performance with an otherwise identical processor using the staggered update order. The consonant test score improved from 79% to 87% correct; the score for the CID test from 53% to 85% correct; and the score for the NU-6 test from 26% to 34% correct.

Note that the improvements across three visits took this subject from zero or near zero levels of open-set recognition with the CA processor to quite high levels with his final CIS processor. This example shows what is possible for at least some patients at the low end of the clinical performance spectrum, and demonstrates dramatically the importance of parameter choices for CIS processors and the potential benefits of parameter optimization.

SPECTRAL PEAK STRATEGY

A number of processing strategies have been used with the Nucleus device since 1982, when the device was introduced for clinical application.[31-33] The SPEAK strategy is the most recent in a line of strategies beginning with a feature extraction approach and ending with a waveform representation approach (see Fig 2). All of the strategies have used pulsatile stimuli.

PRIOR FEATURE EXTRACTION STRATEGIES

The first strategy used with the Nucleus device was designed to represent voicing information and the frequency and amplitude of the second formant (F2). One zero crossings detector was used to estimate the fundamental frequency (F0) of voiced speech sounds from the output of a 270 Hz lowpass filter. A separate zero crossings detector was used to estimate the position of the spectral centroid (or spectral "center of gravity") in the output of a bandpass filter spanning the frequency range of F2 (1,000 Hz to 4,000 Hz in one implementation of the strategy). The amplitude of F2 was estimated by detecting the envelope of the second filter's output with a rectifier and lowpass filter. The cutoff frequency of the lowpass filter was set at 35 Hz. This "F0F2" processor represented voicing information by presenting stimulus pulses at the estimated F0 rate during voiced speech sounds and at quasi-random intervals, with an average rate of around 100/sec, during unvoiced speech sounds. The frequency of the spectral centroid in the F2 band was represented by selecting one position along the electrode array for each successive pulse. High frequencies were represented by stimulation of an electrode or pair of electrodes near the basal end of the array and low frequencies by selecting an electrode or pair of electrodes near the apical end of the array. The estimated amplitude of F2 was represented with the amplitude of each pulse, using a logarithmic transformation of the envelope signal to determine pulse amplitude. Performance with this initial strategy was encouraging in that its use allowed some patients to recognize portions of speech with hearing alone.[31, 33, 34]

In late 1985, the F0F2 strategy was modified to include a representation of the first formant (F1). An additional channel of processing (with bandpass filter, zero crossings detector, and envelope detector) was used to derive estimates of the spectral centroid and amplitude in a band encompassing the range of F1 (300 Hz to 1,000 Hz). For each stimulus cycle the processor selected two electrode positions for stimulation, one corresponding to the estimated frequency of F1 and the other corresponding to the estimated frequency of F2. As in the F0F2 processor, the electrodes were stimulated at a rate equal to the estimated F0 during voiced speech and at quasi-random intervals during unvoiced speech. A stimulus cycle consisted of stimulation of the electrode or electrode pair for F2 followed by stimulation of the electrode or electrode pair for F1.

Within-subject comparisons of the F0F2 and F0F1F2 strategies demonstrated higher levels of speech recognition with the latter.[23, 35, 36] All seven patients in the study of Dowell and co-workers,[35] for instance, enjoyed increases in the recognition of key words in the CID sentences (presented live voice). The average score increased from 30% correct with the F0F2 processor to 63% correct with the F0F1F2 processor ($P < 0.002$).

In the years from 1985 to 1989, Cochlear Pty. Ltd. (a subsidiary of Nucleus Ltd.), in collaboration with investigators at the University of Melbourne, developed new hardware for the speech processor to be used with the Nucleus device.[33, 37, 38] Analog components were replaced by digital components, and various aspects of signal processing were refined in the new processor hardware. Use of a custom integrated circuit for much of the processing allowed substantial reductions in the size and weight of the new "Mini Speech Processor" (MSP) compared to the previous "Wearable Speech Processor" (WSP III). These reductions helped to make the processor more suitable for use by young children.

The MSP could be programmed to implement versions of the F0F2 and F0F1F2 strategies, with the refinements provided by the MSP hardware. In addition, a new strategy, MPEAK, could be implemented through software choices. The MPEAK strategy was intended to augment the F0F1F2 strategy by adding a representation of envelope variations in high-frequency bands of the input signal. The bands were from 2,000 Hz to 2,800 Hz ("band 3," as distinguished from the two bands for F1 and F2), 2,800 Hz to 4,000 Hz (band 4), and 4,000 Hz to 7,000 Hz (band 5).

In the MPEAK strategy four pulses are delivered in each stimulus cycle. During voiced speech these cycles (sets of four pulses) are presented at a rate equal to the estimated F0, and during unvoiced speech at quasi-random intervals, but now with an average rate in the range of 200/sec to 300/sec. Fixed electrode positions at the basal end of the array are reserved for representation of the amplitudes of envelope signals in the upper three bands, and the remaining (more apical) electrode positions are used for representation of F1 and F2. During voiced speech the electrodes for bands 4 and 3, and for F2 and F1, are selected for stimulation. During unvoiced speech the electrodes for bands, 5, 4, and 3, and for F2, are selected. Stimulation of the four electrodes (or electrode pairs) for each cycle is in a base-to-apex order. Manipulations of both pulse amplitude and pulse duration are used to code loudness (through changes in the total amount of charge phase, the product of amplitude and duration), primarily to reduce the time required for the receiver in the transcutaneous transmission system to specify the characteristics of each pulse (specification of a high intensity, short duration pulse requires much less time than specification of a low intensity, long duration pulse of the same charge[39, 40]). This allows higher rates of stimulation, in excess of 400/sec.

Studies have been conducted to compare the F0F1F2 strategy as implemented in the WSP III, the F0F1F2 strategy as implemented in the MSP or a prototype version of the MSP, and the MPEAK strategy as implemented in the MSP.[38, 41] In within-subject comparisons with five patients, Dowell and co-workers found significant increases in open set recognition of speech when the MSP implementation of the F0F1F2 strategy was substituted for the WSP III implementation of that strategy.[23] In within-subject comparisons with a separate set of five patients, Skinner and co-workers[38] found no significant differences in open set scores for the two implementations of the F0F1F2 strategy but, like Dowell and co-workers, did find significant increases in scores when the MPEAK strategy was used. Average scores for recognition of NU-6 words, for example, increased from 13% correct with the F0F1F2 strategy to 29% correct with the MPEAK strategy ($P < 0.01$). Thus, the MPEAK strategy was superior to the tested alternatives and, in one of the studies, the MSP implementation of the F0F1F2 strategy was superior to the WSP III implementation.

SPECTRAL MAXIMA SOUND PROCESSOR

The direct antecedent to the SPEAK strategy was the *spectral maxima sound processor* (SMSP) strategy. It and SPEAK mark a departure from the feature extraction approach of prior strategies used with the Nucleus device.

In the SMSP strategy[42, 43] the input was directed to a bank of 16 bandpass filters covering the range from 250 Hz to 5,400 Hz. Envelope signals were derived for each of the bandpass outputs with a rectifier and lowpass filter. The corner frequency of the lowpass filter for each detector was set at 200 Hz. Each bandpass channel was assigned to an electrode position in the implant. Bandpass channels with lower center frequencies were assigned to more apical electrodes (or closely spaced pairs of electrodes), whereas channels with higher center frequencies were assigned to more basal electrodes. A microprocessor scanned the outputs of the envelope detectors for each cycle of stimulation and identified the channels with envelope signals above a preset noise threshold. If more than six signals exceeded the threshold, then the microprocessor identified the six signals with the greatest amplitudes. If fewer than six signals exceeded the threshold, then all such signals were identified. The identified signals were used to determine pulse amplitudes (through a logarithmic mapping function) for the corresponding bandpass channels. The electrodes assigned to those channels then were stimulated in a nonsimultaneous sequence starting with the highest envelope signal and ending with the lowest envelope signal. In general, six "maxima" were selected for each cycle of stimulation, and cycles were repeated at the rate of 250/sec.

Tests with a small number of subjects at the University of Melbourne indicated that the SMSP strategy might offer substantial improvements in speech recognition over the MPEAK and F0F1F2 strategies.[42, 43] For example, recognition of key words in sentence material presented with multitalker speech babble at the SNR of 10 dB was significantly higher with SMSP than with MPEAK for each of four subjects.

DESIGN AND EVALUATION OF THE SPECTRAL PEAK STRATEGY

Following these encouraging results with the SMSP, Cochlear Pty. Ltd. and the University of Melbourne developed the SPEAK strategy, which is modeled after the SMSP. New hardware also was developed to implement the SPEAK strategy in a small package suitable for widespread clinical use.

In the SPEAK strategy[44] the inputs filtered into as many as 20 bands rather than the 16 of the SMSP strategy. A number of maxima are selected for each stimulus cycle, depending on details of the input such as the distribution of energy across frequencies ("spectral complexity") and the number of envelope signals exceeding a preset noise threshold. In most cases, six maxima are selected, as in the SMSP strategy. However, the number of selected maxima can range from one to a maximum that can be set as high as ten. Sets of the selected maxima are presented at rates between 180/sec and 300/sec, depending on the number of maxima and pulse amplitudes and durations. Presentation of relatively few maxima in a cycle allows relatively high rates, whereas presentation of many maxima in a cycle reduces the rate. The average rate is about 250/sec. In the SPEAK strategy, electrodes or electrode pairs are stimulated in a base-to-apex order.

The new hardware, called the "Spectra 22" processor, includes a custom integrated circuit to perform the functions of bandpass filtering and envelope detection. The design of the integrated circuit provides flexibility in specifications of the corner frequencies and gains for the bandpass filters. In a typical implementation, 20 bandpass filters span a range from 150 Hz to 10,823 Hz, with a linear spacing of corner frequencies below 1,850 Hz and a logarithmic spacing of corner frequencies above 1,850 Hz. The filter gains normally are all set to a single value. Alternative settings may be specified, such as when fewer than 20 electrode positions are available for a given patient.

Within-subject comparisons of the SPEAK and MPEAK strategies have been conducted with 63 English-speaking patients at various centers in Australia, the United States, Canada and England.[44] Some of the principal results, along with key features of processing in the SPEAK strategy, are presented in Figure 11. Subjects were tested with an ABAB design, in which subjects used their clinical MPEAK processor during an initial 3-week period, then used the SPEAK processor for 6 weeks, then returned to the MPEAK processor for 3 weeks, and then used the SPEAK

Spectral Peak Strategy

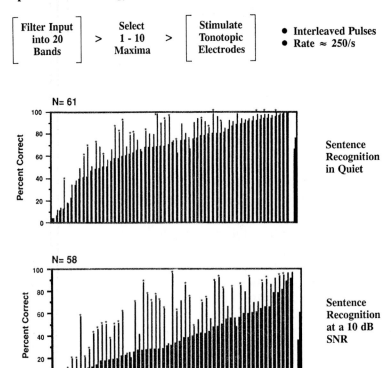

$$\left[\begin{array}{c}\text{Filter Input}\\ \text{into 20}\\ \text{Bands}\end{array}\right] > \begin{array}{c}\text{Select}\\ \text{1 - 10}\\ \text{Maxima}\end{array} > \left[\begin{array}{c}\text{Stimulate}\\ \text{Tonotopic}\\ \text{Electrodes}\end{array}\right]$$

- Interleaved Pulses
- Rate ≈ 250/s

Sentence Recognition in Quiet

Sentence Recognition at a 10 dB SNR

FIGURE 11.

Design of the SPEAK strategy (top panel) and principal results from comparisons of that strategy with the MPEAK strategy in a multicenter study (lower panels). The middle panel shows percent correct scores for recognition of key words in City University of New York or Speech Intelligibility Test for Deaf Children sentences presented in quiet conditions, for each of 61 subjects. The bottom panel shows scores for sentences presented with multitalker speech babble at a signal-to-noise ratio of 10 dB, for each of 58 subjects. Asterisks identify scores that are significantly different ($P < 0.05$) for individual subjects. (Organization of figure and top panel adapted from Rabinowitz WM: *J Acoust Soc Am* 95:2904–2905, 1994. Lower panels are from Skinner MW, Clark GM, Whitford LA, et al: *Am J Otol*, 15(suppl 2):15–27, 1994. All panels and figure organization used by permission.)

processor during a final 3-week period. The processors were tested at the end of each period. All subjects had at least 8 months of daily experience with the MPEAK processor prior to the study.

Averages of the scores for each subject and processor are presented in the middle and lower panels of Figure 11. The middle panel shows scores for the recognition of key words in the City University of New York or Speech Intelligibility Test for Deaf Children sentences presented in quiet conditions. The bottom panel shows scores for those sentences when presented with multitalker speech babble at the SNR of 10 dB.

Among the 61 subjects who were tested with sentences in quiet conditions, 24 had significantly higher scores with the SPEAK processor and 2 had significantly higher scores with the MPEAK processor. Many of the subjects obtained high scores on this relatively easy test and therefore possible differences between processors for those subjects may have been masked by ceiling effects. Among the 58 subjects who were tested with sentences in noise (for the 10 dB condition), 41 had significantly higher scores with the SPEAK processor and none had a significantly higher score with the MPEAK processor.

The principal advantage of the SPEAK processor, at least for the tests conducted to date, is in producing higher scores for recognition of speech in the presence of interfering noise. This advantage may be the result of an improved representation of envelope cues, as mentioned before in connection with the CIS processor. It also may be the result of a high sensitivity of the feature extraction circuits in the MPEAK processor to noise. The accuracy of such extraction can be severely degraded by even modest amounts of noise. Zero crossings circuits in particular are susceptible to deleterious effects of noise interference.[45]

CONVERGENCE OF FINDINGS

The developments outlined in this chapter are good news for implant recipients. The CIS strategy has produced immediate improvements over the clinical CA strategy across a wide range of patients. Comparisons of the SPEAK strategy with the MPEAK strategy have indicated better performance with SPEAK for some subjects when listening to speech in quiet and for a majority of subjects when listening to speech in noise. The processing strategy can have a quite large effect on outcome and general expectations for patient performance can now be higher than was the case just a few years ago.

These recent advances in processor design also demonstrate a certain convergence of ideas and results. In the series using the 22-electrode Nucleus implanted hardware, improvements in performance were found as more information per unit time was added to the representation, and as less reliance was placed on feature extraction and encoding. In our series using the six-electrode Ineraid array, large improvements in performance were found with use of a CIS instead of a CA processor for all tested subjects. Among the pulsatile strategies that have been described to date, the CIS strategy presents the most information per unit time. Finally, the CA/CIS comparisons, along with the simultaneous versus nonsimultaneous comparisons with CIS processors, indicate the value of nonsimultaneous stimulation.

In broad terms, it appears that a waveform representation approach is superior to a feature extraction approach and that use of nonsimultaneous pulses as stimuli is better than use of analog waveforms presented simultaneously on multiple electrodes. In addition, performance may be improved as the total amount of information presented through the implant is increased, either by increasing the number of electrode channels or by increasing the rate of stimulation on each electrode or both.

FUTURE DIRECTIONS

Although the present results are most encouraging, many important questions remain unanswered, and possibilities for further improvement remain unexplored. Such questions and possibilities are being addressed in ongoing studies in our laboratory and elsewhere. In a cooperative study with Cochlear Corporation and Duke University Medical Center, for example, we are evaluating a variety of processing strategies in conjunction with the electrode array used in the present Nucleus 22 implant system. The subjects of this study have percutaneous connectors, allowing direct electrical access to the implanted electrodes. Such access is required for optimized implementations of CIS processors (e.g., with pulse rates in excess of 400/sec for a six-channel processor). Included in the evaluations are within-subject comparisons among CIS processors using 6, 11, and 22 electrodes and between various CIS and SPEAK processors. The results should provide information on the performance potential of CIS processors with more than six electrode channels and on the relative efficacy of CIS and SPEAK processors. A total of six patients will be studied.

Other promising lines of investigation include continued systematic evaluation of parameter choices for CIS processors. Such evaluation may separate choices that produce the best results for most patients from choices whose effects vary widely among patients. Focusing only on those choices most likely to depend on the patient could streamline the fitting of CIS processors in the clinic.

SUMMARY

Major conclusions presented in this chapter include the following:

- CIS processors can produce large gains in speech recognition over clinical CA processors—across a broad range of patients and for a number of different native languages—even when a standardized set of parameters is used.
- CIS performance may be improved substantially by optimizing choices of pulse width, pulse rate, and channel update order for each patient.
- CIS processor performance generally increases with the number of distinct channels used.
- Nonsimultaneous stimulation can convey significantly more information than simultaneous stimulation.
- The addition of speech babble noise to the input degrades the performance of both CA and CIS processors; however, speech recognition scores are substantially better with the CIS processor for all tested subjects and SNRs.
- The SPEAK strategy offers significant advantages over the MPEAK strategy for approximately 40% of a studied population of patients listening to sentences in quiet conditions.
- The addition of speech babble noise to the input degrades the performance of both MPEAK and SPEAK processors; however, the proportion of patients who demonstrate better scores with the SPEAK processor increases to approximately 70%.

- Similarities in the CIS and SPEAK strategies indicate the efficacy of multichannel processors using a waveform representation of speech sounds and nonsimultaneous pulses as stimuli.
- Differences in the CIS and SPEAK strategies indicate the need for future studies to evaluate the effects of each difference.

ACKNOWLEDGMENTS

We thank the subjects of studies conducted in our laboratory for their enthusiastic participation. We also are pleased to acknowledge the important scientific contributions of many colleagues, including for the studies reviewed here, Michael F. Dorman, Donald K. Eddington, Charles C. Finley, James F. Patrick, William M. Rabinowitz, Robert V. Shannon, Margaret W. Skinner and Richard S. Tyler.

REFERENCES

1. Shannon RV: Psychophysics, in Tyler RS (ed): *Cochlear Implants: Audiological Foundations*. San Diego, Calif, Singular Publishing Group, 1993, pp 357–388.
2. Wilson BS, Lawson DT, Finley CC, et al: Importance of patient and processor variables in determining outcomes with cochlear implants. *J Speech Hear Res* 36:373–379, 1993.
3. Dorman MF: Speech perception by adults, in Tyler RS (ed): *Cochlear Implants: Audiological Foundations*. San Diego, Calif, Singular Publishing Group, 1993, pp 145–190.
4. Gantz BJ: Cochlear implants: An overview. *Adv Otolaryngol Head Neck Surg* 1:171–200, 1987.
5. Millar JB, Blamey PJ, Tong YC, et al: Speech perception, in Clark GM, Tong YC, Patrick JF (eds): *Cochlear Prostheses*. Edinburgh, Churchill Livingstone, 1990, pp 41-67.
6. Millar JB, Tong YC, Clark GM: Speech processing for cochlear implant prostheses. *J Speech Hear Res* 27:280–296, 1984.
7. Moore BCJ: Speech coding for cochlear implants, in Gray RF (ed): *Cochlear Implants*. San Diego, Calif, College-Hill Press, 1985, pp 163–179.
8. Parkins CW: Cochlear prostheses, in Altschuler RA, Hoffman DW, Bobbin RP (eds): *Neurobiology of Hearing: The Cochlea*. New York, Raven Press, 1986, pp 455–473.
9. Pfingst BE: Stimulation and encoding strategies for cochlear prostheses. *Otolaryngol Clin North Am* 19:219–235, 1986.
10. Tyler RS, Tye-Murray N: Cochlear implant signal-processing strategies and patient perception of speech and environmental sounds, in Cooper H (ed): *Cochlear Implants: A Practical Guide:* San Diego, Calif, Singular Publishing Group, 1991, pp 58–83.
11. Wilson BS, Finley CC, Lawson DT, et al: Better speech recognition with cochlear implants. *Nature* 352:236–238, 1991.
12. Wilson BS, Lawson DT, Zerbi M, et al: Recent developments with the CIS strategies, in Hochmair-Desoyer IJ, Hochmair ES (eds): *Advances in Cochlear Implants*. Vienna, Manz, 1994, pp 103–112.
13. Pfingst BE: Operating ranges and intensity psychophysics for cochlear implants. *Arch Otolaryngol Hear Neck Surg* 110:140–144, 1984.
14. Shannon RV: Multichannel electrical stimulation of the auditory nerve in man. I. Basic psychophysics. *Hear Res* 11:157–189, 1983.

15. Shannon RV: Threshold and loudness functions for pulsatile stimulation of cochlear implants. *Hear Res* 18:135–143, 1985.

16. White MW, Merzenich MM, Gardi JN: Multichannel cochlear implants: Channel interactions and processor design. *Arch Otolaryngol Head Neck Surg* 110:493–501, 1984.

17. Zeng F-G, Shannon RV: Loudness balance between acoustic and electric stimulation. *Hear Res* 60:236–238, 1992.

18. Dorman MF, Smith L, Parkin JL: Loudness balance between acoustic and electric stimulation by a patient with a multichannel cochlear implant. *Ear Hear* 14:290–292, 1993.

19. Eddington DK: Speech discrimination in deaf subjects with cochlear implants. *J Acoust Soc Am* 68:885–891, 1980.

20. Tyler RS, Preece JP, Lowder MW: *The Iowa Audiovisual Speech Perception Laser Videodisc.* Iowa City, University of Iowa Hospitals and Clinics, Department of Otolaryngology—Head and Neck Surgery, 1987.

21. Owens E, Kessler DK, Raggio M, et al: Analysis and revision of the Minimal Auditory Capabilities (MAC) battery. *Ear Hear* 6:280–287, 1985.

22. Miller GA, Nicely PE: An analysis of perceptual confusions among some English consonants. *J Acoust Soc Am* 27:338–352, 1955.

23. Dowell RC, Seligman PM, Blamey PJ, et al: Evaluation of a two-formant speech-processing strategy for a multichannel cochlear prosthesis. *Ann Otol Rhinol Laryngol* 96(suppl 128):132–134, 1987.

24. Tyler RS, Preece JP, Lansing CR, et al: Previous experience as a confounding factor in comparing cochlear-implant processing schemes. *J Speech Hear Res* 29:282–287, 1986.

25. Gantz BJ, McCabe BF, Tyler RS, et al: Evaluation of four cochlear implant designs. *Ann Otol Rhinol Laryngol* 96(suppl 128):145–147, 1987.

26. Hall JW, Haggard MP, Fernandes MA: Detection in noise by spectro-temporal pattern analysis. *J Acoust Soc Am* 76:50–56, 1984.

27. Boëx C, Pelizzone M, Montandon P: Improvements in speech recognition with the CIS strategy for the Ineraid multichannel intracochlear implant, in Hochmair-Desoyer IJ, Hochmair ES (eds): *Advances in Cochlear Implants.* Vienna, Manz, 1994, pp 136–140.

28. Boëx C, Pelizzone M, Montandon P: Improvements in speech recognition with the CIS strategy for the Ineraid multichannel intracochlear implant. An update of patient results. Presented at the *1993 Conference on Implantable Auditory Prostheses,* Smithfield, RI, July, 1993 (data cited with permission of the authors).

29. Lawson DT, Wilson BS, Finley CC: New processing strategies for multichannel cochlear prostheses. *Prog Brain Res* 97:313–321, 1993.

30. Wilson BS, Lawson DT, Zerbi M: Speech processors for auditory prostheses. *Fifth Quarterly Progress Report, NIH project N01-DC-2-2401.* Bethesda, Md, National Institutes of Health, Neural Prosthesis Program, 1993.

31. Clark GM: The University of Melbourne-Nucleus multi-electrode cochlear implant. *Adv Otorhinolaryngol* 38:1–189, 1987.

32. Clark GM, Tong YC, Patrick JF: *Cochlear Prostheses.* Edinburgh, Scotland: Churchill Livingstone, 1990.

33. Patrick JF, Clark GM: The Nucleus 22-channel cochlear implant system. *Ear Hear* 12(suppl 1):3S–9S, 1991.

34. Dowell RC, Mecklenberg DJ, Clark GM: Speech recognition for 40 patients receiving multichannel cochlear implants. *Arch Otolaryngol Head Neck Surg* 112:1054–1059, 1986.

35. Dowell RC, Seligman PM, Blamey PJ, et al: Speech perception using a two-formant 22-electrode cochlear prosthesis in quiet and in noise. *Acta Otolaryngol (Stockh)* 104:439–446, 1987.

36. Tye-Murray N, Lowder M, Tyler RS: Comparison of the F0F2 and F0F1F2 processing strategies for the Cochlear Corporation cochlear implant. *Ear Hear* 11:195–200, 1990.
37. Patrick JF, Seligman PM, Money DK, et al: Engineering, in Clark GM, Tong YC, Patrick JF (eds): *Cochlear Prostheses*. Edinburgh, Churchill Livingstone, 1990, pp 99–124.
38. Skinner MW, Holden LK, Holden TA, et al: Performance of postlinguistically deaf adults with the Wearable Speech Processor (WSP III) and Mini Speech Processor (MSP) of the Nucleus multi-electrode cochlear implant. *Ear Hear* 12:3–22, 1991.
39. Shannon RV, Adams DD, Ferrel RL, et al: A computer interface for psychophysical and speech research with the Nucleus cochlear implant. *J Acoust Soc Am* 87:905–907, 1990.
40. Crosby PA, Daly CN, Money DK, et al: Cochlear implant system for an auditory prosthesis. U.S. Patent No. 4532930, 1985.
41. Dowell RC, Dawson PW, Dettman SJ, et al: Multichannel cochlear implantation in children: A summary of current work at the University of Melbourne, *Am J Otol* 12(suppl 1):137–143, 1991.
42. McDermott HJ, McKay CM, Vandali AE: A new portable sound processor for the University of Melbourne/Nucleus Limited multielectrode cochlear implant. *J Acoust Soc Am* 91:3367–3391, 1992.
43. McKay C, McDermott H, Vandali A, et al: Preliminary results with a six spectral maxima sound processor for the University of Melbourne/Nucleus multiple-electrode cochlear implant. *J Otolaryngol Soc Australia* 6:354–359, 1991.
44. Skinner MW, Clark GM, Whitford LA, et al: Evaluation of a new spectral peak coding strategy for the Nucleus 22 channel cochlear implant system. *Am J Otol* 15 (suppl 2):15–27, 1994.
45. Rabiner LR, Shafer RW: *Digital Processing of Speech Signals*. Englewood Cliffs, NJ, Prentice-Hall, 1978, pp 129–130.

Management of Caustic Ingestion in Children

Keith H. Riding, F.R.C.S.C.

Clinical Professor, Division of Otolaryngology, Department of Surgery, University of British Columbia; Head of the ENT Department, British Columbia's Children's Hospital, Vancouver, British Columbia, Canada

CAUSTIC INGESTION

INCIDENCE

It has been estimated that there are as many as 5,000 accidental lye ingestions per year by children younger than 5 years of age in the United States.[1-3] Children in the first decade of life constitute the largest group affected, with an especially high incidence in the first three years. Children who are developmentally delayed form another group. Some teenagers (females outnumber males) use caustic ingestion as a suicide attempt.

In all reported series, the substances causing burns most frequently were the alkalis (60% to 80%). The remainder were caused by such substances as Lysol (phenol), Clorox, and acids.[4-9] These substances are all readily available in stores. Common household products that may contain caustic substances are listed in Table I.

TYPES OF CORROSIVES

Alkalis are bases that dissolve in water. They contain a positive radical and a hydroxyl group. The common alkalis are sodium, potassium, and ammonium hydroxides ($NaOH$, KOH, NH_4OH).

Acids are compounds that contain hydrogen and at least one non-metal. Most are soluble in water. Common acids are hydrochloric, sulphuric, and nitric (HCl, H_2SO_4, HNO_3).

Other corrosives commonly encountered are *Phenol* or hydroxybenzene (C_6H_5OH). It is a crystalline, acidic compound that is very caustic. When a little water or alcohol is added to it, it is sold as carbolic acid or Lysol in drugstores. The active ingredient in *bleach* is hypochlorous acid ($HClO$). Usually it is sold as a salt (e.g., Clorox) that is 5.25 percent sodium hypochlorite. When it gives up its oxygen, hydrochloric acid is formed. Other substances, such as *kerosene, creosote, potassium permanganate*, and *sodium dichromate* are also available commercially.

DISC BATTERIES

There have been several reports with regard to esophageal burns from disc batteries.[10] Of 125 batteries ingested during 114 ingestion episodes

Advances in Otolaryngology—Head and Neck Surgery®, vol. 9
© 1995, Mosby–Year Book, Inc.

TABLE 1.
Composition of Some of the More Commonly Used Drain Cleaners*

Name of Product	Manufacturer	Active Ingredient	Concentrated %
Granular			
Plumite	Simoniz Co., Chicago, Ill	NaOH	92%
Rooto Heavy-Duty Drain Cleaner	Roota Corp., Farmington, Mich	KOH	72%
Mitee	DAP Inc., Dayton, OH	NaOH	>10%
Drano	Drackett Prod. Co., Cincinnati, Ohio	NaOH	54%
Liquid			
Liquid Drano	Drackett Prod. Co., Cincinnati, Ohio	NaOH	9.5%
Glamorene Drain Powder	Glamorene Prod. Corp., Clifton, NJ	KOH	35%
Mister Plumber	National Solvent Corp., Cleveland, Ohio	Concentrated H_2SO_4	99.5%
Plunge	Drackett Prod. Co., Cincinnati, Ohio	NaOH	9.5%
Down the Drain	Lehn & Fink Prop., Montvale, NJ	KOH	36.5%
Liquid Plumr	Clorox Corp., Oakland, Calif	NaOH	12%

*From Riding KH, Bluestone CD: Burns and acquired strictures of the esophagus, in Bluestone CD, Stool SE, Kenna MA (eds): *Pediatric Otolaryngology,* ch 61. Philadelphia, WB Saunders, 1994. Used by permission.

between August 1982 and June 1983, one-third (33.9%) were ingested by hearing-impaired children from their own hearing aids. Most batteries pass through the gastrointestinal tract without causing any harm, but if they do become lodged in the esophagus, they can cause severe burns. Apparently, an electrochemical current develops across the battery's seal when the battery becomes lodged in the esophagus, and leakage of the contents occurs. Usually, the battery contains a 45% solution of potassium or sodium hydroxide. Immediate endoscopic removal is indicated. Attempts at retrieval from the stomach are not recommended.

EMERGENCY MANAGEMENT

In the emergency room, it is important to find out the type of substance that was ingested or suspected to have been ingested. Most often, the parents or the people accompanying the patient can provide only the name of the substance. In this case, the information as to the constitution and concentration of the substance can be obtained from the nearest poison center. An attempt should be made to estimate how much of the substance was ingested. In children, this is usually very difficult. It should be emphasized that even small amounts of caustic products can cause severe damage to the esophagus and that once a substance has touched a child's tongue, the natural reflex leads to swallowing. Thus, parents should not be reassured that no damage has been done until the child has been fully examined. It is important to know whether the patient vomited after ingestion or was made to vomit, since this would increase the length of time the esophagus was exposed to the agent.

Examination of the child may reveal that there are burns on the lips, chin, hands, or chest caused by manipulation of the substance and possible regurgitation. The child may be in severe pain and unable to swallow even his or her own saliva. There may be burns in the mouth. The presence of burns in the mouth has been shown to correlate very poorly with burns in the esophagus; thus, it should not be assumed that because of the absence of burns in the mouth, esophageal burns are improbable and vice versa.

The complications of acute laryngitis that lead to airway obstruction, such as stridor, hoarseness, and cough, should be searched for. Mediastinitis from rupture of the esophagus may cause severe chest pains, especially on respiration. The abdomen should also be examined for signs of peritonitis from perforation of the stomach.

From the history and examination, Riding and Bluestone suggest that it may be possible to place the patient into one of three categories.[11]

Category 1. The first category would be the child who is relatively asymptomatic.

Category 2. The second category would include the child who shows definite evidence of ingestion with burns of the mouth and/or surrounding skin and pain on swallowing or refuses to swallow.

Category 3. In the third category would be children with severe burns with complications such as mediastinitis, peritonitis, or laryngitis.

Aim of Management
The aim of management is to prevent strictures forming in the esophagus. Any management modality that reduces the amount of granulation tissue, the number and activity of fibroblasts, or both, will contribute to this end.

Dilemmas in Acute Management
A dilemma is knowing whether to treat all children with a history of caustic ingestion or just those that have symptoms. Most of the children who are in category one (i.e., are asymptomatic) may have either no burn or a first-degree burn and it is possible that most (or even all) of these patients would not develop strictures later. Some physicians would opt not to treat these children.

To be effective, steroids must be given within the first 24 hours of the injury. The extent of the injury cannot be judged until an esophagoscopy is performed, usually 24 to 48 hours later. Some physicians, therefore, might opt to treat all patients with steroids initially, stopping them if no burn is found during esophagoscopy.

ACUTE MANAGEMENT (FIG 1)

Category 1
After careful evaluation has found that there are no signs or symptoms then no treatment is given.

Category 2
Having once established that there is no airway obstruction, mediastinitis, or peritonitis present the following measures are undertaken.

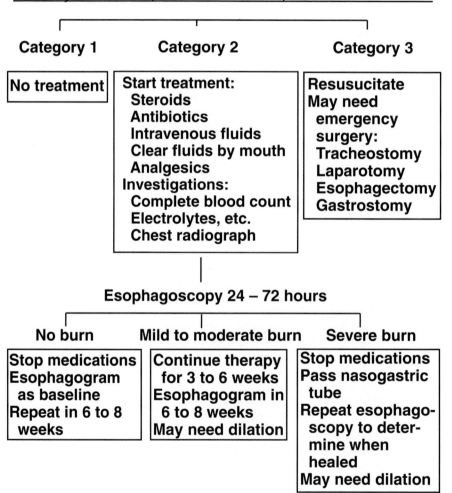

Algorithm for Management of Caustic Burn

Identify substance, estimate amount, and examine child.

Category 1	Category 2	Category 3
No treatment	**Start treatment:** Steroids Antibiotics Intravenous fluids Clear fluids by mouth Analgesics **Investigations:** Complete blood count Electrolytes, etc. Chest radiograph	**Resusucitate** **May need** **emergency** **surgery:** Tracheostomy Laparotomy Esophagectomy Gastrostomy

Esophagoscopy 24 – 72 hours

No burn	Mild to moderate burn	Severe burn

Stop medications
Esophagogram
  as baseline
Repeat in 6 to 8
  weeks
	Continue therapy
	  for 3 to 6 weeks
	Esophagogram in
	  6 to 8 weeks
	May need dilation
		Stop medications
		Pass nasogastric
		  tube
		Repeat esophago-
		  scopy to deter-
		  mine when
		  healed
		May need dilation

FIGURE 1.

Algorithm for management of caustic burn. (From Riding KH, Bluestone CD: Burns and acquired strictures of the esophagus, in Bluestone CD, Stool SE, Kenna MA (eds): *Pediatric Otolaryngology*, ed 3, ch 61. Philadelphia, WB Saunders, 1994. Used by permission.)

ANALGESICS.—Intramuscular or intravenous narcotics may be administered appropriate to age and weight. Acetaminophen might be given by suppository.

ALIMENTATION AND FLUID BALANCE.—The patient, if able to swallow, should be allowed only clear liquids. Krey showed that particles of food become caught up in necrotic tissue and produce more granulation tissue.[12] If the patient is unable to swallow, fluids are given intravenously. At the same time as the intravenous line is being established, blood should be taken for electrolyte estimation.

CHEST RADIOGRAPH.—Posteroanterior and lateral views should be obtained in all cases as a baseline and also to detect evidence of mediastinitis or aspiration pneumonia.

ANTIBIOTICS.—Krey also showed that epithelialization occurred more quickly when animals were treated with antibiotics.[12] By reducing the number of bacteria present in the burn tissue, granulation tissue can be reduced. It is common to use ampicillin, 50 to 100 mg/kg/day, either intravenously or, if the patient can swallow, amoxycillin by mouth, where it has a local effect as well as a systemic effect.

STEROIDS.—Prednisone 2 mg/kg/day to a maximum of 60 mg/day is given intravenously, initially, then orally after a few days as swallowing starts again. This dosage is continued for 21 days and then tapered over the next 21 days, so that the total time on steroids is 6 weeks.

ESOPHAGOSCOPY.—Most physicians would advocate performing a rigid esophagoscopy of the symptomatic patient between 24 and 72 hours after ingestion. Direct visualization is the only accurate way to diagnose esophageal burns. The esophagoscope should not be advanced beyond the first area of a severe burn, since the danger of perforation is greater in these cases than normally. However, advancement of an esophagoscope with a telescope or fiberoptic flexible esophagoscope may be performed when a mild burn is visualized in the proximal esophagus, since a severe burn may be present in the distal esophagus.

LATER MANAGEMENT

No Burn
If no burn is seen on esophagoscopy, medication is discontinued, and an esophagogram is performed before the patient is discharged from the hospital, both as a baseline and as a precaution in case of an overlooked lesion. The patient is discharged from the hospital but should be seen again in 6 to 8 weeks, when a second esophagogram is performed. If the patient is still asymptomatic and the esophagogram is normal, there is no follow-up necessary.

Mild or Moderate Burn
If, on the basis of the esophagoscopic results, the patient is considered to have either a mild or a moderate ulcerative esophagitis, the combination of antibiotic and steroid therapy should be continued for 3 to 6 weeks

(see above). The child should be maintained on clear liquids or intravenous fluids for the first few days, but then may begin a soft diet. At this stage, the child may be nursed at home. After about 3 weeks, the steroids can be tapered. An esophagogram should be performed in 6 to 8 weeks, and the patient should be seen every 3 months for 1 year. If the child has difficulty in swallowing or the esophagogram shows evidence of early stricture formation then dilatation may have to be undertaken. Initially, this should be performed with the patient under general anesthesia and through an esophagoscope using dilators such as Jackson silk woven bougies, although more often nowadays the Gruntzig balloon technique is being used (see below).

Severe Burn
Initially, these patients are treated the same as less severely burned patients, but as soon as the extent of the burn is realized by esophagoscopy, the steroids are discontinued. To continue steroid treatment would increase the danger of perforation in cases where the whole wall of the esophagus is necrotic. Insertion of nasogastric tube or stent together with gastrostomy and insertion of jejunal feeding tube is recommended.

Category 3
Management of severe, complicated esophageal burn. The mortality of patients in this group is very high.

Shock and Metabolic Acid-Base Disturbance
This is treated along basic surgical principles with intravenous replacement therapy and correction of acid-base balance.

Upper Airway Obstruction
The larynx may have been burned to a varying degree. Edema and inflammation may cause an upper airway obstruction, which is relieved by tracheostomy. The larynx may be affected in the same way as the esophagus with a good deal of tissue destruction leading to stricture formation later on. This may require laryngeal surgery at a later date.

Mediastinitis
This occurs because of perforation of the esophagus. It may lead to the development of small, localized abscesses around the esophagus or to full-blown mediastinitis. In instances of small, localized abscesses, the help of a thoracic surgeon may be necessary to place a drain in the chest. Severe mediastinitis may require immediate esophagectomy. Ritter and co-workers recommended radical treatment for these cases, leaving the patient with a cervical esophagostomy and gastrostomy, since the mortality is so high.[13] This means a colon interposition would be required at a later date. However, radical surgery is reserved for the most severely perforated esophagus.

Peritonitis
A burn of severity sufficient to cause mediastinitis may also cause perforation of the stomach, duodenum, or both, leading to peritonitis. In these cases, again, immediate esophagogastrectomy is recommended to remove dead and necrotic tissue in order to reduce the morbidity and mortality rates.

CONTROVERSIES

There are many controversies in management of esophageal burns.

Esophagoscopy

It is difficult to predict which children have burns and so all symptomatic patients (Categories 2 and 3) are treated until esophagoscopy makes the diagnosis.

TIMING.—Suggestions concerning timing of the initial esophagoscopy vary from within 24 hours to 36 to 72 hours later. If esophagoscopy is performed within the first 24 hours, a lesion may be overlooked, since in nearly all animal experiments it took at least 24 hours for lesions to become visible to the naked eye. However, Wijburg and colleagues advocate flexible fiberoptic esophagoscopy within the first 24 hours.[14, 15] Esophagoscopy performed later than 72 hours may cause the patient to have had unnecessary medical treatment and hospitalization, if no burns of the esophagus are found.

CORRELATION WITH MOUTH BURNS.—Daly and Cardona have emphasized the poor correlation between oral or pharyngeal ulcerations and esophageal ulcerations.[16] More recently Crain and co-workers confirmed this and suggested that patients with two or more serious signs such as drooling, vomiting, or stridor may be more reliably predicted to have esophageal burns.[17] Gorman and co-workers concluded that esophagoscopy was not required in asymptomatic patients and agreed that patients with two or more signs of oral burns, dysphagia, pain, or vomiting were more likely to have esophageal burns.[18]

TYPE OF INSTRUMENT.—There is also controversy regarding the instrument to use for esophagoscopy. Some physicians prefer rigid esophagoscopes and some prefer flexible esophagoscopes. Each group claims that the nonpreferred instrument is more likely to perforate the esophagus.

CONCLUSIONS ABOUT ESOPHAGOSCOPY.—Most physicians seem to agree that the presence of burns in the esophagus can be established definitely only by direct visualization and that esophagoscopy should be carried out within 24 to 72 hours after ingestion. Most otolaryngologists prefer rigid esophagoscopes (usually with the Storz-Hopkins telescopes).

Steroids

Neither the use, the dose, nor the length of treatment has general agreement.

USE AND TIMING.—Spain and associates showed that when cortisone was given to a group of mice with wounds on their backs, they exhibited an almost complete lack of exudate and fibrin in the wounds, together with marked diminution of cellular elements as compared with a group of control mice.[19] However, if the steroids were given more than 48 hours after the wound occurred, there was no significant difference between the group receiving the drug and the control group. Johnson experimented on dogs and showed that steroid therapy, if started early, definitely inhibited the inflammatory response and granulation tissue formation, with a subsequent decrease in stricture formation.[20] Since that time, many patients with caustic burns of the esophagus have been treated with steroids combined with antibiotics. Haller and Bachman,[21] Middelkamp and co-workers,[22] Ray and Morgan,[23] Ritter and colleagues,[24] Rosenberg and associates,[25, 26] Yarington and Heatley,[27] Yarington and co-workers,[28] and Weisskopf[29] all treated patients with a combination of antibiotics and steroids, finding the incidence of stricture formation much lower than that previously reported.

CONCLUSIONS ABOUT STEROIDS.—In a review of 214 cases, Hawkins and co-workers concluded that steroids were effective in preventing strictures in moderately severe burns.[30] Anderson and associates concluded in a controlled study that there appears to be no benefit from the use of steroids to treat children who have ingested a caustic substance.[31] In a statistical analysis of past studies, Howell and co-workers concluded that "steroids were not indicated for children with first-degree burns and that further trials were needed to answer the question regarding their efficacy in children with second- or third-degree burns."[32]

Nasogastric Intubation

Contrary to all the aforementioned methods, nasogastric intubation is advocated by some groups as the sole method of treatment of caustic burns.

"SPECIAL NASOGASTRIC TUBE."—Wijburg and co-workers inserted nasogastric tubes under endoscopic control and decided when to remove them by endoscopy.[33] They intubated when deep, circular esophageal burns were encountered and state that of 32 patients so treated, only 2 developed strictures. More recently, Wijburg and co-workers have advocated the passage of a "special" nasogastric tube after esophagoscopy, within 24 hours of the ingestion.[34]

STENT.—Coln and Chang[35] and Estrera and co-workers[36] advocate passing an esophageal "stent," creating a gastrostomy and passing a transgastric jejunal tube at the time of assessment by esophagoscopy. They emphasize leaving the stent in until healing is complete. This may have to be assessed by weekly esophagoscopy.

GASTROSTOMY AND STRING.—Krey found that the best results were obtained in reducing stricture formation by resting the esophagus, which may be accomplished by performing a gastrostomy and using antibiotics.[12] He advocated passing a string through the esophagus and bringing it out through the gastrostomy. The upper end of the string is brought out through the nose and tied to the lower end so that there is a continuous loop of string through the esophagus. If possible, the patient should facilitate placement of the string by swallowing it. If not, than it can be done during esophagoscopy. After 2 or 3 weeks, retrograde bougienage may commence.

CONCLUSION ABOUT NASOGASTRIC TUBES.—Passage of a "special" nasogastric tube or stent may be beneficial for those children who have severe burns.

SUMMARY

The severity of burns of the esophagus caused by a caustic agent depends on the type, concentration, and amount of agent, as well as the length of time of contact. It should be possible clinically to place a patient into one of three categories. In category 1, or asymptomatic patients, no treatment is given. In category 2, or symptomatic patients, therapy is started immediately. The aim of therapy is to reduce the amount of granulation tissue and, hence, the likelihood of stricture formation, by resting the esophagus and administering antibiotics and steroids. Esophagoscopy determines the severity of the burn and further decisions are made regarding treatment. Splinting of the esophagus with a special nasogastric tube seems to be a successful management option and may be all that is necessary. For category 3 patients with complications and severe burns, more drastic measures are necessary.

MANAGEMENT OF ACQUIRED STRICTURES

There are several ways of managing esophageal strictures. One of the more popular and successful ways is the use of the Gruntzig balloon under radiographic control. McLean and LeVeen point out that dilation in a radial direction should be less likely to tear the esophagus than prograde or retrograde dilation, which generates longitudinal forces.[37]

DILATION BY GRUNTZIG BALLOON

A significant change in the ability of physicians to treat esophageal strictures has occurred since 1974, when a balloon dilatation catheter was described by Gruntzig and Hopff, originally to dilate atheromatous narrowing of arteries.[38] The dilatation is performed under radiographic control, with the child under general anesthetic or local anesthetic and heavy sedation. The technique is well described by Dawson and associates.[39] Balloon dilatation catheters are available in a range of sizes: from 10 mm in diameter and 4 cm in length to 20 mm in diameter and 8 cm in length. The advantage of using this form of dilatation is that the catheter can be passed through a narrow stricture and the balloon, when inflated, dilates in a radial direction. Several dilations may be necessary depending on return of symptoms of obstruction, which in turn depend on the length and density of the stricture.

PROGRADE DILATION

There are several types of dilator used for prograde dilation. The Jackson silk woven bougies are passed through a rigid esophagoscope under direct vision with the patient under general anesthetic. Emerson described Teflon dilators which are used the same way.[40] Other methods require the use of a string with a gastrostomy under general anesthetic. For example, the Plummer method uses metal olives passed over a string. Hine and co-workers[41] compared the Eder-Puestow method with the Celestin Neoplex dilator. Both methods require passage of a guide wire first, either under fluoroscopic control or through the biopsy channel of a flexible esophagoscope. Fogarty vascular balloon catheters have also been used and the Gruntzig balloon dilation method has been described above.

Hurst Mercury Bougies

Dilatation may be carried out without the patient under general anesthesia, using Hurst mercury bougies. Hurst or Maloney dilators can be used without general anesthetic. This dilatation may be done in very young children, who must, however, usually be wrapped in a blanket and held upright on the lap of an assistant. A bougie of suitable size may be selected at the time of esophagoscopy. The tip of the dilator should be inserted into the patient's mouth and held high above his or her head so that the weight of the mercury encourages the passage of the tube down the esophagus. It is unfortunate that in some of the smaller-sized bougies, the weight of the mercury is not great enough to carry the bougie down the esophagus, so gentle insertion of the bougie by the operator may be necessary. The size of the dilator is then increased until one size is found that will not pass down the esophagus. The intervals between dilatations are governed by how well the patient can swallow food. The patient will probably need dilatation for the rest of his or her life, but the length of time between dilatations should increase as the patient grows. Periodically throughout this time, esophagograms and esophagoscopy should be performed in order to follow the extent of the disease.

Retrograde Bougienage

Only when prograde dilatation fails to maintain a lumen should retrograde dilatation with gastrostomy be considered. Retrograde bougienage may be done while the patient is awake, even in a very young child, although it is generally very distressing for both the child and the operator. The technique, described by Tucker,[42] should be such that the string is always present in the esophagus. The loop is first cut, and two pieces of string are tied to the lower end. By pulling on the upper end, two new pieces are pulled out through the nose. The upper end of one of these pieces of string is tied to the lower end of the same string. This will be the loop that remains in the esophagus after dilatation. The second loop is brought out through the mouth using forceps. A Tucker dilator is tied to the lower end of the string, and by a combination of pulling on the upper string and pushing the dilator, it can be passed up the esophagus and into the mouth. Dilators of increasing size can be tied end to end like a string of sausages, and the whole string can be pulled right out through the mouth. Alternatively, the first dilator can be pulled through the gastrostomy, and the string should be reattached to the second dilator. This procedure can be undertaken daily at first, and after a while it may be possible to progress to dilatation. Prograde dilatation may continue for the rest of the patient's life, at varying intervals. Periodic esophagoscopy and esophagograms will be necessary to follow the course of the disease.

Prograde vs. Retrograde Dilation

Hawkins compared antegrade versus retrograde dilation of strictures and emphasizes the greater degree of safety using Tucker dilators in a retrograde fashion.[43]

STEROID INJECTION

Mendelsohn and Maloney suggested injection of steroids into the stricture at esophagoscopy.[44] They found that this was useful if the stricture was resistant and if progress toward increasing the lumen was slow by prograde dilatation. They used 1.5 to 2 ml of hydrocortisone acetate or triamcinolone acetonide (40 mg/ml) injected through the esophagoscope with a long needle. One ml of hyaluronidase is mixed with this steroid to act as a spreading agent. This is followed by immediate dilatation, using dilators two or four French sizes greater than those used in previous dilatations. Bleeding is a warning sign to stop the dilatation. The researchers had no problems with infection, abscess, or perimediastinitis and felt that the stricture was softened and dilatation was able to be carried out more rapidly.

COLON INTERPOSITION

If dilatation fails, colon interposition may be the only alternative. Every effort should be made to maintain esophageal function for as long as possible. Campbell and co-workers[45] report on cases who had colon interposition. They stressed that achievement of good functional results with low complication rates depends on experience and the technique employed rather than whether stomach or colon was used. They favored intrathoracic colon interposition.

JEJUNUM INTERPOSITION

McCaffrey and Fisher report three cases of repair of cervical esophageal stenosis using microvascular free jejunum transfer.[46]

Strictures of the esophagus may develop from other causes apart from damage due to caustic burns. Attempts at surgical repair of the strictured esophagus either by direct end-to-end anastomosis (after excising the stenotic segment), gastric pull-up and esophagogastric anastomosis or esophagocolic anastomosis (from colon interposition) may also lead to stricturing at the repair site. Holinger and Johnston[47] and Morrison[48] point out that one of the major problems following repair of congenital esophageal atresia is stenosis at the site of anastomosis.

CONCLUSION

It would seem to be preferable to retain the esophagus, if at all possible, using different methods to keep strictures dilated. It is recognized, however, that children who have severe burns with complications may need emergency esophagectomy or esophagogastrectomy.

OTHER TOPICS RELATED TO CAUSTIC INGESTION
PSYCHIATRIC CONSULTATION

Sobel studied 367 families whose children had been involved in accidental poisonings.[49] In this study, he found that the frequency of poisoning was unrelated to the accessibility of toxic substances, which, he pointed out, was contrary to common sense. There was also found to be no relation between the level of motor development, intelligence of the child, birth complications, or parental accident-proneness. There was, however, significant association between accidental poisoning and measures of maternal psychopathology, such as the mother's marital dissatisfaction, mental illness, poor ego strength, and sexual dissatisfaction. His data suggested the hypothesis that a negative role performance on the mother's part generates a power struggle with the child, which may eventually result in the ingestion of forbidden substances by the child as an act of defiance and rebellion. Accidental poisoning, therefore, should always be treated as a symptom of family disturbance. It is felt that psychiatric consultation is essential for giving emotional support to the mothers who are unable to cope with the stress placed on them by their maternal and marital roles.

The mental trauma, both for the child and the family, in a severe case of poisoning would also warrant psychiatric support. The prolonged treatment necessary if a stricture develops, with frequent and often unpleasant visits to the hospital will also necessitate psychiatric support. In cases in which suicide has been attempted by an older child, psychiatric consultation is mandatory.

LATHYROGENS

Lathyrogens are chemicals that inhibit the covalent cross-links between collagen. These cross-links are thought to be important in the physical characteristics of newly formed collagen. It might be possible either to prevent dense scarring or to soften well-established scarring, using these chemicals. Butler and colleagues[50] and Madden and associates[51] used beta-aminopropionitrile in dogs and showed greater benefit from its use than from using steroids in reducing scarring. This drug is not approved for human clinical trials. Penicillamine has been shown by Gehanno and Guedon to have good results in rats.[52] Liu and Richardson point out that N-acetyl-L-cysteine, another lathyrogen, is commercially available and is approved for clinical use in the treatment of various bronchopulmonary disorders for its mucolytic properties, and in acetaminophen and arsenic overdosage.[53] They report a study using N-acetyl-L-cysteine in caustic burns of the esophagus in a few rats.

CARCINOMA OF THE ESOPHAGUS

Appelqvist and Salmo[54] and Hopkins and Postlethwait[55] point out that up to 7% of patients with esophageal carcinoma have a history of caustic ingestion in childhood. It is estimated that after caustic ingestion there is a thousand-fold increase in the likelihood of developing esophageal carcinoma. The interval between injury and development of the squamous cell carcinoma varies between 13 and 71 years.

REFERENCES

1. Sobel R: The psychiatric implications of accidental poisoning in childhood. *Pediatr Clin North Am* 17:653–685, 1970.
2. Leape LL, Ashcraft KW, Scarpelli DG, et al: Hazard to health—liquid lye. *N Engl J Med* 284:578–581, 1971.
3. Moore WR: Caustic ingestions. Pathophysiology, diagnosis and treatment. *Clin Pediatr (Phila)* 25:192–196, 1986.
4. Alford BR, Harris HH: Chemical burns of the mouth, pharynx, and esophagus. *Ann Otol Rhinol Laryngol* 68:122–128, 1959.

5. Bikhazi HB, Thompson ER, Shumrick DA: Caustic ingestion: Current status, a report of 105 cases. *Arch Otolaryngol Head Neck Surg* 89:112–115, 1969.
6. Daly JF, Cardona JC: Acute corrosive esophagitis. *Arch Otolaryngol Head Neck Surg* 74:41–46, 1961.
7. Yarington CT Jr, Bales GA, Frazer JP: A study of the management of caustic esophageal trauma. *Ann Otol Rhinol Laryngol* 73:1130–1135, 1964.
8. Holinger PH, Johnston KC: Caustic strictures of the esophagus. *Illinois Medical Journal* 98:246–250, 1950.
9. Owens H: Chemical burns of the esophagus: The importance of various chemicals as etiologic agents in stricture formation. *Arch Otolaryngol Head Neck Surg* 60:482–486, 1954.
10. Litovitz TL: Battery ingestions: Product accessibility and clinical course. *Pediatrics* 75:469–476, 1985.
11. Riding KH, Bluestone CD: Burns and acquired strictures of the esophagus, in Bluestone CD, Stool SE, Kenna MA (eds): *Pediatric Otolaryngology*, ed 3, ch 61. Philadelphia, WB Saunders, 1994.
12. Krey H: On the treatment of corrosive lesions in the esophagus, an experimental study. *Acta Otolaryngol (Stockh)* (suppl)102; 1952.
13. Ritter FN, Gago O, Kirsh M, et al: The rationale of emergency esophagogastrectomy in the treatment of liquid caustic burns of the esophagus and stomach. *Arch Otolaryngol Head Neck Surg* 80:513–520, 1971.
14. Wijburg FA, Beukers MM, Bartelsman JF, et al: Nasogastric intubation as sole treatment of caustic esophageal lesions. *Ann Otol Rhinol Laryngol* 94:337–341, 1985.
15. Wijburg FA, Heymans HSA, Urbanus NAM: Caustic esophageal lesions in childhood: Prevention of stricture formation. *J Pediatr Surg* 24:171–173, 1989.
16. Daly JF, Cardona JC: Acute corrosive esophagitis. *Arch Otolaryngol Head Neck Surg* 74:41–46, 1961.
17. Crain EF, Gershel JC, Mezey AP: Caustic ingestions. Symptoms as predictors of esophageal injury. *Am J Dis Child* 138:863–865, 1984.
18. Gorman RL, Khin-Maun-Gyi MT, Klein-Schwartz W, et al: Initial symptoms as predictors of esophageal injury in alkaline corrosive ingestions. *Am J Emerg Med* 10:189–194, 1992.
19. Spain DM, Molomut N, Haber A: The effect of cortisone on the formation of granulation tissue in mice. *Am J Pathol* 261:710–711, 1950.
20. Johnson EE: A study of corrosive esophagitis. *Laryngoscope* 73:1651–1695, 1963.
21. Haller JA, Bachman K: The comparative effect of current therapy on experimental caustic burns of the esophagus. *Pediatrics* 34:236–245, 1964.
22. Middelkamp JN, Ferguson TB, Roper CL, et al: The management of problems of caustic burns in children. *J Thorac Cardiovasc Surg* 57:341–347, 1969.
23. Ray ES, Morgan DL: Cortisone therapy of lye burns of the esophagus. *J Pediatr* 49:394–397, 1956.
24. Ritter FN, Newman MH, Newman DE: A clinical and experimental study of corrosive burns of the stomach. *Ann Otol Rhinol Laryngol* 67:830–842, 1968.
25. Rosenberg N, Kunderman PJ, Vroman L, et al: Prevention of experimental lye strictures of the esophagus by cortisone. *Arch Surg* 63:147–151, 1951.
26. Rosenberg N, Kunderman PJ, Vroman L, et al: Prevention of experimental esophageal stricture by cortisone. *Arch Surg* 66:593–598, 1953.
27. Yarington CT Jr, Heatley CA: Steroids, antibiotics, and early esophagoscopy in caustic esophageal trauma. *N Y State J Med* 63:2960–2963, 1963.
28. Yarington CT Jr, Bales GA, Frazer JP: A study of the management of caustic esophageal trauma. *Ann Otol Rhinol Laryngol* 73:1130–1135, 1964.

29. Weisskopf A: Effects of cortisone on experimental lye burn of the esophagus. *Ann Otol Rhinol Laryngol* 61:681–691, 1952.

30. Hawkins DB, Demeter MJ, Barnett TE: Caustic ingestion: Controversies in management. A review of 214 cases. *Laryngoscope* 90:98–109, 1980.

31. Anderson KD, Rouse TM, Randolph JG: A controlled trial of corticosteroids in children with corrosive injury of the esophagus. *N Engl J Med* 233:637–640, 1990.

32. Howell JM, Dalsey WC, Hartsell FW, et al: Steroids for the treatment of corrosive esophageal injury: A statistical analysis of past studies. *Am J Emerg Med* 10:421–425, 1992.

33. Wijburg FA, Beukers MM, Bartelsman JF, et al: Nasogastric intubation as sole treatment of caustic esophageal lesions. *Ann Otol Rhinol Laryngol* 94:337–341, 1985.

34. Wijburg FA, Heymans HSA, Urbanus NAM: Caustic esophageal lesions in childhood: Prevention of stricture formation. *J Ped Surg* 24:171–173, 1989.

35. Coln D, Chang JHT: Experience with esophageal stenting for caustic burns in children. *J Pediatr Surg* 21:588–591, 1986.

36. Estrera A, Taylor W, Mills LJ, et al: Corrosive burns of the esophagus and stomach: A recommendation for an aggressive surgical approach. *Ann Thorac Surg* 41:276–283, 1986.

37. McLean GK, LeVeen RF: Shear stress in the performance of esophageal dilation: Comparison of balloon dilation and bougienage. *Radiology* 172:983–986, 1989.

38. Gruntzig A, Hopff H: Perkutane Rekanalisation chronischer arterieller Verschlusse mit einen neuen Dilatationskatheter. Modification der Dotter-Technik. *Dtsch Med Wochenschr* 99:2502–2507, 1974.

39. Dawson SL, Mueller PR, Ferrucci JT, et al: Severe esophageal strictures: Indications for balloon catheter dilatation. *Radiology* 153:631–635, 1984.

40. Emerson EB: Teflon esophageal dilators. *Arch Otolaryngol Head Neck Surg* 81:213–215, 1965.

41. Hine KR, Hawkey CJ, Atkinson M, et al: Comparison of the Eder-Puestow and Celestin techniques for dilating benign esophageal strictures. *Gut* 25:1100–1102, 1984.

42. Tucker G: Cicatricial stenosis of the esophagus with particular reference to treatment by continuous string, retrograde bougienage with the author's bougie. *Ann Otol Rhinol Laryngol* 69:1180–1214, 1924.

43. Hawkins DB: Dilation of esophageal strictures: Comparative morbidity of antegrade and retrograde methods. *Ann Otol Rhinol Laryngol* 97:460–465, 1988.

44. Mendelsohn HJ, Maloney WH: The treatment of benign strictures of the esophagus with cortisone injection. *Ann Otol Rhinol Laryngol* 79:900–906, 1970.

45. Campbell JR, Webber BR, Harrison MW, et al: Esophageal replacement in infants and children by colon interposition. *Am J Surg* 144:29–34, 1982.

46. McCaffrey TV, Fisher J: Repair of traumatic cervical esophageal stenosis using microvascular free jejunum transfer. *Ann Otol Rhinol Laryngol* 93:512–516, 1984.

47. Holinger PH, Johnston KC: Postsurgical endoscopic problems of congenital esophageal atresia. *Ann Otol Rhinol Laryngol* 72:1035–1049, 1963.

48. Morrison LE: Experiences with dilatation of the esophagus following surgery for esophageal atresia. *Ann Otol Rhinol Laryngol* 68:581–594, 1959.

49. Sobel R: The psychiatric implications of accidental poisoning in childhood. *Pediatr Clin North Am* 17:653–685, 1970.

50. Butler C, Madden JW, Davis WM, et al: Morphologic aspects of experimental

esophageal lye strictures. II. Effect of steroid hormones, bougienage and induced lathyrism on acute lye burns. *Surgery* 81:431–435, 1977.

51. Madden JW, Davis WM, Butler C, et al: Experimental esophageal lye burns. II. Correcting established strictures with beta-aminopropionitrile and bougienage. *Ann Surg* 178:277–284, 1973.
52. Gehanno P, Guedon C: Inhibition of experimental esophageal lye strictures by penicillamine. *Arch Otolaryngol Head Neck Surg* 107:145–147, 1981.
53. Liu AJ, Richardson MA: Effects of N-acetylcysteine on experimentally induced esophageal lye injury. *Ann Otol Rhinol Laryngol* 94:477–482, 1985.
54. Appelqvist P, Salmo M: Lye corrosion carcinoma of the esophagus—a review of 63 cases. *Cancer* 45:2655–2658, 1980.
55. Hopkins RA, Postlethwait RW: Caustic burns and carcinoma of the esophagus. *Ann Surg* 194:146–148, 1981.

Practical Aspects of Intraoperative Cranial Nerve Monitoring

Aage R. Møller, Ph.D.

Professor, Department of Neurological Surgery, University of Pittsburgh School of Medicine, Pittsburgh, Pennsylvania

I ntraoperative neurophysiologic monitoring is a technique the use of which throughout the past 10 years to 15 years has been increasing during operations in which neural tissue is at risk of being injured. The primary goal of intraoperative neurophysiologic monitoring is to provide information that can help to reduce the risk of postoperative neurological deficits. This goal is generally accomplished by recording neuroelectric potentials in response to appropriate stimulation.

The use of neurophysiologic monitoring to help to reduce the risk of neurological deficits is based on the assumption that it is possible to detect injury to neural tissue before it becomes so severe that it causes permanent neurological deficits, and that it is possible to reverse the injury by appropriate surgical intervention. This presumes that it is possible to detect related changes in some recordable neuroelectric potentials before the injury has reached a level that implies that permanent neurological deficits will result.

Various techniques have been described that make it possible to continuously monitor neural conduction in several of the cranial nerves. Of all the sensory nerves, it has mainly been the auditory nerve that has been possible to monitor intraoperatively, and it has been shown in several studies that such monitoring can help to reduce hearing impairment as a complication to operations in which the auditory vestibular nerve has been manipulated.[1, 2] Methods have also been described to identify motor nerves that are not visible in the operative field.[3-11] This is important for preserving neural function in such nerves when they are affected by tumor or are otherwise at risk of being injured from surgical manipulations. Identification of motor nerves is most often done by recording and observing neuroelectric electromyographic (EMG) potentials from the muscles that are innervated by the respective nerve while using an electrical stimulating electrode to probe the surgical area.

Intraoperative neurophysiologic monitoring can help the surgeon carry out the operation with a minimum risk of causing permanent neurological deficits. In a few cases it is possible to use intraoperative recordings to determine if the therapeutic goal of an operation has been achieved.[12, 13]

Advances in Otolaryngology—Head and Neck Surgery®, vol. 9
© 1995, Mosby–Year Book, Inc.

Intraoperative neurophysiologic monitoring can also, in some cases, provide prognostic information about the likelihood of acquiring permanent neurological deficits. This may be of practical importance if the question should arise during the operation about whether or not to graft a nerve that has been injured.

PRINCIPLES OF INTRAOPERATIVE NEUROPHYSIOLOGIC MONITORING

Intraoperative neurophysiologic monitoring uses essentially the same methods for recording sensory evoked potentials and for recording EMG potentials that have been in use for many years in the clinical testing laboratory and in physiological research laboratories. The way that the recorded sensory evoked potentials are utilized in the operating room, however, differs from the way the results of recordings in clinical testing are used. Thus, in the operating room it is important to be able to interpret the recorded potentials immediately, and it is only the changes from the patient's own baseline recording that are important. In the clinic, however, it is the deviations in the patient's recorded potentials from a laboratory standard of evoked potentials that is important, and interpretation usually does not need to be done immediately and can thus be done by a different person than the one that does the testing.

The operating room is usually regarded as being a hostile environment with regard to electrical interference, because a host of other electronic equipment is either connected to the patient or is near the patient.

Sensory evoked potentials normally cannot be observed directly. Only after a number of responses have been averaged does the response appear as a clear waveform. This is because the recorded potentials have a much smaller amplitude than ongoing electroencephalographic (EEG) activity or electrical interference. The number of responses that need to be collected before an interpretable record can be obtained increases with increasing noise or electrical interference. Since it is important to be able to obtain an interpretable record in the shortest possible time, reducing the electrical interference is important, as is optimal processing (filtering and signal averaging) of the recorded responses.

Electromyographic potentials can usually be viewed directly on an oscilloscope screen without averaging the responses, because such potentials normally have amplitudes that are much greater than the background noise. While intraoperative monitoring using neurophysiologic recordings in the operating room does not require any specialized techniques or equipment, it does require expertise in interpreting the recorded potentials and knowledge about reducing electrical interference and quickly solving technical problems, such as the appearance of unexpected interference and equipment failure.

It is advantageous to have optimal display of the recorded potentials so that the interpretation of the recorded potentials is facilitated. Monitoring of cranial motor nerves may be facilitated by making the EMG recorded from muscles audible so that changes in the response can be made known to all members of the operating team.

There are now several companies that offer equipment for the recording and display of neuroelectric potentials that is specialized for use in the operating room, and equipment is constantly under development.

MONITORING SENSORY NERVES

The use of intraoperative neurophysiologic monitoring of the auditory portion of the eighth cranial nerve (CN VIII) for the purpose of reducing the risk of hearing loss was first described more than a decade ago.[9, 14-19] Intraoperative recording of the brain stem auditory evoked potentials (BAEP) was one of the first examples to show that intraoperative neurophysiologic monitoring of a sensory cranial nerve can help reduce postoperative complications in the form of neurological deficits (in this case, hearing loss). More recently, the changes in the recorded BAEP and their relationship to surgical manipulations have been analyzed in detail,[20, 21] and a few studies have described the reduction in postoperative hearing loss from intraoperative monitoring of auditory evoked potentials.[1, 2] Intraoperative monitoring of other sensory cranial nerves is not as common as that of the auditory nerve and, so far, no descriptions of intraoperative neurophysiologic monitoring of the vestibular portion of CN VIII has been described in the literature. Methods for monitoring the sensory part of the trigeminal nerve have been described[22, 23] but such monitoring has not been generally utilized to date. Technical problems in presenting adequate stimuli have been a hindrance to the use of visual evoked potentials (VEP) in intraoperative monitoring.[24]

MONITORING THE AUDITORY NERVE

Intraoperative recording of sound-evoked auditory potentials, such as the BAEP, can be used for intraoperative monitoring of the function of the ear and of neural conduction in the auditory portion of the CN VIII.[1-3, 9, 15, 16, 20, 21, 25] The BAEP, recorded from electrodes placed on the scalp in response to click stimuli, have a very low amplitude and it is necessary to average the responses to many stimuli in order to obtain an interpretable record. This makes it rather time consuming to use BAEP in intraoperative monitoring, and the information about injury to the auditory nerve, for instance, becomes correspondingly delayed by about 1 minute or, more likely, 2 to 3 minutes.

The recording of click-evoked potentials directly from the exposed eighth nerve (compound action potentials [CAP]) offers the possibility to obtain evoked potentials of much higher amplitudes, and such responses provide nearly real-time information about injuries to the auditory nerve.[3, 9, 19, 25, 26, 27] These methods are therefore valuable in operations in which there is a high risk of injuring the auditory nerve, as they provide a possibility to obtain an interpretable record almost instantaneously because of the high amplitude of such potentials. The disadvantage of using these methods is that the CN VIII must be surgically exposed and the recording electrode may be in the surgeon's way during the operation.

It has been shown that evoked potentials of a high amplitude can be recorded from the vicinity of the cochlear nucleus by placing a recording electrode in the lateral recess of the fourth ventricle,[28] and recently this method has been applied to intraoperative monitoring in operations of the cerebellopontine (CP) angle.[29, 30] This can provide, in many instances, a more practical way of monitoring intraoperatively neural conduction in the auditory nerve, particularly in operations on acoustic tumors.

Directly recorded CAP from CN VIII using a bipolar recording electrode can also make it possible to determine the location of the demarcation between the auditory and vestibular nerves.[31, 32] This is important for hearing preservation in operations in which the vestibular nerve is to be severed selectively.

RECORDING BRAIN STEM AUDITORY EVOKED POTENTIALS

The recording of BAEP is the method most commonly used for intraoperative monitoring of the auditory nerve. Brain stem auditory evoked potentials are commonly recorded differentially from electrodes placed on the vertex (C_z, according to the International 10–20 system for EEG recordings) and the ipsilateral mastoid or earlobe (A_1 or A_2).[1, 3, 9, 15, 16, 25] Some investigators have chosen to record BAEP on two channels, one recording differentially between electrodes placed on the vertex and the upper neck, and the other between electrodes placed in the earlobes.[3] The recorded responses are usually evoked by click sounds presented through insert earphones, miniature stereo earphones, or earphones that are connected through a plastic tube.

The amplitude of the BAEP is much smaller than the ongoing brain activity (EEG) that is also picked up by the recording electrodes. In order to be able to observe the BAEP it is therefore necessary to average many responses. This process is time consuming and delays the reflection of surgically induced changes in the neural conduction of the auditory nerve.

There are several factors that can facilitate obtaining an interpretable record within the shortest possible time:

1. The stimulus intensity should be sufficiently high (but not so high that it poses the risk of permanent hearing loss).
2. The stimuli should be presented at the optimal (high) rate.
3. Optimal filtering of the recorded responses should be used so that maximum noise suppression is achieved at the same time as the peaks of the BAEP are enhanced.
4. A method for quality control that does not require replication of the responses should be used.

A suitable stimulus intensity is about 105 dB peak equivalent sound pressure level (Pe SPL), corresponding to about 65 dB normal hearing level when the clicks are presented at a rate of 20 clicks/sec. The time required to collect a certain number of responses decreases with increasing repetition rate, but above a certain repetition rate the amplitude of the responses decreases. There is, therefore, an optimal repetition rate of the click stimulation at which an interpretable record is obtained within the shortest time. The amplitudes of early peaks (I-III) are more affected by increased repetition rate than is that of peak V. For BAEP, the optimal rate is probably as high as 60 to 80 clicks/sec if only peak V is to be observed.

Adequate filtering of the responses reduces the noise so that fewer responses need to be collected to obtain an interpretable record. Such filtering should be carried out using computer programs instead of electronic filters[3, 33–35] because the use of digital filters makes it possible to perform a more adequate optimal filtering than that done using electronic filters. This is mainly because digital filters can be designed so that they do not shift the peaks in time (zero-phase filters). Different kinds of digital filters have been described by several investigators and are now implemented in some commercially available equipment. Examples of the effects of different kinds of digital filtering on recorded BAEP are illustrated in Figure 1.

If digital filters are used, the electronic filters on the physiological amplifiers should be set at 10 to 3,000 Hz. If digital filters are not available, suitable settings for the electronic filters are 150 to 1,500 Hz.

It is usually advantageous to use a relatively low amplification (50,000 times) because it reduces the effect of transients that may overload the amplifiers (such as strong electrical interference). Artifact rejection should be included in the recording system so that electrical artifacts that have a high amplitude can be eliminated from the averaged response. It is beneficial to use a time-extended artifact rejection system that is activated by electrocoagulation, because the amplifiers are usually not functioning properly immediately after the heavy overload that occurs during electrocoagulation. Interference from periodic signals may be reduced by having the stimulus repetition rate vary randomly by a few percent.[3]

Traditionally, quality control of the recorded BAEP (and for that matter, other sensory evoked potentials) is performed by replicating a record to see if the two records are similar. Naturally, this takes twice as much time as it takes to obtain one interpretable record, and this is a disadvantage in the operating room where it is important to be able to interpret the responses as soon as possible. Several methods have been described for performing quality control without replicating the record. One method is based on a comparison between the averaged response and similar averaged responses in which every other record is inverted.[3, 36–38] Other more complex methods have been described for quality control as well as for making signal averaging more effective, particularly when the interference is periodic in nature.[39] However, these methods have not been applied in practical monitoring to date, except in a few places using custom designed systems.

HOW TO INTERPRET THE RECORDED BRAIN STEM AUDITORY EVOKED POTENTIALS

Brain stem auditory evoked potentials are characterized by a series of peaks, of which the vertex-positive peaks (shown by some investigators as downward deflections, while by others as upward deflections) are usually identified by Roman numerals.[40] The different components of the BAEP are generated by the auditory nerve and some of the nuclei and fiber tracts of the ascending auditory pathway. The vertex-positive peaks

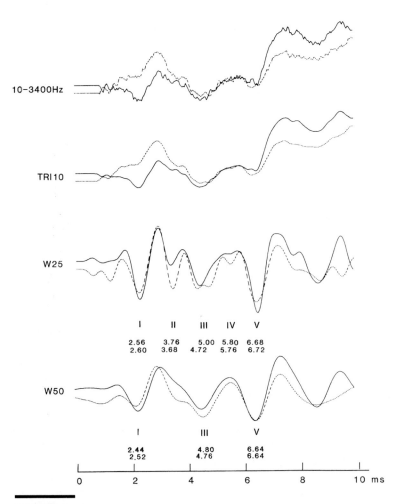

FIGURE 1.
Effects of different types of digital filters. The upper tracing is filtered with electronic filters only; the second tracing from top (TRI10) shows the same recordings after low-pass filtering with a digital filter that had a triangular weighing function with a base length of 0.4 milliseconds. The two lower tracings show the effects of filtering of the same record with two different digital band-pass filters (W25 and W50) that had W-shaped weighing functions (similar to a truncated sin(x)/x function) with the duration of the base length being 1 and 2 milliseconds, respectively. The numbers on the two bottom curves are the latency values obtained using computer programs. The two tracings (solid and dashed) show replications.

(specifically their latencies) have mainly been used for diagnostic purposes, as well as for the detection of intraoperative injuries. However, recent studies have pointed out the importance of vertex-negative peaks.[29, 41, 42]

The two earliest vertex-positive peaks (I and II) are generated by the auditory nerve distally (I) and near the brain stem (II).[26, 43] The subsequent peaks have more complex origins and are generated by the various nuclei and fiber tracts of the ascending auditory pathway. In general, it seems that different structures contribute to more than one peak, and that one peak may receive contributions from more than one structure.

The use of BAEP to detect surgically induced injuries to the auditory nerve is mainly based on the assumption that an injury is associated with a prolonged conduction time in the auditory nerve. A prolonged conduction time will result in a shift (increase in latency) of the peaks of the BAEP that are generated by neural structures located central to the entrance of the auditory nerve in the brain stem.

It is supposedly unimportant to know the exact generators of the peaks that are used to detect changes in the function of the ear when using BAEP to monitor the function of the auditory nerve (and the ear). However, if the intracranial portion of CN VIII is being manipulated, for instance, it is important to detect prolongation of neural conduction in that part of the auditory nerve. For this purpose, the latency of peaks of the BAEP that originate from structures located central to the entrance of CN VIII into the brain stem should be used. Thus, any peak that is generated by structures that are located central to CN VIII can theoretically be used to detect changes in neural conduction of the auditory nerve and to detect changes in the function of the ear. Since peak V usually has the largest amplitude of all the peaks, it is usually used for intraoperative monitoring of the auditory nerve. Some investigators, however, have advocated the use of peak III, which is usually assumed to be generated by the cochlear nucleus.[3] The vertex-negative peak between peak III and peaks IV to V may be even more suitable. The reason for using peak III instead of peak V is that peak V is known to be less affected by a decrease in stimulus intensity and, therefore, peak V may also be less sensitive to injuries of the auditory nerve. This, however, is an assumption that has not been substantiated by research.

If peaks III or V are affected and peak I is unchanged, the cause can be assumed to be manipulations of the intracranial portion of the auditory nerve. If peak I is also affected (or disappears), it is a sign of a compromised blood supply to the cochlea (peak I is generated in the auditory nerve where it leaves the cochlea) (Fig 2).

It is, therefore, important in some operations to be able to identify peak I. This can be done by recording differentially between the two earlobes. If the BAEP is recorded on two channels, one between the vertex and the neck and the other between the earlobes, then the first channel will display peaks III and V clearly and the second channel will display a clear peak I.

Changes in the amplitude of the different peaks of the BAEP may also be of value in detecting injury to the auditory nerve, and they may be even better than utilizing changes in latency for this purpose. However, changes in amplitude have not been utilized to the same extent as changes in latency, mainly because the normal variability of the amplitude is large. (The normal variations of the latency of peak III or peak V in the same individual are usually less than 0.5 milliseconds, whereas as much as a 50% change in amplitude may be seen.) Additionally, there will be a change in the amplitude of the peaks of the BAEP whenever the latency of the peaks changes during the time when the responses are being averaged. This makes amplitude changes more difficult to interpret than changes in latencies.

Intraoperative changes in the BAEP can be easily detected by com-

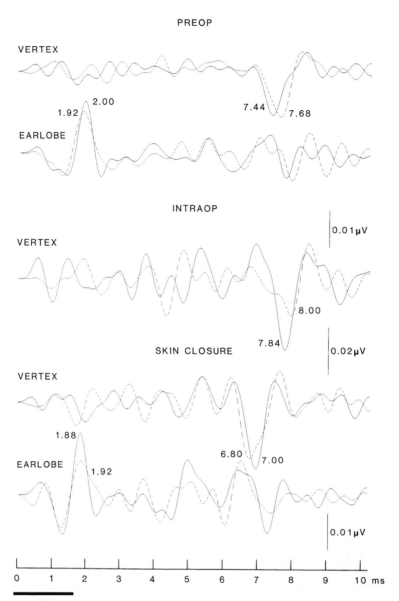

FIGURE 2.

BAEP recorded between electrodes placed at the vertex and the neck (*VERTEX*) and between the two earlobes (*EARLOBE*), obtained in a patient who was operated on to remove an acoustic tumor. The recordings were obtained before the operation began but after the patient was anesthetized (top tracings), during the operation (middle tracings), and at the end of the operation (lower tracings). The dashed lines show replications, and the numbers below the peaks are the latency values obtained using computer programs that automatically detected the various peaks. Each recording was the average of 2,048 responses. Note the clear peak I in the earlobe-earlobe recording.

paring the BAEP with a baseline BAEP that is obtained after the patient is anesthetized but before the operation begins. This baseline BAEP should be displayed so that it appears overlaid on the subsequently obtained averaged responses. All subsequent recordings can thus easily be compared with the baseline.

RECORDING OF COMPOUND ACTION POTENTIALS FROM THE EIGHTH CRANIAL NERVE

Even when optimal stimulus and recording parameters are used, recording of BAEP requires collection of data for 1 to 2 minutes in order to obtain an interpretable record. This time will be longer in patients with hearing loss, which can be associated with deterioration of the BAEP. Therefore, investigators have been searching for better ways to obtain evoked potentials that can provide information about changes in neural conduction in the auditory nerve. Recordings of the CAP from the exposed CN VIII were described more than a decade ago,[26, 44, 45] and such recordings have been in routine use in connection with operations on acoustic tumors for the past decade,[3, 9, 25, 27] as well as in other operations in the CP angle.[3, 19]

Recording directly from the exposed auditory nerve yields responses with amplitudes as high as several microvolts. These potentials can therefore be immediately viewed directly on an oscilloscope or after only a few responses have been averaged. Thus, an interpretable record can be obtained almost instantaneously, and this permits detection of changes in neural conduction in the auditory nerve without delay.

Recording from the intracranial portion of CN VIII can be done conveniently by placing an electrode directly in contact with the exposed intracranial portion of CN VIII. One electrode, which has been previously described, is made from a malleable, Teflon-insulated, multistrand, silver wire, and a small wick of cotton or Teflon is sutured to the uninsulated tip.[3, 19, 46] Such a wick electrode (Fig 3) provides little risk of injuring the auditory nerve, and its performance is not affected by small movements of the electrode or if it is covered by cerebrospinal fluid. Such factors are likely to produce large artifacts in the recording if a bare metal electrode is used. When using recordings made directly from CN VIII to detect changes in neural conduction in the auditory nerve it is important that the recording electrode is placed at a more central location on the nerve than where surgical manipulations may affect the function of the nerve.

It is not necessary to filter these potentials as drastically as suggested for BAEP (Fig 4). A filter setting of 10 to 3,000 Hz is suitable and digital filtering is not necessary. An amplification of 20,000 times is suitable. The same click stimuli used to elicit BAEP can be used to elicit CAP.

INTERPRETATION OF COMPOUND ACTION POTENTIALS RECORDED FROM THE EXPOSED EIGHTH CRANIAL NERVE

Typically, direct recordings from the exposed CN VIII in response to click stimulation yield a CAP with a triphasic waveform in individuals with normal hearing (see Fig 4).[26, 47] The main negative peak is generated when the volley of depolarization passes under the recording electrode, and the initial positive deflection is caused by the approaching volley. In patients with hearing loss the waveform can be considerably different.[48, 49]

Because click-evoked potentials that are recorded directly from the exposed CN VIII can immediately be visualized directly on an oscilloscope or after only a few responses have been averaged, these potentials can be interpreted immediately. This makes it possible to detect changes

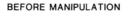

BEFORE MANIPULATION

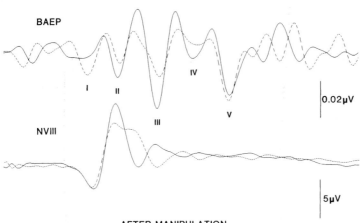

AFTER MANIPULATION

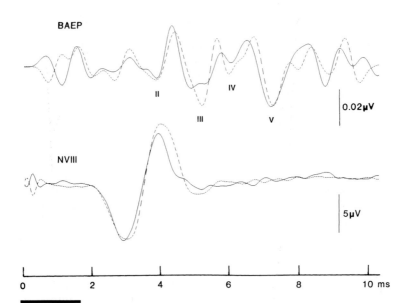

FIGURE 3.

Comparison between the BAEP and the CAP recorded from the exposed eighth nerve before (top tracing) and after the eighth nerve was stretched (bottom tracing).

in neural conduction of the auditory nerve practically at the time they occur.

The latency of the CAP becomes prolonged as a result of a decrease in conduction velocity of the portion of the auditory nerve that is distal to the recording site. This may typically be caused by stretching of CN VIII (see Fig 4). If heat spreads to the auditory nerve from electrocoagulation near CN VIII, a more complex pattern of change may occur (Fig 5). There is typically a decrease in the amplitude of the main negative peak, and this is an indication of a conduction block in a fraction of the nerve fibers in the auditory nerve.

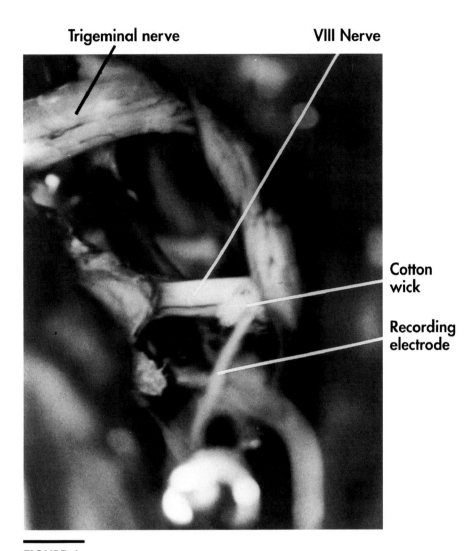

FIGURE 4.

Placement of a wick recording electrode on CN VIII in an operation to relieve hemifacial spasm. (From Møller, AR: *Evoked Potentials in Intraoperative Monitoring.* Baltimore, Williams & Wilkins, 1988. Used by permission.)

RECORDING FROM THE VICINITY OF THE COCHLEAR NUCLEUS

It may be difficult to place a recording electrode on the appropriate location on CN VIII in operations of acoustic tumors and to keep it there during the operation. It has been described earlier how recordings made from the vicinity of the cochlear nucleus can yield evoked potentials of an amplitude similar to those recorded directly from the eighth nerve.[28] Because the evoked potentials that may be recorded from the cochlear nucleus originate from structures located central to the auditory nerve, these potentials are suitable for monitoring neural conduction over the entire course of the auditory nerve.

Practically, recording from the cochlear nucleus may be accomplished by placing a recording electrode in the lateral recess of the fourth

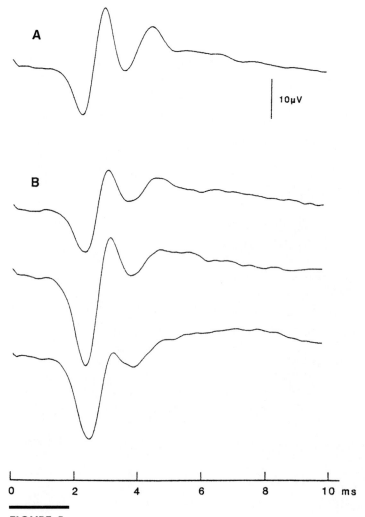

FIGURE 5.

CAP recorded from the exposed CN VIII in response to click stimulation. **A,** when the eighth nerve was exposed. **B,** successive recordings obtained during and immediately after electrocoagulation near the eighth nerve. (From Møller AR: *Evoked Potentials in Intraoperative Monitoring.* Baltimore, Williams & Wilkins, 1988. Used by permission.)

ventricle (Fig 6).[29] The wick electrode previously described in this chapter used for recording from CN VIII is also suitable for recording from the vicinity of the cochlear nucleus. This electrode can be introduced through the foramen of Luschka in a caudal-to-medial-rostral direction to a depth of about 2 mm to 3 mm into the lateral recess of the fourth ventricle.[50] When using a retromastoid (or retrosigmoid) approach to the CP angle the recording electrode can usually be inserted under the choroid plexus that normally protrudes from the foramen of Luschka, just above the entrance/exit of CN IX and CN X into the brain stem (see Fig 6).[28, 29, 50] To place the recording electrode deep in the lateral recess so that it is close to the cochlear nucleus, it should be inserted in a rostral-medial direction.[50] It may be advantageous to shrink the choroid plexus, if it is large, by coagulation.

Recordings from the lateral recess of the fourth ventricle can conveniently be done in operations on acoustic tumors, because in most cases the placement of the recording electrode will be located away from the tumor and the wire of the recording electrode can be placed at the caudal wall of the wound (see Fig 6), thus located where there is much less of a risk of its being dislodged by surgical manipulations or accidentally caught by the drill used to drill the bone of the porous acusticus.

There is no need for the recorded potentials to be filtered more than that done by the physiological amplifier (settings of 10 to 3,000 Hz are suitable), unless only the fast components are to be viewed selectively, in which case digital filters may be used or setting the electronic filters to 150 to 3,000 Hz is suitable (Fig 7). An amplification of 20,000 times is suitable when recording from the cochlear nucleus.

INTERPRETATION OF RECORDINGS FROM THE COCHLEAR NUCLEUS

Recording from the vicinity of the cochlear nucleus in the way described above will normally yield potentials with large enough amplitudes to be interpreted after only a few responses have been averaged. The response contains a few early sharp peaks that are most likely generated by the termination of the auditory nerve in the cochlear nucleus, followed by a slow negative deflection that is likely to originate in the cochlear nucleus. When the stimulus intensity is lowered, the amplitude of the slow negative potential decreases much less rapidly than do the initial peaks (see Fig 7).[30, 41] It may, therefore, be expected that this slow component of the response may also be less affected by changes in neural conduction of the auditory nerve, such as those induced by surgical manipulations (see Fig 7C), than are the early sharp peaks. Thus, it seems advisable to use the early and fast components of the response to monitor changes in neural conduction of the auditory nerve, at least until more experience has been gained regarding how the slow component changes according to changes in neural conduction of the auditory nerve.

OTHER METHODS OF MONITORING HEARING IN OPERATIONS IN THE CEREBELLOPONTINE ANGLE

It has been previously described by various investigators how auditory evoked potentials that are recorded from the ear or its vicinity (ECoG potentials) may be used in monitoring during removal of acoustic tumors.[51-53] However, the value of ECoG potentials for monitoring during operations in the CP angle is rather limited, because all of the components of the recorded ECoG potentials originate in the ear or the most distal portion of the auditory nerve. These ECoG potentials will be affected if the blood supply to the cochlea is compromised, but they will remain largely unaffected by injury to the intracranial portion of the auditory nerve because they depend on the response from the most distal portion of the auditory nerve, which is not affected by injury in opera-

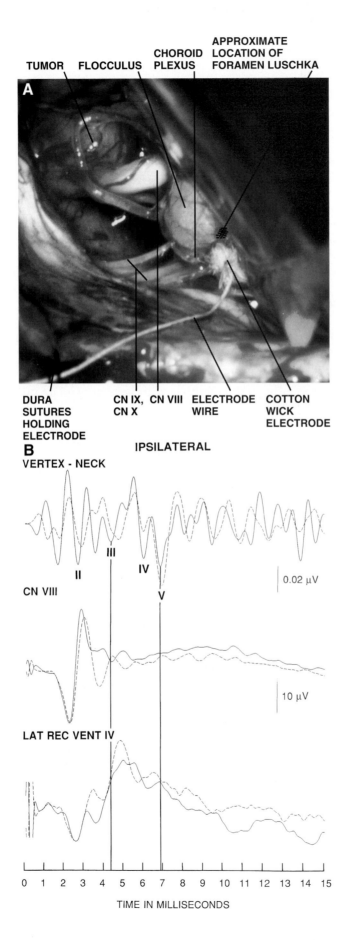

A

TUMOR FLOCCULUS CHOROID PLEXUS APPROXIMATE LOCATION OF FORAMEN LUSCHKA

DURA SUTURES HOLDING ELECTRODE CN IX, CN X CN VIII ELECTRODE WIRE COTTON WICK ELECTRODE

B

IPSILATERAL

VERTEX - NECK

II III IV V

0.02 μV

CN VIII

10 μV

LAT REC VENT IV

0 1 2 3 4 5 6 7 8 9 10 11 12 13 14 15

TIME IN MILLISECONDS

tions in the CP angle unless the blood supply to the cochlea is compromised by surgical manipulations. ECoG recording will detect if the blood supply to the cochlea is compromised, but this can just as well be detected by recording differentially between the earlobes (see page 153 and Fig 2).

WHICH CHANGES SHOULD BE REPORTED TO THE SURGEON?

There is disagreement among investigators who are involved in intraoperative neurophysiologic monitoring as to how large a change in evoked potentials such as BAEP or CAP from the auditory nerve or cochlear nucleus should be before it is reported to the surgeon. Some investigators have advocated that only large changes, such as a total obliteration of the wave pattern of the BAEP, should be reported because such large changes are assumed to be an indication that there is a noticeable risk of postoperative hearing loss.[21] However, other investigators have presented the view that any change that is larger than those small changes that occur when no manipulation of CN VIII is done should be reported to the surgeon.[3] The justification for the latter is that information about small changes in the evoked potentials that are definite indications of surgically induced changes in neural conduction is of value to the surgeon. Information about such small changes makes the surgeon aware that CN VIII has been surgically manipulated to an extent that has caused a measurable change in neural function (although it may not represent any noticeable risk of postoperative hearing loss). The question is whether the result of monitoring auditory evoked potentials is regarded as a source of information that may be valuable to the surgeon in any way or whether it should be regarded as a warning only.

There are several reasons to report small changes in evoked potentials to the surgeon. Changes in the evoked potentials that are caused by stretching of CN VIII from retraction, for instance, often develop slowly. If the surgeon is not informed until the change has reached a level of a large latency shift or a total obliteration of the wave pattern, it may be difficult for the surgeon to determine what caused the greater change and he or she would then have limited options of how to correct the problem.

Such early information about changes in neural conduction gives the surgeon the option to intervene immediately or wait to see if the changes increase, in which case the surgeon will know exactly what caused the change and can thus take appropriate intervention. Such use of intraop-

---

FIGURE 6.

A, placement of the recording electrode in the lateral recess of the fourth ventricle. **B,** comparison of the BAEP (digitally filtered as in Figure 1, W50), together with the responses recorded from the exposed eighth nerve (middle tracings) and the responses recorded from an electrode placed in the lateral recess of the fourth ventricle, as shown in **A.** The dashed lines are replications, and all recordings were obtained at about the same time during an operation for hemifacial spasm. (From Møller AR, Jho HD, Jannetta PJ: Neurosurgery 34:668–693, 1994. Used by permission.)

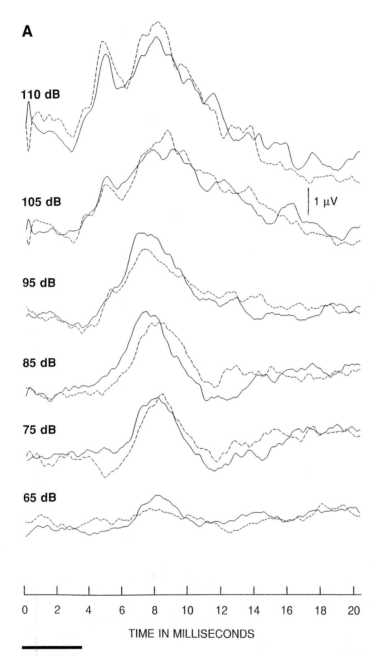

A

110 dB

105 dB

1 μV

95 dB

85 dB

75 dB

65 dB

0   2   4   6   8   10   12   14   16   18   20

TIME IN MILLISECONDS

FIGURE 7.

A, click-evoked responses recorded from the lateral recess of the fourth ventricle. The different records were obtained at different stimulus intensities (given in dB Pe SPL; 105 dB Pe SPL corresponds to 65 dB above normal hearing level). *Solid line:* response to rarefaction clicks; *dashed line:* response to condensation clicks. (From Møller AR, Jannetta PJ, Jho HD: *Electroencephalogr Clin Neurophysiol* 92:215–224, 1994. Used by permission.)   *(Continued.)*

Moving?

I'd like to receive my *Advances in Otolaryngology* without interruption.
Please note the following change of address, effective:

Name: _____

New Address: _____

_____

City: _____ State: _____ Zip: _____

Old Address: _____

_____

City: _____ State: _____ Zip: _____

Reservation Card

Yes, I would like my own copy of *Advances in Otolaryngology* . Please begin my subscription with the current edition according to the terms described below.* I understand that I will have 30 days to examine each annual edition. If satisfied, I will pay just $xx.95 plus sales tax, postage and handling (price subject to change without notice).

Name: _____

Address: _____

City: _____ State: _____ Zip: _____

Method of Payment
O Visa   O Mastercard   O AmEx   O Bill me   O Check (in US dollars, payable to Mosby, Inc.)

Card number: _____ Exp date: _____

Signature: _____

ls-0909

---

*Your Advances Service Guarantee:

When you subscribe to *Advances*, we'll send you an advance notice of future volumes about two months before they publish. This automatic notice system is designed to take up as little of your time as possible. If you do not want *Advances*, the advance notice makes it quick and easy for you to let us know your decision, and you will always have at least 20 days to decide. If we don't hear from you, we'll send you the new volume as soon as it's available. And, of course, *Advances* is yours to examine free of charge for 30 days (postage, handling and applicable sales tax are added to each shipment.).

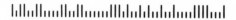

BUSINESS REPLY MAIL

FIRST CLASS MAIL   PERMIT No. 762   CHICAGO, IL

NO POSTAGE
NECESSARY
IF MAILED
IN THE
UNITED STATES

POSTAGE WILL BE PAID BY ADDRESSEE

Chris Hughes
Mosby-Year Book, Inc.
200 N. LaSalle Street
Suite 2600
Chicago, IL 60601-9981

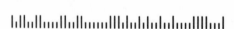

BUSINESS REPLY MAIL

FIRST CLASS MAIL   PERMIT No. 762   CHICAGO, IL

NO POSTAGE
NECESSARY
IF MAILED
IN THE
UNITED STATES

POSTAGE WILL BE PAID BY ADDRESSEE

Chris Hughes
Mosby-Year Book, Inc.
200 N. LaSalle Street
Suite 2600
Chicago, IL 60601-9981

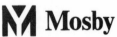

Mosby

Dedicated to publishing excellence

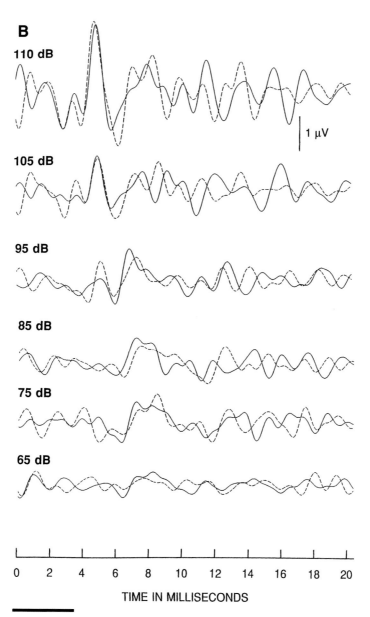

B

110 dB

1 μV

105 dB

95 dB

85 dB

75 dB

65 dB

0 2 4 6 8 10 12 14 16 18 20

TIME IN MILLISECONDS

FIGURE 7 (cont'd).
B, same records as in **A** but after digital filtering to enhance the narrow peaks and suppress the broad peaks.

erative neurophysiologic monitoring emphasizes its value as a source of information rather than a simple warning to the surgeon that there is a noticeable risk of postoperative deficit if the change is not reversed promptly.

If the results of intraoperative monitoring should only be used as a warning, it would be necessary to establish criteria for what changes the surgeon can ignore and what changes imply a noticeable risk of postoperative hearing loss. Such criteria have not been established, and the information that is necessary for the establishment of such criteria is not available. Thus, it is not known what changes in auditory evoked potentials can be tolerated without a risk of causing postoperative permanent hearing loss. It should also be noted that tolerance levels for such changes would also most likely differ among individuals, which adds to the difficulty in using recorded auditory evoked potentials as warning signs. It also seems likely that factors such as the length of time that certain changes in the evoked potentials have been sustained are important to the risk of permanent postoperative hearing loss.

In a case in which a sudden and unexpected large change in the recorded potentials occurs (or the waveform of the evoked potentials totally disappears), some investigators also advocate that the neurophysiologist who is responsible for monitoring should first ascertain whether or not the change was caused by a technical failure. Other investigators[3] have pointed out that if the cause of such dramatic changes in the evoked potentials was surgical manipulations, then precious time for surgical intervention would have been wasted by taking time to check for technical problems. It would seem more beneficial to first assume that the change in the recorded evoked potentials was caused by surgical manipulation, alert the surgeon appropriately, and only then begin to check the equipment. If it should be determined that the cause was indeed a technical failure of some kind, the only loss would be a few minutes of the surgeon's time, but the patient would not have been exposed to any risk. However, if the change was caused by a serious surgical event and intervention was delayed for a period of time to check equipment, then the patient could have been exposed to a risk of postoperative neurological deficit because by then it may not have been possible to reverse the change in neural function because of the delay in intervention.

AUDITORY NERVE RECORDINGS IN OPERATIONS FOR VESTIBULAR NERVE SECTION

Recording CAP from CN VIII may be useful to distinguish between the auditory and vestibular nerves in operations in which the vestibular nerve is to be severed. Because the vestibular nerve is a good conductor of electrical current, it is also possible to record auditory evoked potentials when a monopolar recording electrode is placed on it. It has therefore been suggested that a bipolar recording electrode be used instead.[31, 54] Such a bipolar electrode may consist of two wires with bare tips that are placed in contact with the nerve (Fig 8,B) and connected to the two inputs of a differential amplifier. Such an electrode is supposed to only record propagated neural activity, because it senses only the difference between the electrical potentials that are recorded from the two tips.[32] Thus, passively conducted potentials are theoretically not recorded by such a bipolar electrode. However, because it is difficult to make the size of the electrode and the distance between its two tips small compared to the diameter of CN VIII, bipolar recordings from the auditory nerve can usually not be regarded as ideal.[32] Figure 9 shows how the amplitude of the recorded CAP changes when the recording electrode is moved around the circumference of the intracranial portion of CN VIII.[32]

This above mentioned study[32] also showed that a sharp-tipped mo-

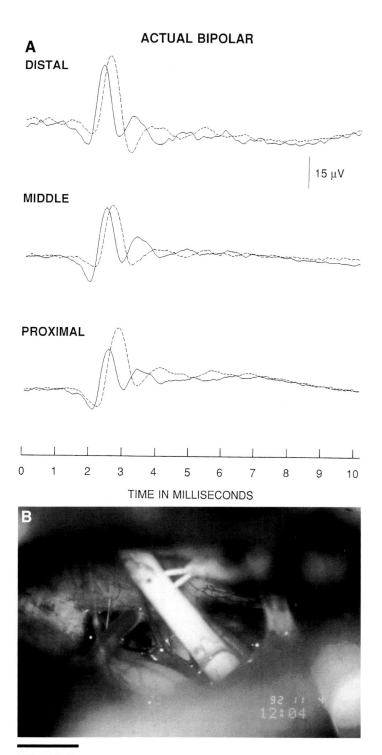

FIGURE 8.
A, recordings from CN VIII using a bipolar recording electrode obtained from the distal (near the porus acusticus), middle, and proximal (near the brain stem) portions of the intracranial portion of CN VIII. **B,** bipolar recording electrode placed on the exposed intracranial portion of CN VIII. (From Møller AR, Colletti V, Fiorino F: *Electroencephalogr Clin Neurophysiol* 92:17–29, 1994. Used by permission.)

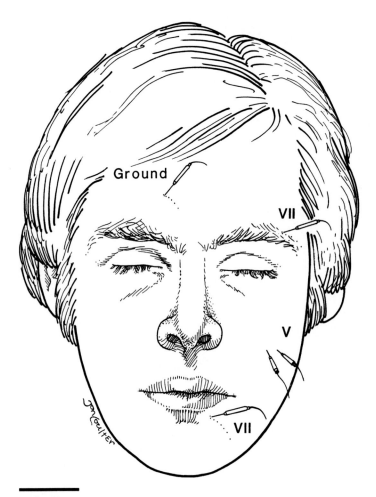

FIGURE 9.
Placement of recording electrodes for EMG recordings from face muscles. Also shown is how recording can be done from the masseter muscle.

nopolar recording electrode that is in contact with the nerve also has a high degree of spatial selectivity and offers a valid alternative to the bipolar recording technique, provided that the nerve is not immersed in fluid. Such a monopolar electrode, however, will also record electrical potentials that are passively conducted to the recording site, not only propagated activity as is supposedly the case for a bipolar recording electrode. Using a recording electrode with sharp tips that have to be placed in direct contact with the auditory-vestibular nerve may easily injure the very fragile CN VIII, and therefore such recordings should be done with great caution.

PREOPERATIVE AND POSTOPERATIVE TESTS

Although it is only the changes in the recorded responses during the operation that are important when BAEP are used in the operating room, it is vital that the patient's hearing be properly tested before an operation in which auditory evoked potentials are to be monitored. A BAEP record should also be obtained preoperatively in such patients.

If a patient does not have any hearing preoperatively or if it is not possible to obtain an interpretable BAEP preoperatively, then it will probably not be possible to obtain an interpretable BAEP in the operating room. If BAEP are not tested preoperatively and if BAEP cannot be obtained intraoperatively, it would then be impossible to determine whether the cause of the failure to obtain BAEP intraoperatively was technical or that the patient had inadequate hearing at the time of intraoperative testing or, for that matter, before the operation began. If it is not possible to obtain an interpretable record during the operation, but the patient had a readable BAEP before the operation, then it may be concluded that the cause of failure to obtain BAEP intraoperatively was technical in nature.

It is also important to have precise records of a patient's preoperative hearing status to be able to determine if any postoperative impairment of hearing has occurred as a result of surgical manipulations. The patient's hearing should therefore be tested several times after the operation in the same way as done before the operation (for instance, at the time of discharge and 3 months postoperatively) to ascertain if any damage to the patient's hearing has occurred as a result of the operation.

MONITORING OF OTHER SENSORY NERVES

THE TRIGEMINAL NERVE

Only a few reports have been published in the literature that describe methods for intraoperative monitoring of the trigeminal nerve. It has been shown how the response to electrical stimulation of peripheral branches of the sensory portion of the trigeminal nerve can be recorded either directly from the intracranial portion of the trigeminal nerve[22] using a technique similar to that described for the auditory nerve (see page 155), or from electrodes placed on the scalp (far-field potentials). Short-latency components that originate in the trigeminal nerve have been identified in such recordings from electrodes placed on the scalp,[22] but different investigators have obtained conflicting results with regard to longer latency trigeminal evoked potentials (TEP).[22, 55, 56] It seems that long-latency components of the TEP recorded from electrodes placed on the scalp are not generally present in anesthetized patients,[23] and it seems doubtful at this time whether any noticeable far-field TEP that have intra-axial neural generators can be recorded in the anesthetized individual.

Some investigators[57] have promoted the use of mechanical stimulation (in the form of air puffs) instead of electrical stimulation to elicit TEP. Far-field TEP evoked by such stimulation seem to be of a higher amplitude, and there are no electrical artifacts, as there are for electrically evoked TEP. However, we have at present inadequate experience in the use of such mechanically (air puff) evoked TEP, and this method does not seem to have been evaluated for use in anesthetized patients.

THE OPTIC NERVE

The use of intraoperative monitoring of the visual system has been limited because of problems associated with presenting an adequate stimulation to the anesthetized patient.[24] It is known from clinical studies that flash stimulation does not reveal pathologies that are related to vision as well as pattern reversal stimulation does, such as the commonly used reversing checkerboard stimuli.[58] This method is difficult to use in the anesthetized patient because it requires that a pattern be focused on the patient's retina, and to date, no method has been described that makes this possible. The only way to elicit visual evoked potentials (VEP) intraoperatively, therefore, is to use flash stimulation. At present, this can best be accomplished using light-emitting diodes. The best response is obtained while the eye is light-adapted. Since red light flashes cannot easily keep the eye light-adapted, a different color of light should be used, such as green,[3] and the light stimuli should be left on, even throughout the time during an operation when it may not be required to record VEP.

Recordings of VEP can be made from electrodes placed on the scalp as well as directly on the optic nerve or optic tract.[3] Again, since the specificity of such flash-evoked potentials is rather poor, intraoperative monitoring of VEP is at present regarded as having only limited value.

MONITORING OF THE SENSORY PORTION OF MIXED CRANIAL NERVES

Although CN V carries both motor and sensory fibers, it may not commonly be regarded as a mixed nerve because the motor and sensory fibers of CN V are separated into two anatomically distinct parts (portio minor and portio major, respectively). Monitoring of the sensory part (by eliciting TEP) was discussed above. Intraoperative monitoring of the sensory parts of CN IX and CN X has not yet been found to have any practical use.

MONITORING OF CRANIAL MOTOR NERVES

Of all the cranial motor nerves, it is mainly monitoring of the function of the facial nerve that has been described most extensively.[3-7, 9-11, 59-61] This is probably because of the importance of preserving facial function during operations in the CP angle, such as those to remove acoustic tumors, during which the facial nerve is often injured to an extent that postoperative facial palsy or facial weakness results. Only recently has interest been directed to the use of intraoperative monitoring as an aid to preserve the function of other cranial motor nerves, such as those innervating the extraocular muscles,[3, 62-64] and methods for intraoperative monitoring of lower cranial motor nerve have also been described recently.[7, 8, 65]

The general technique of monitoring cranial motor nerves intraoperatively makes use of recording contractions of the muscles that are innervated by respective motor nerves upon electrical stimulation of the respective nerves intracranially with a hand-held stimulating electrode. This makes it possible to test neural conduction in a motor nerve, and it also makes it possible to find a motor nerve when it is not directly visible in the surgical field. Monitoring of surgically induced neural activity in such motor nerves is also important and this can also be done by recording muscle activity.

MONITORING OF FACIAL FUNCTION IN PATIENTS UNDERGOING OPERATIONS FOR ACOUSTIC TUMORS

Loss or impairment of facial function is a noticeable handicap for practical as well as social reasons. Intraoperative neurophysiologic monitoring of the function of the facial nerve is very rewarding, because it can contribute to the preservation of facial function following operations in the CP angle, such as those to remove acoustic tumors.

Intraoperative neurophysiologic monitoring of the facial nerve was one of the first kinds of intraoperative neurophysiologic monitoring of cranial nerves that came into general use and, in fact, it was the first type that won the approval of a representative national organization.[66] Thus, intraoperative monitoring of facial nerve function in operations to remove acoustic tumors is now officially recognized as a valuable adjunct to such operations. A recent "Consensus Statement" of the National Institutes of Health, Consensus Development Conference stated that "There is a consensus that intraoperative real-time neurologic monitoring improves the surgical management of vestibular schwannoma,* including the preservation of facial nerve function and possibly improves hearing preservation by the use of intraoperative auditory brainstem response monitoring. New approaches to monitoring acoustic nerve function may provide more rapid feedback to the surgeon, thus enhancing their usefulness. Intraoperative monitoring of cranial nerves V, VI, IX, X, and XI also has been described, but the full benefits of this monitoring remain to be determined."[66] In the "Conclusion and Recommendation" of this report it is stated, "The benefit of routine intraoperative monitoring of the facial nerve has been clearly established. This technique should be included in surgical therapy of vestibular schwannoma. Routine monitoring of other cranial nerves should be considered."[66]

The primary purposes of intraoperative neurophysiologic monitoring of the facial nerve are to identify the facial nerve in the operative field when it is not directly visible or when it is not possible to visually distinguish it from other nerves in the CP angle, and to detect when surgical manipulations have caused injury to the facial nerve. Secondly, such monitoring can provide information about the degree of injury to the facial nerve and thereby help in the decision about whether or not to perform a nerve graft at the end of a tumor operation.

PRINCIPLES OF FACIAL NERVE MONITORING

The methods used to identify the facial nerve consist of electrical stimulation with a hand-held stimulating electrode using one of several methods for detecting when such stimulation is causing a contraction of facial muscles. This can be done by visually observing the face[67] or by placing sensors of one kind or another on the face.[6, 60, 68, 69] Recording of EMG activity from facial muscles is now the most common way to detect contractions of facial muscles.[3, 5, 7–11, 61, 70]

---

*Vestibular schwannoma is now the official name for tumors of the eighth nerve that previously were (and still are) called acoustic tumors. We have in this article retained the old name, acoustic tumors.

When a hand-held stimulating electrode is used, it is possible to map a tumor within a very short time so that the location of the facial nerve becomes known, even when it is not directly visible. The use of such electrical stimulation to assure that the portion of the tumor that is to be removed *does not* contain any part of the facial nerve is of great value, particularly during the first stage of the removal of large tumors. Any portion of a tumor that is to be removed should be probed with the hand-held electrical stimulating electrode before attempting to remove it.

The most suitable stimulating electrode for such probing of a tumor is a hand-held monopolar electrode that has a form similar to that of the commonly used surgical microdissection instruments.[3, 7, 10, 65] The use of a bipolar stimulating electrode has been advocated by some investigators[71, 72] because of its greater spatial selectivity. There is no doubt that a bipolar stimulating electrode is more suitable for the purpose of distinguishing between two different nerves that are located close to each other. However, the fact that the ability of a bipolar stimulating electrode to stimulate nervous tissue depends on its orientation makes it less suitable for use in connection with the removal of acoustic tumors, for testing a region of a tumor for the presence of any part of the facial nerve.

It would, therefore, seem ideal to have both monopolar and bipolar stimulating electrodes available. When the stimulus strength is properly adjusted, however, a monopolar stimulating electrode becomes rather selective, and when the stimulus intensity is low then such an electrode will only stimulate the facial nerve when it is close to the stimulating electrode. A monopolar electrode can also be used to distinguish between two nerves that are located close together, such as CN VII and CN VIII, provided that the stimulus strength is properly chosen.

It has been debated whether the electrical stimulation should be of a constant-voltage or constant-current type.[3, 7, 8, 10, 65, 73] These two forms of stimulation are affected differently when external factors change. Thus, if the electrode impedance changes, a constant-current stimulus source tends to deliver stimulation that is little dependent on changes of the electrode impedance. When the shunting of stimulus current occurs, such as in a situation in which the surgical field changes from relatively dry to wet, a constant-voltage stimulus source will deliver a stimulus that is relatively independent of such changes in shunting of current.[3, 7, 8, 10, 65, 74]

The reason that the electrical stimulators commonly used for stimulation of peripheral nerves through electrodes placed on the skin have traditionally been the constant-current type is that most changes in such situations are in the electrode impedance. A constant-current source is most adequate in such situations, because it will keep the stimulation of a nerve relatively unaffected by changes in electrode impedance. In the CP angle the situation is different. Here it is the shunting of electrical current that is likely to vary, as the operative field will fluctuate from wet to dry and vice versa, which is why the most appropriate stimulator would be one that delivers a constant voltage.

It is not practically possible to realize an absolute constant-voltage stimulation because of the unavoidable electrical resistance in the electrode itself. We have preferred to use a semiconstant voltage stimulus source[3, 10, 74] as have others.[7, 8, 65] Other investigators[61, 73] have advocated a constant-current source in connection with a "flush" tip electrode. This stimulating electrode's entire shaft is electrically insulated, with only a small area of stimulating surface left uninsulated.

RECORDING OF MUSCLE CONTRACTIONS

At present, the most commonly used method for detecting contractions of the facial muscles is by recording EMG potentials. This can be accomplished by placing recording electrodes into facial muscles.[4, 5, 7, 10, 11, 74–76] This makes it possible to visualize the muscle responses on an oscilloscope screen as well as makes the potentials audible so that all personnel in the operating room can know when electrical stimulation is causing a muscle contraction.[3–5, 10, 74] The stimulus artifact should be electronically suppressed before the EMG signal is made audible, but it should be present in the oscillographic display because it is an indication that stimulus current is passing through tissue.

One should, however, be somewhat cautious in relying on the stimulus artifact as an indication that the EMG amplifiers and the stimulator are working perfectly. It is advisable to test the stimulus and recording systems as early as possible in an operation. This can be done by stimulating the facial nerve wherever it becomes visible early in the operation.

It has been described how EMG potentials are recorded separately from muscles from different portions of the face. Usually two recording channels are used, one recording from the upper face and the other recording from the lower face. Since the facial nerve may be split and different parts located at a distance from each other within the operative field, stimulation of one part of the facial nerve may cause contractions of muscles in one part of the face while stimulating other portions of the facial nerve may cause contractions of muscles in other parts of the face. There is, however, no need to make a distinction between which part of the face is activated, because it is important to preserve all parts of the facial nerve. We therefore attempt to record from the entire face using only one recording channel for the sake of simplicity (see Fig 9).

In cases involving large tumors it may be difficult to distinguish between the facial nerve and the motor portion of CN V (portio minor) on the basis of visual observations. Electrical stimulation of CN V will cause contractions of the mastication muscles. Electrodes placed in the face to record EMG potentials, as shown in Figure 9, will record contractions of not only facial muscles but also of the mastication muscles. The latency of the EMG potentials generated by the mastication muscles elicited by electrical stimulation of portio minor of CN V, however, have a much shorter latency than those generated by facial muscles (1.5 to 2 versus 6 to 7 milliseconds) (Fig 10).[3] When the EMG potentials are displayed on an oscilloscope, this difference in latency can be used to determine which nerve, CN VII or CN V, has been stimulated. If a second recording channel is available, it could be used to record selectively from the masseter muscle, which can be accomplished by placing a pair of recording electrodes (about 1 cm apart) deep into that muscle (see Fig 9). Electromyographic activity on that channel will mainly occur when CN V has been stimulated electrically.

It is not only the muscle activity that is elicited by specific electrical stimulation that is important in intraoperative neurophysiologic monitor-

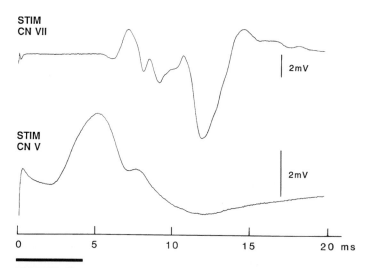

FIGURE 10.

EMG potentials recorded from electrodes placed on the face, as shown in Fig 9, when the intracranial portion of the facial nerve was stimulated electrically (*upper tracing*) and when the portio minor of CN V was stimulated (*lower tracing*). (From Møller AR: *Evoked Potentials in Intraoperative Monitoring.* Baltimore, Williams & Wilkins, 1988. Used by permission.)

ing of the facial nerve to reduce the risks of facial weakness or paresis. Neural activity in the facial nerve may also be generated when the facial nerve is being manipulated or being mechanically stimulated by touching it with surgical instruments.[4, 7, 10, 65, 70, 76, 77] The nature of such activity is different for different kinds of stimulation, and injury to the facial nerve may create ongoing neural activity that can be discriminated from other kinds of facial muscle activity.[5, 76, 77] There are different variations of such activity and different investigators have classified such EMG activity into several different groups to represent activity caused by mechanical stimulation or by injury of difficult severity.[5, 76, 77]

Recording such continuous EMG activity from facial muscles is important, particularly when dissecting tumor off an injured facial nerve when such activity may act as an important feedback to the surgeon when presented in an audible form. Activity that persists for a considerable time (minutes) after the manipulation that caused it is a more serious sign of injury than is activity that is only present when the facial nerve is being manipulated. It may be beneficial to stop all surgical manipulations of the facial nerve until such activity has ceased.

Although mechanical stimulation of the facial nerve, such as that in operations to remove acoustic tumors, often gives rise to facial muscle activity, it should be remembered that it is mainly injured nerves that are mechano-sensitive[78] while normal nerves are not likely to become activated because of mechanical manipulations. Therefore, mechanical stimulation should not be used as a substitute for electrical stimulation when attempting to identify the facial nerve or for finding regions of a tumor where no facial nerve is present.

When removal of an acoustic tumor is completed, recordings of the EMG response to electrical stimulation of the facial nerve near the brain stem have some predictive value regarding the patient's postoperative facial function.[79] Thus, the amplitude of the EMG response is an approximate measure of the number of nerve fibers of the facial nerve that are activated by the stimulation.[80]

It is important to consider that the results of such a test only determine the condition of the nerve at the time it is stimulated. Therefore, a reduced amplitude of electrically evoked EMG potentials that is indicative of neural block in many nerve fibers does not necessarily mean that the patient will have a large degree of permanent loss of facial function. The poor responses may just as well be a result of neuropraxia, a reversible blockage of neural transmission. Therefore, the results of EMG recordings of electrically elicited facial muscle contractions should be considered cautiously when making important decisions, such as whether or not to graft the facial nerve in the same operation. Several other factors, such as, for instance, the anatomic appearance of the facial nerve, are important indicators of the prognosis of postoperative facial function, and these factors should be taken into consideration when making such decisions.

MONITORING OTHER CRANIAL MOTOR NERVES

Cranial nerve III, CN IV, and CN VI may be at risk of injury in operations to remove different kinds of skull base tumors. Cranial nerve III is particularly important, because the loss of CN III results in functional loss of the eye that is affected. Lower cranial motor nerves, such as CN IX, CN X, CN XI, and CN XII, are mixed nerves with noticeable sensory afferent fibers. While the motor fibers of these nerves can be monitored intraoperatively using methods similar to those described for monitoring the facial nerve, it is important to consider the effect of also stimulating the sensory portion of these nerves.

MOTOR NERVES OF THE EXTRAOCULAR MUSCLES

The three nerves that innervate the extraocular muscles can be monitored by recording EMG potentials from respective muscles.[1, 3, 8, 62–64, 81] Intracranial electrical stimulation, as described above for identifying the facial nerve, is also suitable for finding these cranial motor nerves intracranially when they are not directly visible.

Several methods have been described for recording EMG potentials from the extraocular muscles. Sekhar and Møller[62] and Møller[3, 63] described methods to place needle electrodes percutaneously to reach three of the extraocular muscles (lateral rectus, CN VI; inferior rectus, CN III; and superior oblique, CN IV) (Fig 11). The recorded EMG potentials had amplitudes in the microvolt range, and they could be visualized directly on an oscilloscope or after only a few responses were averaged (Fig 12). Other investigators[81] have made use of surface electrodes in the form of small wire loops that were placed under the eyelids, close to the respective muscles. Although this way of recording EMG potentials may result in potentials of slightly lower amplitudes, they could also be visualized on an oscilloscope.

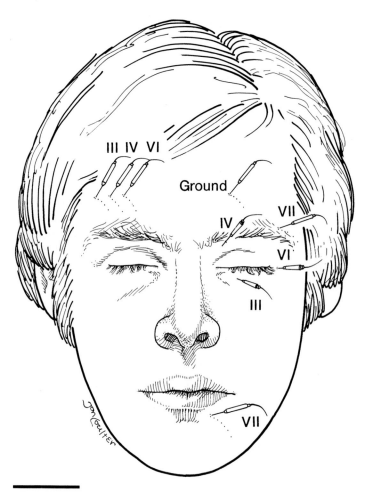

FIGURE 11.

Placement of EMG recording electrodes for monitoring cranial motor nerves (CN III, CN IV, CN VI, CN VII, and CN V). (From Møller AR: *Evoked Potentials in Intraoperative Monitoring*. Baltimore, Williams & Wilkins, 1988. Used by permission.)

MONITORING OF THE MOTOR PORTION OF CRANIAL NERVE V

Monitoring of the motor portion of CN V (portio minor) is important in removal of acoustic tumors. It can be done by recording EMG potentials from the muscles of mastication, such as the masseter muscles. This method has been discussed above in detail.

LOWER CRANIAL MOTOR NERVES

Monitoring of the motor portion of CN IX can be done by recording EMG potentials from muscles in the pharynx, which are innervated by this nerve. This can be done by placing recording electrodes in the soft palate.[8, 65]

Cranial nerve X can be monitored by recording from the laryngeal muscles.[8, 65, 82] It also has been described how the tracheal tube can be equipped with metal rings, from which EMG potentials from laryngeal

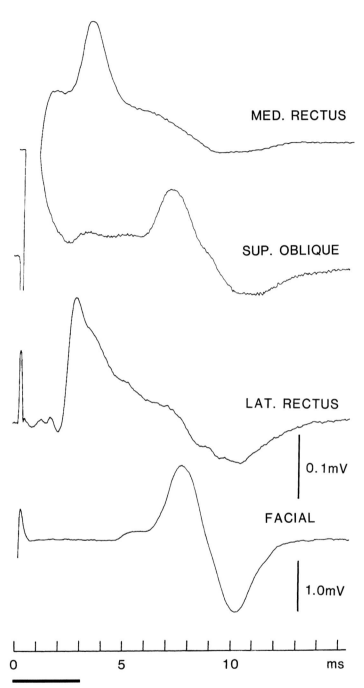

FIGURE 12.
Recordings of EMG potentials from the three extraocular muscles that are innervated by CN III, CN IV, and CN VI. Also shown *(lower tracings)* are recordings
obtained from the facial muscles when the intracranial portion of the facial nerve
was stimulated electrically. (From Møller AR: *Evoked Potentials in Intraoperative Monitoring*. Baltimore, Williams & Wilkins, 1988. Used by permission.)

muscles can be recorded when the rings are placed so that they will be close to the larynx when the tracheal tube is in place. Cranial nerve XI and CN XII can be monitored by recording EMG potentials from muscles of the scapula[65] and the tongue,[3, 65] respectively.

Methods similar to those described above for monitoring facial function may be used for electrical stimulation of all cranial motor nerves for the purpose of intraoperative monitoring. It is also valuable to make the recorded EMG activity audible when monitoring lower cranial motor nerves in a way similar to that described above for monitoring facial function.

It is important to keep in mind that there are specific potential risks associated with electrical stimulation of any of the lower cranial motor nerves. One reason for such specific risks is that these nerves also contain nerve fibers other than those that innervate the muscles from which the recordings are made. Some of these other nerve fibers are afferent fibers, and they will all be stimulated when the nerves are stimulated electrically. Also, these nerves innervate several different organs. Thus, electrical stimulation of CN IX and CN X may affect the cardiovascular system, and electrical stimulation of CN X may also cause contractions of the diaphragm, all of which can have potentially serious consequences. For stimulation of CN IX and CN X the stimulus rate should not exceed 5 pulses per second (pps), and strong stimulation should be avoided and effects on the cardiovascular system should be watched carefully so that the risks are minimized.

Electrical stimulation of CN XI may cause ruptures of tendons and muscles and dislocation of joints, because the normal feedback from tendon and joint receptors does not regulate the strength of contractions when the motor nerves are stimulated electrically.

MONITORING THE PERIPHERAL PORTION OF THE FACIAL NERVE

Monitoring of the peripheral portion of the facial nerve may be important in various operations on the face, from procedures to treat trauma to removal of tumors, such as those in the parotid gland.[83] In the latter case, monitoring may be a valuable aid in identifying if the facial nerve is involved in the tumor. A method of electrical stimulation similar to that described when removing acoustic tumors can be used. The response from facial muscles can be recorded in the form of EMG potentials from the respective muscles that are innervated by the branches of the facial nerve that are embedded in the tumor. In many cases, it is possible to detect muscle contractions by just observing the face by visual inspection. Mechanically evoked or injury-related neural activity may best be detected by recording EMG activity to detect muscle contractions.

REFERENCES

1. Møller AR, Møller MB: Does intraoperative monitoring of auditory evoked potentials reduce incidence of hearing loss as a complication of microvascular decompression of cranial nerves? *Neurosurgery* 24:257–263, 1989.
2. Radtke RA, Erwin W, Wilkins RH: Intraoperative brainstem auditory evoked potentials: Significant decrease in postoperative morbidity. *Neurology* 39:187–191, 1989.

3. Møller AR: *Evoked Potentials in Intraoperative Monitoring*. Baltimore, Williams & Wilkins, 1988.

4. Prass R, Lueders H: Acoustic (loudspeaker) facial electromyographic monitoring. Part I. Neurosurgery 19:392–400, 1986.

5. Prass RL, Kinney SE, Hardy RW, et al: Acoustic (loudspeaker) facial EMG monitoring: Part II. Use of evoked EMG activity during acoustic neuroma resection. Otolaryngol Head Neck Surg 97:541–551, 1987.

6. Silverstein H, Smorha E, Jones R: Routine identification of the facial nerve using electrical stimulation during otological and neurotological surgery. Laryngoscope 98:726–730, 1988.

7. Yingling CD, Gardi JN: Intraoperative monitoring of facial and cochlear nerves during acoustic neuroma surgery. Otolaryngol Clin North Am 25:413–448, 1992.

8. Yingling CD: Intraoperative monitoring in skull base surgery, in Jackler RK, Brackmann D (eds): *Neurotology*. St. Louis, Mosby, 1994, pp 967–1002.

9. Linden RD, Tator CH, Benedict C, et al: Electrophysiological monitoring during acoustic neuroma and other posterior fossa surgery. Le Journal Canadien des Sciences Neurologigues 15:73–81, 1988.

10. Møller AR, Jannetta PJ: Preservation of facial function during removal of acoustic neuromas. Use of monopolar constant-voltage stimulation and EMG. J Neurosurg 61:757–760, 1984.

11. Benecke JE, Calder HB, Chadwick G: Facial nerve monitoring during acoustic neuroma removal. Laryngoscope 97:697–700, 1987.

12. Møller AR, Jannetta PJ: Monitoring facial EMG during microvascular decompression operations for hemifacial spasm. J Neurosurg 66:681–685, 1987.

13. Haines SJ, Torres F: Intraoperative monitoring of the facial nerve during decompressive surgery for hemifacial spasm. J Neurosurg 74:254–257, 1991.

14. Hardy RW Jr, Kinney SE, Lueders H, et al: Preservation of cochlear nerve function with aid of brain stem auditory evoked potentials. Neurosurgery 11:16–19, 1982.

15. Grundy BL: Intraoperative monitoring of sensory evoked potentials. Anesthesiology 58:72–87, 1983.

16. Grundy BL: Evoked potential monitoring, in Blitt CD (ed): *Monitoring in Anesthesia and Critical Care Medicine*. New York, Churchill-Livingstone, 1985, pp 345–411.

17. Raudzens PA: Intraoperative monitoring of evoked potentials. Ann N Y Acad Sci 388:308–326, 1982.

18. Daspit CP, Raudzens PA, Shetter AG: Monitoring of intraoperative auditory brain stem responses. Otolaryngol Head Neck Surg 90:108–116, 1982.

19. Møller AR, Jannetta PJ: Monitoring auditory functions during cranial nerve microvascular decompression operations by direct recording from the eighth nerve. J Neurosurg 59:493–499, 1983.

20. Schramm J, Mokrusch T, Fahlbusch R, et al: Detailed analysis of intraoperative changes monitoring brain stem acoustic evoked potentials. Neurosurgery 22:694–702, 1988.

21. Friedman WA, Kaplan BJ, Gravenstein D, et al: Intraoperative brain-stem auditory evoked potentials during posterior fossa microvascular decompression. J Neurosurg 62:552–557, 1985.

22. Stechison MT, Kralick FJ: The trigeminal evoked potential: Part I. Long-latency responses in awake or anesthetized subjects. Neurosurgery 33:633–638, 1993.

23. Stechison MT: The trigeminal evoked potential: Part II. Intraoperative recording of short-latency responses. Neurosurgery 33:639–644, 1993.

24. Cedzich C, Schramm J, Fahlbusch R: Are flash-evoked visual potentials useful for intraoperative monitoring of visual pathway function? Neurosurgery 21:709–715, 1987.

25. Fischer C: Brainstem auditory evoked potential (BAEP) monitoring in posterior fossa surgery, in Desmedt JE (ed): *Neuromonitoring in Surgery*. Amsterdam, Elsevier Science Publishers, 1989, pp 191–218.

26. Møller AR, Jannetta PJ, Møller MB: Neural generators of brainstem evoked potentials. Results from human intracranial recordings. *Ann Otol Rhinol Laryngol* 90:591–596, 1981.

27. Silverstein H, Norrell H, Hyman S: Simultaneous use of CO_2 laser with continuous monitoring of eighth cranial nerve action potential during acoustic neuroma surgery. *Otolaryngol Head Neck Surg* 92:80–84, 1984.

28. Møller AR, Jannetta PJ: Auditory evoked potentials recorded from the cochlear nucleus and its vicinity in man. *J Neurosurg* 59:1013–1018, 1983.

29. Møller AR, Jho HD, Jannetta PJ: Preservation of hearing in operations on acoustic tumors: An alternative to recording BAEP. *Neurosurgery* 34:688–693, 1994.

30. Møller AR, Jannetta PJ, Jho HD: Click-evoked responses from the cochlear nucleus: A study in humans. *Electroencephalogr Clin Neurophysiol* 92:215–224, 1994.

31. Colletti V, Bricolo A, Fiorino FG, et al: Changes in directly recorded cochlear nerve compound action potentials during acoustic tumor surgery. *Skull Base Surg* 4:1–9, 1994.

32. Møller AR, Colletti V, Fiorino F: Click evoked responses from the exposed intracranial portion of the eighth nerve during vestibular nerve section: Bipolar and monopolar recordings. *Electroencephalogr Clin Neurophysiol* 92:17–29, 1994.

33. Møller AR: Use of zero-phase digital filters to enhance brainstem auditory evoked potentials (BAEPs). *Electroencephalogr Clin Neurophysiol* 71:226–232, 1988.

34. Boston JR, Ainslie PJ: Effects of analog and digital filtering on brain stem auditory evoked potentials. *Electroencephalogr Clin Neurophysiol* 48:361–364, 1980.

35. Doyle DJ, Hyde ML: Analogue and digital filtering of auditory brainstem responses. *Scand Audiol (Stockh)* 10:81–89, 1981.

36. Schimmel H: The (+/−) reference: Accuracy of estimated mean components in average response studies. *Science* 157:92–94, 1967.

37. Hoke M, Ross B, Wickesberg R, et al: Weighted averaging—Theory and application to electrical response audiometry. *Electroencephalogr Clin Neurophysiol* 57:484–489, 1984.

38. Wong PKH, Bickford RG: Brain stem auditory potentials: The use of noise estimate. *Electroencephalogr Clin Neurophysiol* 50:25–34, 1980.

39. Sgro JA, Emerson RG, Pedley TA: Methods for steadily updating the averaged responses during neuromonitoring, in Desmedt JE (ed): *Neuromonitoring in Surgery*. Amsterdam, Elsevier Science Publishers, 1989, pp 49–60.

40. Jewett DL, Williston JS: Auditory evoked far fields averaged from the scalp of humans. *Brain* 94:681–696, 1971.

41. Møller AR, Jho HD, Yokota M, et al: Contribution from crossed and uncrossed brainstem structures to the brainstem auditory evoked potentials (BAEP): A study in humans. *Laryngoscope* 1995, in press.

42. Møller AR, Colletti V, Fiorino FG: Mapping of the exposed intracranial portion of the human intracranial auditory nerve in response to clicks: Recordings during vestibular nerve section. *Laryngoscope* 1994, submitted.

43. Møller AR, Jannetta PJ, Sekhar LN: Contributions from the auditory nerve to the brainstem auditory evoked potentials (BAEPs): Results of intracranial recording in man. *Electroencephalogr Clin Neurophysiol* 71:198–211, 1988.

44. Hashimoto I, Ishiyama Y, Yoshimoto T, et al: Brainstem auditory evoked potentials recorded directly from human brain-stem and thalamus. *Brain* 104:841–859, 1981.
45. Spire JP, Dohrmann GJ, Prieto PS: Correlation of brainstem evoked response with direct acoustic nerve potential, in Courjon J, Manguiere F, Reval M (eds): *Advances in Neurology: Clinical Applications of Evoked Potentials in Neurology*, vol 21. New York, Raven Press, 1982, pp 159–167.
46. Møller AR, Jannetta PJ: Compound action potentials recorded intracranially from the auditory nerve in man. *Exp Neurol* 74:862–874, 1981.
47. Møller AR, Jho HD: Compound action potentials recorded from the intracranial portion of the auditory nerve in man: Effects of stimulus intensity and polarity. *Audiology* 30:142–163, 1991.
48. Møller AR, Jho HD: Effect of high-frequency hearing loss on compound action potentials recorded from the intracranial portion of the human eighth nerve. *Hear Res* 55:9–23, 1991.
49. Møller AR, Møller MB, Jannetta PJ, et al: Auditory nerve compound action potentials and brain stem auditory evoked potentials in patients with various degrees of hearing loss. *Ann Otol Rhinol Laryngol* 100:488–495, 1991.
50. Kuroki A, Møller AR: Microsurgical anatomy around the foramen of Luschka with reference to intraoperative recording of auditory evoked potentials from the cochlear nuclei. *J Neurosurg* 1995, in press.
51. Levine R: Surgical monitoring application of brainstem auditory evoked response and electroencephalography. *Clin Atlas Auditory Evoked Potentials* 6:103–116, 1988.
52. Levine RA, Ojemann RG, Montgomery WW, et al: Monitoring auditory evoked potentials during acoustic neuroma surgery. Insights into the mechanism of the hearing loss. *Ann Otol Rhinol Laryngol* 93:116–123, 1984.
53. Sabin HI, Bentivoglio P, Symon L, et al: Intraoperative electrocochleography to monitor cochlear potentials during acoustic neuroma excision. *Acta Neurochir (Wien)* 85:110–116, 1987.
54. Colletti V, Fiorino FG: Electrophysiologic identification of the cochlear nerve fibers during cerebellopontine angle surgery. *Acta Otolaryngol (Stockh)* 1993; 113:746–754.
55. Soustiel JF, Hafner H, Guilburd JN, et al: A physiological coma scale: Grading of coma by combined use of brain-stem trigeminal and auditory evoked potentials and the Glasgow Coma Scale. *Electroencephalogr Clin Neurophysiol* 87:277–283, 1993.
56. Bennett MH, Jannetta PJ: Evoked potentials in trigeminal neuralgia. *Neurosurgery* 13:242–247, 1983.
57. Hashimoto I: Trigeminal evoked potentials following brief air puff: Enhanced signal-to-noise ratio. *Ann Neurol* 23:332–338, 1988.
58. Chiappa KH: Evoked potentials in clinical medicine, in Baker AB, Baker LH (eds): *Clinical Neurology*, vol 1. Philadelphia, JB Lippincott, 1983, pp 1–55.
59. Harner SG, Daube JR, Beatty CW, et al: Intraoperative monitoring of the facial nerve. *Laryngoscope* 98:209–212, 1988.
60. Sugita K, Kobayashi S: Technical and instrumental improvements in the surgical treatment of acoustic neurinomas. *J Neurosurg* 57:747–752, 1982.
61. Kartush JM, Bouchard KR: Intraoperative facial nerve monitoring. Otology, neurotology, and skull base surgery, in Kartush JM, Bouchard KR (eds): *Neuromonitoring in Otology and Head and Neck Surgery*. New York, Raven Press, 1992, pp 99–120.
62. Sekhar LN, Møller AR: Operative management of tumors involving the cavernous sinus. *J Neurosurg* 64:879–889, 1986.

63. Møller AR: Electrophysiological monitoring of cranial nerves in operations in the skull base, in Sekhar LN, Schramm VL (eds): *Tumors of the Cranial Base: Diagnosis and Treatment.* Mt. Kisco, New York, Futura Publishing, Inc., 1987, pp 123–132.

64. Møller AR: Neuromonitoring in operations in the skull base. *Keio J Med* 40:151–159, 1991.

65. Lanser MJ, Jackler RK, Yingling CD: Regional monitoring of lower (ninth through twelfth) cranial nerves, in Kartush JM, Bouchard KR (eds): *Neuromonitoring in Otology and Head and Neck Surgery.* New York, Raven Press, 1992, pp 131–150.

66. National Institutes of Health (NIH) Consensus Development Conference (held December 11–13, 1991): *Consensus Statement* 9:1–24, 1991.

67. Rand RW, Kurze TL: Facial nerve preservation by posterior fossa transmeatal microdissection in total removal of acoustic tumours. *J Neurol Neurosurg Psychiatry* 28:311–316, 1965.

68. Hilger J: Facial nerve stimulator. *Trans Am Acad Ophthalmol Otolaryngol* 68:74–76, 1964.

69. Jako G: Facial nerve monitor. *Trans Am Acad Ophthalmol Otolaryngol* 69:340–342, 1965.

70. Møller AR, Jannetta PJ: Synkinesis in hemifacial spasm: Results of recording intracranially from the facial nerve. *Experientia* 41:415–417, 1985.

71. Babin RW, Jai HR, McCabe BF: Bipolar localization of the facial nerve in the internal auditory canal, in Graham MD, House WF (eds): *Disorders of the Facial Nerve: Anatomy, Diagnosis, and Management.* New York, Raven Press, 1982, pp 3–5.

72. Shibuya M, Mutsuga N, Suzuki Y, et al: A newly designed nerve monitor for microneurosurgery: Bipolar constant current nerve stimulator and movement detector with pressure sensor. *Acta Neurochir (Wien)* 125:173–176, 1993.

73. Prass RL, Lueders H: Constant-current versus constant-voltage stimulation. *J Neurosurg* 62:622–623, 1985.

74. Møller AR, Jannetta PJ: Monitoring of facial nerve function during removal of acoustic tumor. *Am J Otol* November Suppl:27–29, 1985.

75. Delgado TE, Buchheit WA, Rosenholtz HR, et al: Intraoperative monitoring of facial muscle evoked responses obtained by intracranial stimulation of the facial nerve: A more accurate technique for facial nerve dissection. *J Neurosurg* 4:418–421, 1979.

76. Daube JR, Harper CM: Surgical monitoring of cranial and peripheral nerves, in Desmedt JE (ed): *Neuromonitoring in Surgery.* Amsterdam, Elsevier Science Publishers, 1989, pp 115–138.

77. Prass R: Intraoperative electromyographic recording, in Kartush JM, Bouchard KR (eds): *Neuromonitoring in Otology and Head and Neck Surgery.* New York, Raven Press, 1992, pp 81–97.

78. Howe JF, Loeser JD, Calvin WH: Mechanosensitivity of dorsal root ganglia and chronically injured axons: A physiological basis for the radicular pain of nerve root compression. *Pain* 3:25–41, 1977.

79. Beck DL, Aitkins JS, Benecke JE, et al: Intraoperative facial nerve monitoring: Prognostic aspects during acoustic tumor removal. *Otolaryngol Head Neck Surg* 104:780–782, 1991.

80. Goldstein MH: A statistical model for interpreting neuroelectric responses. *Inf Contr* 3:1–17, 1960.

81. Sekiya T, Hatayama T, Iwabuchi T, et al: A ring electrode to record extraocular muscle activities during skull base surgery. *Acta Neurochir (Wien)* 117:66–69, 1992.

82. Beck DL, Maves MD: Recurrent laryngeal nerve monitoring during thyroid surgery, in Kartush JM, Bouchard KR (eds): *Neuromonitoring in Otology and Head and Neck Surgery*. New York, Raven Press, 1992, pp 151–162.
83. Schwartz DM, Rosenberg SE: Facial nerve monitoring during parotidectomy, in Kartush JM, Bouchard KR (eds): *Neuromonitoring in Otology and Head and Neck Surgery*. New York, Raven Press, 1992, pp 121–130.

Advances in Neck Dissection

Jesus E. Medina, M.D.

Professor and Chairman, Department of Otorhinolaryngology, University of Oklahoma Health Sciences Center, Oklahoma City, Oklahoma

John R. Houck, M.D.

Associate Professor, Department of Otorhinolaryngology, University of Oklahoma Health Sciences Center, Oklahoma City, Oklahoma

S urgical removal of regional lymph nodes has been a major component in the treatment of patients with cancer of the head and neck region. The concept that only a radical removal of the lymph-node–bearing tissues and adjacent neck structures was appropriate in patients with head and neck cancer has prevailed since the beginning of the century; this concept has been contested during the past few decades. During the 1970s the stage was set, according to Byers, for a "conceptual revolution in the surgical treatment of cervical metastases from squamous carcinoma of the head and neck."[1] Since then attitudes have shifted. The radical neck dissection is no longer used for the surgical treatment of the N0 neck and modifications of the radical operation are more commonly used in patients with palpable metastases. Responsible for these changes have been the realizations that the distribution of lymphatic drainage is not the same for all regions of the head and neck, and that removal of the lymph-node–bearing tissues of the neck without removing the sternocleidomastoid muscle, the spinal accessory nerve, or the internal jugular vein is oncologically sound. Also, a better understanding of the role of surgery, radiation, and the combination of both has had a significant influence on the evolution of the surgical treatment of the neck in patients with cancer. It is the intent of this monograph to review these advances and their effect on the principles that are currently followed in the surgical treatment of the neck in patients with head and neck cancer.

STANDARDIZATION OF NOMENCLATURE

An important recent advance in the area of neck dissection has been the classification of neck dissections recently put forth by the American Academy of Otolaryngology-Head and Neck Surgery, Inc., and the American Society for Head and Neck Surgery.[2] It has brought order to the confusion that existed in the late 1980s, when surgeons were performing different types of neck dissections, typically using diverse names to refer to the same operation. Based, primarily, on the lymph node groups of the neck that are removed and, secondarily, on the anatomic structures that may be preserved, such as the spinal accessory nerve and the internal

Advances in Otolaryngology—Head and Neck Surgery®, vol. 9
© 1995, Mosby–Year Book, Inc.

jugular vein, this classification groups neck dissections in four categories: radical, modified radical, selective, and extended (Table 1).

The *radical neck dissection* consists of the removal of all five lymph node groups of one side of the neck including the sternocleidomastoid muscle, the internal jugular vein, and the spinal accessory nerve.

The *modified radical neck dissection* category includes those modifications of the radical neck dissection that were developed with the intention of reducing the morbidity of this operation by preserving one or more of the following structures: the spinal accessory nerve, the internal jugular vein, or the sternocleidomastoid muscle. Like the radical neck dissection, the modified radical neck dissections remove all five nodal groups in one side of the neck. The three neck dissections that can be included in this category differ from each other only in the number of neural, vascular, and muscular structures that are preserved. Therefore, Medina suggested subclassifying these neck dissections into a Type I in which only "one" structure, the spinal accessory nerve, is preserved; Type II in which "two" structures, the spinal accessory nerve and the internal jugular vein, are preserved; and Type III in which all "three" structures, the spinal accessory nerve, the internal jugular vein, and the sternocleidomastoid muscle are preserved.[3]

The *selective neck dissection* consists of the removal of only the lymph node groups that are at highest risk of containing metastases, according to the location of the primary tumor; the spinal accessory nerve, the internal jugular vein, and the sternocleidomastoid muscle are preserved. There are four different neck dissections that can be included in this category:

1. The "lateral neck dissection," in which the lymph node groups removed are groups II, III, and IV
2. The "supraomohyoid neck dissection," in which the lymph node groups removed are group I, II, and III
3. The "posterolateral neck dissection," in which the suboccipital and retroauricular nodes are removed in addition to lymph node groups II, III, IV, and V

TABLE 1.
Classification of Neck Dissections

Radical
Modified radical
Type I
Type II
Type III
Selective
Lateral
Supraomohyoid
Posterolateral
Anterior
Extended

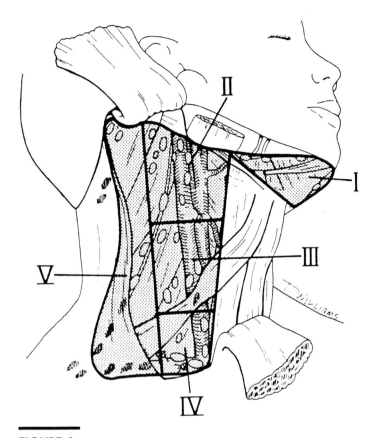

FIGURE 1.
Diagrammatic division of the lymph nodes of the neck, in groups, or levels, I to V.

4. The "anterior neck dissection," which consists of the removal of the pretracheal and paratracheal nodes.

The term *extended neck dissection* is used, in addition to any of the above designations, when a given neck dissection is "extended" to include either lymph node groups or structures of the neck that are not routinely removed, such as the retropharyngeal nodes or the carotid artery. Fundamental to this classification is the acceptance of a uniform nomenclature for the lymph node groups of the neck. The diagrammatic division of the lymph nodes of the neck in groups or levels I through V is ideal for this purpose (Fig 1).

ADVANCES IN THE TREATMENT OF THE N0 NECK

ADVANCES IN PREOPERATIVE EVALUATION

The likelihood of survival of patients with squamous cell carcinoma of the head and neck decreases by at least one-half when palpable lymph node metastases are present, particularly when the tumor involves multiple lymph nodes and extends beyond the nodal capsule.[4-7] The prognostic impact of occult, i.e., nonpalpable, nodal metastases in the neck clinically staged N0, is less clear.[8-11] However, extracapsular spread of tumor (ECS) has recently been shown to occur in nonpalpable lymph nodes. Furthermore, the number of nodes involved by tumor and their location in the N0 neck also has a distinct bearing on prognosis. For instance, Kalnins and associates found that patients with squamous cell carcinoma of the oral cavity and uninvolved neck nodes had a 75% 5-year survival rate.[12] The survival rate decreased to 49% when one node was histopathologically involved, to 30% when two nodes were involved, and to 13% when three or more nodes were involved by tumor. Similar observations have been reported by other clinicians.[14-17]

It is imperative, therefore, to assess the status of the lymph nodes when the likelihood of occult metastases is reasonably high. To date, reliable assessment of the status of the lymph nodes in the N0 neck requires histopathological examination of the lymph nodes surgically removed by means of a neck dissection. Ideally, a neck dissection would be performed only when occult metastases are present. Unfortunately, the accuracy of palpation in the detection of cervical lymph node metastases is often hampered by normal structures, such as a tortuous carotid and the transverse process of the second cervical vertebra, the patient's body habitus, and previous treatment to the neck with surgery or radiation therapy. It is not surprising that the reported error rate in assessing the presence or absence of cervical lymph node metastases by palpation ranges from 20% to 51%.[18-20] Reported false-negative rates vary between 0% and 77%, averaging 20% to 40%. False-positive rates of up to 35% have been reported.[21]

Hopes that recent advances in imaging technology would allow restricting elective neck dissections to only those patients in whom occult metastases are certain, or at least highly probable, have not materialized. Computed tomography (CT), magnetic resonance imaging (MRI), and ultrasonography (US) have a higher sensitivity and specificity than clinical examination in the detection of lymph nodes larger than 1 or 1.5 cm in diameter.[22-24] Multidirectional US scanning can now easily depict lymph nodes as small as 3 mm in diameter, a level of resolution better than that of CT. However, neither of these techniques can distinguish reactive enlargement of a node from metastatic deposits. Although there is a correlation between the size of a lymph node and the probability of it containing metastasis, not all enlarged lymph nodes contain metastatic deposits. Equally important is the observation that in patients with head and neck cancer, a large number of nodes that are found to contain metastatic tumor measure less than 1 cm.[25] Furthermore, even the presence of a central area of lucency within a node shown on CT, which was once considered pathognomonic of tumor necrosis within a node,[26] can be mimicked by an artery with plaque formation or a fatty inclusion in a lymph node.[24]

Ultrasonically directed fine needle biopsy of neck nodes appears promising for a better preoperative evaluation of the N0 neck.[27] Material for cytopathological examination can be obtained from lymph nodes with a minimal axial diameter of 3 mm. In a recent study, van den Brekel and co-workers found that positive cytopathology in a random sampling of the nodes at highest risk was always associated with histologically proven metastases (25/25 cases). However, negative cytopathology was reported in 8 (17.7%) of 45 histologically positive nodes.[28]

ADVANCES IN SURGICAL TREATMENT

One of the most consequential recent advances in the surgical treatment of the N0 neck has been the development and acceptance of the concept of selective neck dissection. As a result, the radical and modified radical neck dissections are no longer indicated in the treatment of the N0 neck. Unlike these operations, which remove all lymph node groups in one side of the neck, the selective neck dissections remove en bloc only the lymph node groups that are most likely to contain metastases, depending upon the location of the primary tumor.

These neck dissections are predicated on the basis of the following observations:

1. Anatomic and radiographic studies of the lymphatics of the head and neck have demonstrated that the lymphatic drainage of this region follows predictable pathways.[29, 30]
2. Multiple clinical studies have demonstrated that the distribution of cervical lymph node metastases is indeed predictable in patients with previously untreated squamous cell carcinoma of the upper aerodigestive tract.[31–33]
3. En bloc removal of only the lymph node groups at highest risk of harboring metastases appears to have the same therapeutic value and provide the surgeon with the same "staging" information as the more extensive radical and modified radical neck dissections.[34–36]
4. The morbidity associated with these operations is minimal and potentially reversible.[37, 38]

There are four operations in this category of neck dissections:

The *lateral neck dissection* consists of the en bloc removal of nodal regions II, III, and IV (Fig 2). It is now indicated in patients with tumors of the larynx, oropharynx, and hypopharynx staged T2-T4, N0. Because the lymphatic drainage of these regions is such that metastases are frequently bilateral, the operation is often done on both sides of the neck.

The *supraomohyoid neck dissection* consists of the en bloc removal of nodal regions I, II, and III (Fig 3). It is the preferred procedure for the surgical management of patients with squamous cell carcinoma of the oral cavity staged T2-T4, N0. The procedure is performed in both sides of the neck in patients with cancers of the anterior tongue and floor of the mouth. This type of dissection is performed when an elective neck dissection is indicated in the management of patients who have squamous cell carcinoma of the lip or skin of the mid-portion of the face. A bilateral dissection is performed when the lesion is located at or near the midline. Using the supraomohyoid and the lateral neck dissections in this manner, the rate of recurrence in the neck, in a prospective analysis of our practice, ranged from zero when the nodes removed were histologically negative to 12.5% when there were multiple positive nodes or extracapsular spread.[39] Similar results have been reported by Byers[36] (5% to 15%) and Spiro[34] (5% to 21%). In a more recent prospective study, a recurrence in the neck following supraomohyoid neck dissection occurred in 4 (11.7%) of 34 patients with T1-T2 squamous cell carcinomas of the oral cavity.[40]

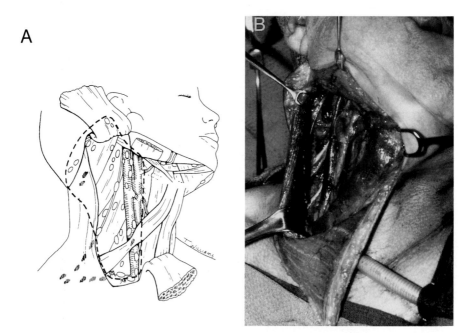

FIGURE 2.

A, diagrammatic photograph of lateral neck dissection. **B,** intraoperative photograph of lateral neck dissection.

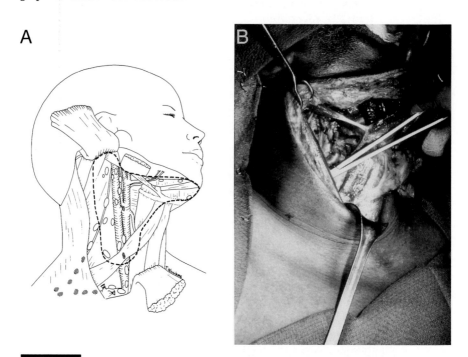

FIGURE 3.

A, diagrammatic photograph of supraomohyoid neck dissection. **B,** intraoperative photograph of supraomohyoid neck dissection. Tip of clamp marks posterior extent of the dissection.

A

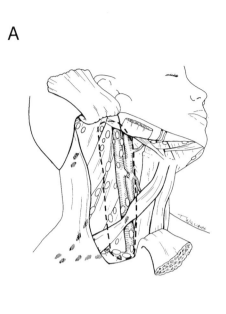

B

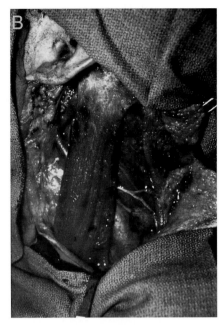

FIGURE 4.

A, diagrammatic photograph of posterolateral neck dissection. **B,** intraoperative photograph of posterolateral neck dissection.

The *posterolateral neck dissection* consists of the removal of the suboccipital and retroauricular lymph node groups and nodal regions II, III, IV, and V (Fig 4). It is indicated in the treatment of melanomas, squamous cell carcinomas, or other skin tumors with metastatic potential such as the Merckle cell carcinomas that originate in the posterior and posterolateral aspects of the neck and the occipital scalp. It is rarely indicated in the treatment of squamous cell carcinoma of the upper aerodigestive tract.

The *anterior compartment dissection* consists of the removal of the pretracheal and paratracheal lymph nodes (Fig 5). It is indicated as part of the surgical treatment of tumors of the thyroid, subglottic larynx, trachea, and cervical esophagus.

ADVANCES IN THE SURGICAL TREATMENT OF THE N+ NECK

With few exceptions, surgery continues to be the mainstay in the treatment of patients with palpable cervical lymph node metastases. Interestingly, several notable advances have occurred in the surgical treatment of these patients in recent years.

ADVANCES IN PREOPERATIVE EVALUATION

Preoperative assessment of the resectability of extensive metastases in the neck has been enhanced by CT and MRI. This technology has enabled surgeons to define more clearly the relationship of a metastatic tumor to critical structures, such as the common and the internal carotid arteries,

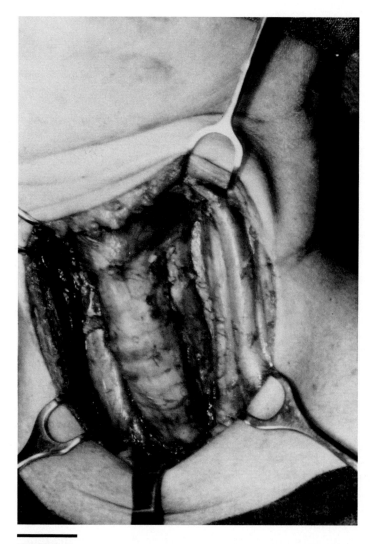

FIGURE 5.
Intraoperative photograph of anterior compartment dissection and total thyroidectomy.

the cervical spine and the vertebral artery, and the brachial plexus. The advantages of having such information in advance are obvious, particularly when tumor involvement of the common or the internal carotid artery is suspected. In that case it is desirable to assess accurately the structural and functional status of the contralateral carotid and the collateral intracerebral circulation. Angiography is now routinely complemented by measuring carotid back-pressure and using balloon occlusion techniques, while monitoring the patient for evidence of neurological deficits under normotensive and hypotensive conditions.[41]

ADVANCES IN SURGICAL TREATMENT

The surgical treament of the N+ neck is quickly becoming a matter of surgical judgement as more surgeons accept the premise that it is surgically feasible and oncologically sound to remove lymph nodes obviously involved by tumor, with the surrounding fibrofatty tissue of the neck, and without removing important uninvolved structures, such as the spinal accessory nerve. In addition, with the judicious combination of surgery and radiation therapy, excellent tumor control in the neck can be obtained while preserving function and cosmesis.[36] It cannot be overemphasized, however, that the main goal of the neck dissection is to *adequately* remove the tumor in the neck and that radiation therapy does not compensate for poor surgical judgement and technique. Preservation of adjacent structures should be pursued *only* when a clearly identifiable plane exists between the tumor and such structure. Creation of a plane by cutting into the tumor and tumor spillage must be avoided. It should also be emphasized that the timing and dose of radiation therapy are crucial, if good regional control is to be achieved. Based on the results of a recent prospective clinical trial, it is recommended that patients with advanced head and neck cancer treated with daily fractions of 1.8 Gy, receive a minimum postoperative dose of 57.6 Gy to the entire operative bed. Sites of increased risk for recurrence, such as areas of the neck where ECS of tumor was found, should be boosted to 63 Gy. Radiation therapy should be started as soon as possible after surgery.[42] Other studies have suggested that a delay in the initiation of radiotherapy beyond 6 weeks may compromise tumor control.[43]

In patients with stage N1 disease, the results obtained with the selective neck dissections when the node is less than 3 cm in diameter, is mobile and, particularly, if it is located in the first echelon of lymphatic drainage, are outlined in Table 2. For more advanced nodal metastases the rates of tumor control in the neck reported with the modifications of the radical neck dissection are shown in Table 3. These results appear to be comparable to those obtained with the radical neck dissection. Andersen and associates have recently reviewed the results of 378 neck dissections performed in 366 patients with clinically and pathologically positive nodal metastases from squamous cell carcinoma of the upper aerodigestive tract.[44] The study compared survival and tumor recurrence in the neck in patients who had radical neck dissection to those who had modified radical neck dissection with preservation of the spinal accessory nerve. The authors found that preservation of the spinal accessory

TABLE 2.

Recurrence Rates in the N1 Neck After Selective Neck Dissection*

Neck Dissection		Neck Recurrence (%)		
Type	Total	Surgery	Surgery + xRT	Other
Supraomohyoid	92	10/44 (23)	13/46 (28)	1/2 (50)
Lateral	26	3/8 (38)	2/18 (11)	
Total	118	13/52 (25)	15/64 (23)	1/2 (50)

*Data from Byers, R: The MD Anderson Experience, 1994. Unpublished information.
xRT = radiation therapy.

TABLE 3.

Range of Reported Recurrence Rates in the Neck After
Modified Radical Neck Dissection

Neck Dissection Type	Author	Recurrence (%)
Type I	Skolnik et al.[51]	0
	Pearlman et al.[52]	20
Type III	Molinari et al.[53]	3.7
	Bocca et al.[54]	30.4

nerve does not affect survival and tumor control in the neck (Table 4).
Interestingly, the pattern of failure in the neck was similar for the two
operations.

The extent of the tumor in the neck may dictate the need to extend
the neck dissection to include structures that are not routinely removed
by this operation, such as the hypoglossal nerve, the carotid, the overlying skin, and others. Unfortunately, at the time of this writing the controversy about the advisability of resecting the common or the internal carotid artery has not been resolved. Even in 1994, some surgeons feel that
carotid resection in patients with advanced squamous cell carcinoma of
the neck does not improve long-term survival,[45] even though improved
techniques for vascular and soft tissue reconstruction have made it possible to resect the carotid with acceptable morbidity rates.[46, 47]

TREATMENT OF ADVANCED NECK METASTASES WITH A SMALL PRIMARY TUMOR

The results of a therapeutic approach that may represent an advancement
in the treatment of neck metastases with a small primary tumor have been
reported recently. Treatment of these patients, who frequently have a carcinoma of the oropharynx of hypopharynx, has traditionally consisted of
either excision of the primary tumor, concomitant neck dissection and
postoperative irradiation, or radiation therapy to the primary tumor and
the neck followed by neck dissection 4 to 6 weeks later. The second ap-

TABLE 4.

Modified Radical Neck Dissection With Preservation of the XI Nerve: Results in
the Clinically Positive Neck*

	N	Postop xRT	5-Year Survival	Neck Recurrence
Radical	234	83.8%	62.7%	12.0%
Modified radical	132	93.2%	70.6%	8.1%

*Modified from Andersen PE, et al: Annual Meeting of the Society of Head and Neck Surgeons,
Paris, France, May 11, 1994.
Postop = postoperative; xRT = radiation therapy.

proach is preferred by some surgeons because the primary tumor is small and is usually located in an area where preservation of function is more likely with radiation, such as the soft palate, base of the tongue, or hypopharynx. It has, however, two significant drawbacks: the uncertainty of tumor control at the primary site 4 to 6 weeks after completion of radiation therapy, and the intraoperative and postoperative consequences of the effects of radiation on tissue planes and healing. In search for a better treatment solution, the surgeons at the M.D. Anderson Tumor Institute have performed, in selected patients, a neck dissection first and then radiotherapy: postoperative to the neck and definitive to the primary tumor.[48] They recently reported their results in a group of 35 patients with previously untreated stage IV squamous cell carcinoma of the upper aerodigestive tract with advanced neck disease (median size 5 cm × 4 cm) and primary tumors thought to be amenable to treatment by radiotherapy. Recurrence of tumor in the neck occurred in only 11% of the patients, and the overall 5-year survival rate was 55%. Using a similar treatment protocol in 65 patients with tumors of the larynx and hypopharynx, the French Head and Neck Study Group observed a rate of recurrence in the neck of 4.6%.[49]

It should be noted that successful application of this treatment strategy requires careful assessment of the resectability of the tumor in the neck, and a meticulous surgical technique in order to avoid complications that may delay the initiation of radiation therapy. It also requires a commitment on the part of the radiation oncologist to begin therapy only a few days after the neck dissection. In fact, in this study,[48] a delay in the start of radiation therapy of more than 2 weeks was associated with a significant decrease in survival ($P < .01$).

REFERENCES

1. Byers RM, Wolf PF, Shallenberger R: Indications for modified neck dissection in squamous cancer of the neck, in Larson, Ballantyne, Guillamondegui (eds): *Cancer in the Neck*. New York, Macmillan Publishing, 1986, pp 127–132.
2. Robins KT, Medina JE, Wolfe GT, et al: Standardizing neck dissection terminology. *Arch Otolaryngol Head Neck Surg* 117:604–605, 1991.
3. Medina JE: A rational classification of neck dissections. *Otolaryngol Head Neck Surg* 100:169–176, 1989.
4. O'Brien CJ, Smith JW, Soong SJ, et al: Neck dissection with and without radiotherapy—prognostic factors, patterns of recurrence and survival. *Am J Surg* 152:456–463, 1986.
5. Shah JP, Cendon RA, Farr HW, et al: Carcinoma of the oral cavity: Factors affecting treatment failure at the primary site and neck. *Am J Surg* 132:504–507, 1976.
6. Spiro RH, Alfonso AE, Farr HW, et al: Cervical node metastasis from epidermoid carcinoma of the oral cavity and oropharynx. A critical assessment of current staging. *Am J Surg* 128:562–567, 1974.
7. Whitehurst JO, Droulias CA: Surgical treatment of squamous cell carcinoma of the oral tongue. *Arch Otolaryngol Head Neck Surg* 103:212–215, 1977.
8. Mendelson BC, Woods JE, Beahrs OH: Neck dissection in the treatment of carcinoma of the anterior two thirds of the tongue. *Surg Gynecol Obstet* 143:75–80, 1976.

9. Shah JP, Tollefsen HR: Epidermoid carcinoma of the supraglottic larynx. *Am J Surg* 128:494–500, 1974.
10. Spiro RH, Alfonso AE, Farr HW, et al: Cervical lymph node metastases from epidermoid carcinoma of the oral cavity and oropharynx. *Am J Surg* 128:562–567, 1974.
11. Tulenko J, Priore RL, Hoffmeister FS: Cancer of the tongue. *Am J Surg* 112:562–568, 1966.
12. Kalnins IK, Leonard AG, Sako K, et al: Correlation between prognosis and degree of lymph node involvement in carcinoma of the oral cavity. *Am J Surg* 134:450–454, 1977.
13. Deleted in proof.
14. Fall HW, Goldfarb PM, Farr CW: Epidermoid carcinoma of the mouth and pharynx at Memorial Sloan Kettering Cancer Center 1965–1969. *Am J Surg* 140:563–567, 1980.
15. DeSanto LW, Holt JJ, Beahrs OH, et al: Neck dissection: Is it worthwhile? *Laryngoscope* 92:502–509, 1982.
16. Callery CS, Spiro RH, Strong EW: Changing trends in squamous carcinoma of the tongue. *Am J Surg* 148:449–454, 1984.
17. Shaha AR, Spiro RH, Shah JP, et al: Squamous carcinoma of the floor of the mouth. *Am J Surg* 148:455–459, 1984.
18. Sako K, Pradier RN, Marchetta FC, et al: Fallibility of palpation in the diagnosis of metastases to cervical lymph nodes. *Surg Gynecol Obstet*, 118:989–990, 1964.
19. Medina JE, Johnson D: Selective neck dissection. Presented at the 33rd Annual Meeting of the American Society for Head and Neck Surgery, May 7–9, 1991. Hyatt Regency Waikoloa, Hawaii.
20. Southwick HW: Elective neck dissection for intraoral cancer. *Arch Surg* 80:905–909, 1960.
21. Bocca E, Calearo C, de Vincentiis I, et al: Occult metastases in cancer of the larynx and their relationship to clinical and histological aspects of the primary tumor: A four year multicentric research. *Laryngoscope* 94:1086–1090, 1984.
22. Friedman M, Shelton VK, Mafee MM: Metastatic neck disease: Evaluation by CT. *Arch Otolaryngol Head Neck Surg* 110:443, 1984.
23. Friedman M, Mafee MM, Pacella BL, et al: Rationale for elective neck dissection in 1989. *Laryngoscope* 100:54–59, 1990.
24. Close L, Merkel M, Vuitch MF, et al: CT evaluation for regional lymph node involvement cancer of oral cavity and oropharynx. *Head Neck Surg* 11:309–317, 1989.
25. Cachin, Y: Management of cervical nodes in head and neck cancer, in Evans PH, Robin PE, Fielding JW (eds): *Head and Neck Cancer.* New York, Alan R. Liss, 1983.
26. Mancuso A, Hanafee WN: *Computed Tomography and Magnetic Resonance Imaging of the Head and Neck,* second edition. Baltimore, Williams & Wilkins, 1985, p 185.
27. van den Brekel MW, Castelijns JA, Stel HV, et al: Modern imaging techniques and ultrasound guided aspiration cytology for the assessment of neck node metastases: A prospective comparative study. *Eur Arch Otorhinolaryngol* 250:11–17, 1993.
28. van den Brekel MWM, Stel HV, Castelijns JA, et al: Lymph node staging in patients with clinically negative neck examinations by ultrasound and ultrasound guided aspiration cytology. *Am J Surg* 162:362–366, 1991.
29. Rouviere H: *Anatomy of the Human Lymphatic System.* Ann Arbor, Michigan, Edward Brothers, 1938.

30. Fisch UP, Sigel ME: Cervical lymphatic system as visualized by lymphography. *Ann Otol Rhinol Laryngol* 73:869–882, 1964.
31. Linberg R: Distribution of cervical lymph node metastases from squamous cell carcinoma of the upper respiratory and digestive tracts. *Cancer* 29:1446–1449, 1972.
32. Skolnik EM: The posterior triangle in radical neck surgery. *Arch Otol* 102:1–4, 1976.
33. Shah JP: Patterns of cervical lymph node metastasis from squamous carcinomas of the upper aerodigestive tract. *Am J Surg* 160:405–409, 1990.
34. Spiro JD, Spiro RH, Shah JP: Critical assessment of supraomohyoid neck dissection. *Am J Surg* 156:286–289, 1988.
35. Medina JE, Byers RM: Supraomohyoid neck dissection: Rationale, indications and surgical technique. *Head Neck Surg* 11:111–122, 1989.
36. Byers RM: Modified neck dissection. A study of 967 cases from 1970 to 1980. *Am J Surg* 150:414–421, 1986.
37. Sobol S, Jensen C, Sawyer W II, et al: Objective comparison of physical dysfunction after neck dissection. *Am J Surg* 150:503–509, 1985.
38. Remmler D, Byers RM, Scheetz J, et al: A prospective study of shoulder disability resulting from radical and modified neck dissections. *Head Neck Surg* 8:280–286, 1986.
39. Medina JM: The role of the neck dissection in the treatment of the neck, in Johnson J, Didolkar M (eds): *Head and Neck Surgery*. New York, Elsevier Publishing, 1993.
40. Kligerman J, Lima RA, Soares JR, et al: Supraomohyoid neck dissection in the treatment of T1/T2 squamous cell carcinoma of the oral cavity: A prospective study of 67 cases. Presented at the Annual Meeting of the Society of Head and Neck Surgeons, Paris, France, May 11, 1994.
41. De Vries EJ, Sekhar LN, Janecka IP, et al: Elective resection of the internal carotid artery without reconstruction. *Laryngoscope* 98:960–966, 1988.
42. Peters LJ, Goepfert H, Kiang Ang K, et al: Evaluation of the dose for postoperative radiation therapy of head and neck cancer: First report of a prospective randomized trial. *Int J Radiat Oncol Biol Phys* 26:3–11, 1993.
43. Vikram B, Strong EW, Shah JP: Failure in the neck following multimodality treatment for advanced head and neck cancer. *Head Neck* 6:724–729, 1984.
44. Andersen PE, Shah JP, Cambronero E, et al: The role of comprehensive neck dissection with preservation of the spinal accessory nerve in the clinically positive neck. Presented at the Annual Meeting of the Society of Head and Neck Surgeons, Paris, France, May 11, 1994.
45. Brennan JA, Jafek BW: Elective carotid artery resection for advanced squamous cell carcinoma of the neck. *Laryngoscope* 104:259–263, 1994.
46. Reilly MK, Perry MO, Netterville JL, Meacham PW: Carotid artery replacement in conjunction with resection of squamous cell carcinoma of the neck: Preliminary results. *J Vasc Surg* 15:324–330, 1992.
47. McIvor NP, Willinsky RA, TerBrugge KG, et al: Validity of test occlusion studies prior to internal carotid artery sacrifice. *Head Neck* 16:11–16, 1994.
48. Byers RM, Clayman GL, Guillamondegui OM, et al: Resection of advanced cervical metastasis prior to definitive radiotherapy for primary squamous carcinomas of the upper aerodigestive tract. *Head Neck* 14:133–138, 1992.
49. French Head and Neck Study Group. Early pharyngolaryngeal carcinomas with palpable nodes. *Am J Surg* 162:377–380, 1991.
50. Byers R: Recurrence rates for the N1 neck after selective neck dissection. The MD Anderson Experience, 1994. Unpublished information.
51. Skolnik EM, Tenta LT, Wineinger DM: Preservation of XI cranial nerve in neck dissection. *Laryngoscope* 77:1304–1314, 1967.

52. Pearlman NW, Meyers AD, Sullivan WG: Modified radical neck dissection for squamous cell carcinoma of the head and neck. *Surg Gynecol Obstet* 154:214–216, 1982.
53. Molinari R, Chiesa F, Cantu G: Retrospective comparison of conservative and radical neck dissection in laryngeal cancer. *Ann Otol* 89:578–581, 1980.
54. Bocca E, Pignataro O, Oldini C: Functional neck dissection: An evaluation and review of 843 cases. *Laryngoscope* 94:942–945, 1984.

Current Role of Chemotherapy in the Management of Head and Neck Cancer

Herbert E. Jacob, M.D.

Assistant Professor of Critical Care Medicine, Department of Anesthesia and Critical Care Medicine; Assistant Professor of Medicine, Division of Medical Oncology, University of Pittsburgh, Pittsburgh Cancer Institute, Pittsburgh, Pennsylvania

INTRODUCTION

Overall, cancer occurring primarily in the head and neck, excluding skin, accounts for 5% of the malignancies diagnosed in the United States yearly. The vast majority of these will be of the squamous cell histology but several other histologies occur in the head and neck region and will be mentioned separately. Of the squamous cell carcinomas, approximately 40% will be early stage lesions (American Joint Commission [AJC] stage I and II). Eighty to 90% of these early stage lesions will be cured with conventional surgery and/or radiotherapy.[1] However, at least 60% of the newly diagnosed cases will present with advanced locoregional disease. Of these, only 10% to 30% (Radiation Therapy Oncology Group [RTOG] stage III A–C, stage IV A–C, stage V) will be alive at 3 years after combined modality treatment.[2] Of this group with advanced disease, 60% to 70% will develop locoregional recurrence, usually within 2 years.[3] Despite local therapy, 20% to 30% will develop distant metastases; even in patients who die with distant metastases, 91% also have evidence of locoregional disease.[4, 5] In spite of significant improvements in diagnosis and surgical treatment, long-term (5-year) survival rates have not significantly improved in the last 30 years[3, 6] and are usually put at 30%.[7–9] Of equal concern is the rate of second primary tumors in patients successfully treated for one head and neck squamous cell cancer, reported to be as high as 40% over 5 to 7 years (or an annual rate of 3% to 7%).[10–14] Therefore, one can see that a significant number of patients presenting with head and neck squamous cell carcinoma will have locoregional recurrence, despite aggressive local treatment, and will ultimately die of their disease. Most investigators agree that the "standard" treatment for locally–advanced-stage, operable head and neck cancer should be surgery followed by radiation therapy. Intensive investigations are currently underway to evaluate other approaches within the context of clinical trials. There have been several excellent recent reviews published on the use of chemotherapy in head and neck squamous cell carcinoma and the reader is also referred to these.[6, 15–17]

Chemotherapy has been used regularly for the last 3 decades in an effort to improve these dismal survival statistics. Despite some very encouraging responses in phase II trials, very few large studies have demonstrated a survival advantage to chemotherapy added to surgery or radiation therapy.[18] I suspect, however, that the best results will ultimately come from close cooperative efforts between head and neck surgeons and medical and radiation oncologists in a multidisciplinary attack on this disease. The efforts of multiple specialists in the disciplines of speech, nutrition, psychosocial, prosthetics, and rehabilitation also make up an integral part of the treatment team.

Like other epithelial malignancies of the upper area digestive tract, there are few presently available chemotherapeutic agents that are active. Newer agents continue to be investigated in phase II trials but the studies (some of which will be reviewed here) are in stages too early to make meaningful comment. There has been a consistent difference found in response rates, depending on whether chemotherapy has been given to previously untreated patients with total response rates (complete response and partial response) in the 50% to 80% range, or to previously treated patients whose response rates are in the 15% to 30% range.[19–23] The reasons for this include compromise of the vascular supply and, thus, compromise of drug delivery in previously treated patients, more resistant tumor clones emerging after previous treatment, and many other explanations.

Since the treatment of relapsed or metastatic disease with chemotherapy is currently palliative and the large phase III trials of combined modality treatments have not yet shown survival benefit for chemotherapy arms, it is important to attempt to sort patients for treatment with the highest likelihood of benefit. Some of the yardsticks by which benefit can be measured include response, duration of response, survival, quality of life, convenience, and toxicity of therapy.

Several factors have been identified as having a role in predicting overall prognosis including continued use of alcohol and tobacco (as it relates to ongoing risk of additional primary tumors), performance status at presentation,[24, 25] stage of the primary tumor with complete response to chemotherapy decreasing as stage increases (i.e., 23% for a T1 lesion and 5% for a T3 or T4 lesion),[26] nodal stage[27] with N3 necks having a 4% complete response rate compared with a 25% complete response noted in N1 necks,[26] overall stage,[28, 29] tumor DNA content,[30] presence of extracapsular spread in regional nodes,[31–34] and the location of the primary tumor,[35, 36] with nasopharynx and larynx primaries having the best outcomes. Several of these factors, in addition to others, also predict for the response to chemotherapy in some studies. These include performance status prior to therapy, site of disease,[37] DNA content, p53 expression,[38] as well as certain immunologic parameters.[39, 40] Performance status has been found by many studies to be a major factor in response to therapy.[24]

Before reviewing the active drugs for squamous cell carcinoma of the head and neck and some basic therapeutic concepts for their use, it is important to generally review the clinical trials by phase. Phase I trials explore the feasability and toxicity of new treatments typically using a dose-escalating method in a heterogenous population of patients. Phase II trials attempt to determine the efficacy of a new therapy in a more homogenous patient population (i.e., only patients with head and neck squamous cell cancer). Phase III trials compare promising regimens or agents from phase II trials in a prospectively randomized fashion against "standard therapy" for a specific patient group (i.e., inoperable squamous cell carcinoma, for example). It is through this process that "standard therapy" is continually tested and hopefully improved. Because the role of chemotherapy in head and neck cancer is still being defined, it is my belief that all patients with head and neck cancer should be viewed from the multidisciplinary perspective. Those patients believed to be candidates for chemotherapy in whatever mode (i.e., adjuvant, palliative, organ preservation, concurrent) should be offered enrollment in clinical trials.

CHEMOTHERAPY OF RELAPSED DISEASE

There are a limited number of well-studied chemotherapeutic agents with activity in this disease. Agents with activity in the 15% to 40% range in relapsed disease when used alone include methotrexate,[41-45] cisplatin,[46-50] bleomycin,[18, 51-53] infusional 5-fluorouracil,[23, 54-56] carboplatin[57-63] and perhaps taxol.[64-67] Of these agents, cisplatin and methotrexate are the most studied and have the highest consistently reported response rates from several trials and different centers. There have been two trials where methotrexate and cisplatin have been compared in a prospective randomized fashion. Hong and colleagues found in 22 patients treated with cisplatin and 20 patients treated with methotrexate, a total response rate (complete and partial) of 29% versus 24%, a response duration of 3.1 months versus 2.8 months, and a survival rate of 6.3 months versus 6.1 months, respectively.[68] Grose and colleagues, in a larger trial (50 patients per arm) presented similar results, although the response rates reported for each agent, 8% for cisplatin and 16% for methotrexate, are lower than usually reported.[69] It is important to note here that methotrexate is, from both a patient and physician perspective, a much better tolerated agent than cisplatin. The ranges of response rates reported are 10% to 35% for methotrexate,[41-43, 59, 70-72] 15% for 5-fluorouracil by infusion,[55] 14% for bleomycin,[52, 53] 14% to 40% for cisplatin,[46-50, 73-76] and 25% for carboplatin.[62] These studies represent meaningful numbers of patients with relapsed disease who were treated. In these studies, however, the response duration for single agent therapy in recurrent disease has ranged from 1.4 months to 7.6 months with a median of 3.8 months and a mean of 4 months. Morton and colleagues reported on a randomized multi-arm trial that included a no treatment arm.[75] Each arm of the trial contained from 22 to 25 patients. The no treatment arm had a survival rate of 2.1 months while the cisplatin arm alone and the cisplatin and bleomycin arm had survival rates of 4.2 months and 4.0 months, respectively. This did represent a statistically significant difference in survival but toxicity of therapy was not directly discussed.

To attempt to improve on these results, several studies over the past decade have compared single agent versus combination chemotherapy in relapsed disease. Response rates for combination chemotherapy have been generally higher using combinations of the above mentioned agents, but few studies have shown a statistically significant difference in response rate and only one study has shown a survival advantage. Campbell and colleagues compared two combinations (cisplatin with 5-fluorouracil and cisplatin with methotrexate) against single agent methotrexate or cisplatin, and showed a statistically significant survival advantage for the cisplatin with 5-fluorouracil over the methotrexate alone (6.7 months versus 2.7 months), but not over cisplatin alone (6.7 months for the combination and 8.7 months for the cisplatin alone).[71] There were 124 total patients treated in this study. When the data from this trial are analyzed, two things may be significant: the first is that the survival duration of patients on the methotrexate arm is shorter (2.7 months) compared with other methotrexate only trials (usually in the 4 month to 6 month range), and second, there were more previously untreated patients in the cisplatin arms. As will be seen when response rates in previously untreated patients are discussed, this may have created an unintended bias towards the combination.

Studies of combinations that have shown a statistically significant increased response rate compared to single agents in recurrent or metastatic disease include those of Clavel, Forastiere and colleagues, and Jacobs and colleagues.[76, 59, 50] Clavel and colleagues, in a randomized trial, compared three groups of patients.[76] Eighty patients treated with cisplatin alone had a 15% response rate compared with 83 patients treated with the combination of cisplatin and 5-fluorouracil who had a 31% response rate (a statistically significant difference). In the same study, the third arm was a multi-drug combination of cisplatin, methotrexate, bleomycin, and vincristine in 87 patients with a 34% response rate. This four drug response rate is not different than the two drug cisplatin and infusional fluorouracil for this study. Jacobs and colleagues showed a higher rate of response and longer time to progression when they compared cisplatin with fluorouracil against cisplatin alone or infusional 5-fluorouracil.[50] Forastiere and the Southwest Oncology Group compared, in relapsed or metastatic disease, three treatments in a prospectively randomized fashion.[59] Eighty-seven patients received cisplatin, 100 mg/m^2 intravenously day 1 with 5-fluorouracil 4,000 mg/m^2 intravenously via a 96-hour infusion every 3 weeks; 86 patients received carboplatin 300 mg/m^2 intravenously day 1 and the same infusional 5-fluorouracil dose every 4 weeks; while 88 patients received methotrexate 40 mg/m^2 intravenously weekly. The total response rates (complete and partial) for the cisplatin with 5-fluorouracil arm was 32%; for the carboplatin with 5-fluorouracil, 21% and for the methotrexate arm, 10%. The response of the cisplatin arm compared to the methotrexate arm reached statistical significance ($p < 0.001$), while the carboplatin with fluorouracil arm compared to methotrexate was of borderline significance ($p = 0.05$). However, as was appropriately pointed out, the hematologic and nonhematologic toxicity of the cisplatin treatment exceeded that of the carboplatin treatment and both were significantly more toxic than the methotrexate arm. Therefore, they concluded that although there was an increased response rate with combination chemotherapy, it was at the expense of higher toxicity. Improvement in overall survival was not shown. Therefore, we still need to look for new treatments with acceptable toxicities to alter the course of recurrent head and neck carcinoma.

Kish and colleagues have reported the highest response rate (74%) with cisplatin and infusional fluorouracil in recurrent disease.[25] Subsequent studies have reported total responses (complete and partial) in the 25% to 70% range with the majority of results in the 30% to 40% level and of these, 15% are complete responses.[20, 77, 78] Additionally, it has been observed that responses to the cisplatin with fluorouracil combination occur early in the treatment course. In the Department of Veterans Affairs cooperative trial for larynx preservation (in previously untreated disease), 85% of responding patients had done so after two cycles of chemotherapy, and after three cycles, 64% had a histologic complete response at the primary.[79] These are similar findings to those of others that most clinical responses in head and neck cancer occur within three courses of cisplatin with infusional fluorouracil treatment.[80–82] Also of relevance to the time to response is an abstract by DiBlasio and colleagues.[83] In a neoadjuvant (chemotherapy first) trial of conventional cisplatinum with infusional fluorouracil, the patients with significant (greater than 80%) partial response after three cycles of chemotherapy went on to complete response if treatment cycles were extended by two before local therapy. Since complete response has been a predictor of prolonged survival, this observation could be tested in a larger phase III trial.

The most common cisplatin with fluorouracil regimen is cisplatin 100 mg/m^2 intravenously day 1 with 5-fluorouracil 1 gm/m^2 continuous infusion for 4 or 5 days every 3 weeks. In patients who have had previous radiation, most investigators give 4-day infusions because of the increased incidence of mucositis in the 5-day group. Despite the increased technical difficulty of infusional 5-fluorouracil (usual need for hospital admission or ambulatory pump), this mode of administration is preferred over bolus 5-fluorouracil because of the higher response rates seen with infusional fluorouracil.[23] This cisplatin dose usually requires admission to the hospital in this patient population for symptom control (acute nausea and vomiting) and forced diuresis in an effort to reduce potential nephrotoxicity of the drug. In terms of the dose of cisplatinum, some work has been done. Similar degrees of activity were seen by Sako and colleagues for doses ranging between 60 mg/m^2 to 120 mg/m^2 delivered every 3 to 4 weeks.[84] Veronesi and colleagues directly compared 60 mg/m^2 with 120 mg/m^2 given every 3 weeks and found no difference in response or survival rates.[49] In this study, the response rates were 10% and 18%, respectively. Additionally, there have been efforts to give cisplatin with fluorouracil in the outpatient setting. Merlano and colleagues reported on an outpatient regimen that gave cisplatin 20 mg/m^2 and fluorouracil 200 mg/m^2 by bolus injection daily for 5 days every 21 days.[85] Their results, in a preliminary study, were a total response rate of 53% in 27 patients treated. Toxicity was manageable, with nephrotoxicity, nausea, and vomiting infrequently seen. Additionally, mild to moderate leukopenia is reported in 60% of patients treated with this combination. Fortunately, severe neutropenic fever and sepsis are unusual as are treatment-related deaths. The other significant expected toxicity alluded to above is mucositis in 40%, but it is usually not of a significant enough grade to require admission for nutritional correction. Other vascular toxicity syndromes, such as Raynaud's phenomenon, cardiac events including ischemia and infarction,[86–88] ototoxicity, and hand-foot syndrome are rare but occur often enough to be considered. There has been little attempt made to vary the delivery of cisplatin doses beyond short infusion. In a nonrandomized neoadjuvant sequential study, Fonseca and colleagues compared three regimens over a 7-year period.[89] Their reported response to conventional cisplatin with fluorouracil, as outlined above, was, in 27 patients, 22% complete response and 48% partial response. The next group, treated between 1986 and 1989, consisted of 79 patients who received cisplatin 25 mg/m^2 with fluorouracil 1,000 mg/m^2, both by continuous infusion daily for 4 days. Here the complete response rate was 49%, the partial response rate was 29%, and the survival was prolonged. This increase in complete response is statistically significant in their historically controlled study. Forastiere and colleagues have documented a pharmacologic advantage of infusional cisplatinum over equivalent bolus doses.[90] Another technique being studied by some investigators is the concept of alternating potentially non–cross resistant or sequential regimens in the hope of increasing complete response rates. Most of this work is being done in patients with unresectable disease.[91–94]

In summary, based on the above information, I agree with Vokes that treatment of recurrent head and neck cancer with methotrexate, cisplatin, infusional 5-fluorouracil, or a combination of cisplatin and infusional fluorouracil is acceptable palliative treatment.[15] This must be based on a response to chemotherapy that translates to an improved quality of life, such that this benefit outweighs the toxicity and hospitalization for treatment. It is for these very reasons that we need to continue an agressive search for more active therapies, particularly for recurrent disease. This can only be done in the context of clinical trials.

With the development of platinum analogs, the use carboplatin has been reported with increased frequency in the treatment of head and neck cancer. Because of the ease of administration and different toxicity profile of this agent compared to that of cisplatin, it has begun to be investigated as a substitute for cisplatinum in a similar fashion as has evolved in the ovarian cancer trials. However, there is reason for caution. In a recently completed Southwest Oncology Group trial in recurrent disease reported by Forastiere and colleagues, the cisplatinum with fluorouracil had a 32% total response rate (5/87 or 6% complete response and 23/87 or 26% partial response rate) and 14/87 or 16% progression on treatment, while the carboplatin with fluorouracil arm demonstrated an overall 21% total response rate (2/86 or 2% complete response and 16/86 or 19% partial response) and 22/86 or 25% progression on treatment.[59] This study was of patients with relapsed or metastatic disease, prospectively randomized and well balanced for known prognostic factors. Nonhematologic toxicities, as previously mentioned, are significantly less with carboplatin. Lopez and colleagues, in a randomized comparison of cisplatinum with fluorouracil versus carboplatin with fluorouracil as neoadjuvant treatment for advanced stage disease preceding radiation therapy in complete responders or surgery in partial responders, showed a statistically significant difference in response rates favoring the cisplatinum with fluorouracil (p < 0.05).[95] In this trial there were 95 evaluable good performance status patients that formed the basis of their results. The nonhematologic toxicities were higher in the cisplatinum group, and the hematologic toxicities were higher in the carboplatin group. For this study, the 5-year actuarial overall and disease-free survival rates for the cisplatinum arm were 45% and 47%, respectively, while for the carboplatin arm they were 24% and 24%, respectively. Both these results are statistically significant (P = 0.02). Both of these studies used meter squared dosing of carboplatinum (300 mg/m^2 and 400 mg/m^2, respectively) and not area under the curve (AUC) carboplatin dosing. Whether a study exploring this dosing approach would show different results is currently unknown, but early phase II work is in progress and will be cited later.

Besides shifting from bolus 5-fluorouracil to infusional fluorouracil, other modifications of the biologic activity of fluorouracil have been explored with the goal of response improvement. From the biochemical perspective, fluorouracil interferes with cellular metabolism in two ways. First, it can be phosphorylated and incorporated into RNA. Second, it can inhibit the enzyme thymidylate synthetase. A metabolite of fluorouracil, 5-FdUMP binds to thymidylate synthetase covalently and, in the presence of reduced folates, forms a stable ternary complex. Since thymidylate synthetase is required for thymidine synthesis, this enzyme inhibition results in depletion of a DNA precursor. This stability of the ternary complex is augmented by an increased availability of reduced folates.[96-98] This biochemistry has been chemically manipulated using leucovorin, hydroxyurea, and interferon.

On the basis of this information and the demonstration, particularly in colorectal cancer, of improved response, Vokes and colleagues evaluated the addition of leucovorum in high dose to cisplatinum with 5-fluorouracil (maximum tolerated dose of fluorouracil was 800 mg/m^2/day for 5 days).[99] In recurrent disease, the total response rate was 56% and mucositis was the dose-limiting toxicity. As induction therapy (in previously untreated patients) this regimen had a 29% complete response rate and a 55% partial response rate for a total response rate of 84%.[100] Lehmann and colleagues, in a small phase II trial comparing cisplatinum with fluorouracil with or without leucovorum showed similar response rates (13% complete, 55% partial) but with significant toxicity (four deaths) in the leucovorin arm.[101] In their study, the cisplatinum with fluorouracil alone arm had a 15% complete response rate and a 50% partial response rate in 24 patients. In a trial in previously untreated patients (where response rates are expected to be higher), Dreyfuss and colleagues found that the addition of leucovorin (500 mg/m^2 continuous infusion daily for 6 days) to 5-fluorouracil (800 mg/m^2 infusion for 24 hours, days 2 to 6) and cisplatin (25 mg/m^2 daily, days 1 to 5) yielded a complete response rate of 66% after three cycles with histologic confirmation of complete response in 75% of these.[29]

Additional mechanisms for fluorouracil enhancement include the use of hydroxyurea which depletes cellular dUMP pools, thus increasing binding of 5-fdUMP to the thymidylate synthetase enzyme.[102] Also, because of the enhancing effects of this compound with ionizing radiation, trials of concurrent radiation and chemotherapy using hydroxyurea are being investigated by Vokes and colleagues.[103] This additive effect of hydroxyurea and radiation has also been initially investigated in small numbers of patients with relapse after irradiation. In two reported pilot studies, the chemotherapy used was infusional fluorouracil in one[104] and bolus fluorouracil in the other.[105] Both studies also gave hydroxyurea concurrently with re-irradiation to tolerance. Mucositis was quite significant (30% grade 3 and 4) in the infusional fluorouracil trial while neutropenia was the predominant dose-limiting toxicity in the bolus fluorouracil trial. Impressive responses were seen in both studies.

Interferon-α has been shown to potentiate both the efficacy and toxicity of fluorouracil in vitro[106] and in vivo[107] in colon cancer. With these observations, Vokes and colleagues[108] have been investigating the addition of interferon-α to cisplatin and fluorouracil with leucovorin. In a group of 70 patients with stage IV disease, without prior therapy, the clinical complete response rate was 51% and the partial response rate was 49% (a total response rate of 99%). This included 46 patients with N2 or N3 neck disease.[108] The toxicity of this induction regimen was quite significant, with severe or life-threatening mucositis in 60% and mylosuppression in 40%. There were four drug-related deaths. The 3-year progression-free survival in this very high risk group was 74%.

In a trial of locoregionally recurrent or metastatic disease, a regimen of cisplatin (20 mg/m^2/day intravenously, days 1 to 4), fluorouracil (750 mg/m^2/day by continuous infusion, days 1 to 4) and interferon-α (9 × 10^6 subcutaneously, days 1, 3, and 5), repeated every 4 weeks, was used.[109] The overall response rate was 24% with only two complete responses and seven partial responses in 40 patients. The median survival rate was 6.5 months. The authors correctly point out that this is no better than the results seen for the combination without interferon-α, although dosing, particularly of cisplatinum, is somewhat different.

Langecker and colleagues have launched a multi-institutional, prospectively randomized trial that compares cisplatin and fluorouracil with or without interferon-α in relapsed (disease-free interval greater than 3 months) and metastatic squamous cell carcinoma. Accrual to this trial has recently closed and should answer the questions of benefit and toxicity of the addition of interferon-α in this setting.

Because the response rate of previously treated patients with recurrent disease is limited both in percentage of response and duration, there is a need to identify new agents or combinations. Ifosfamide with MESNA (uroepithelial protectant) has been reported by several groups in small phase II trials.[91, 110-113] As an example, Cervellino and colleagues, of the GETLAC group, reported on the use of ifosfamide with MESNA in 28 patients, most of whom were previously treated.[110] Their regimen, which could be used on an outpatient basis, yielded a total response rate of 43%, with 14% complete and 29% partial responses. The median survival was greater than 11 months, and the toxicity was acceptable with no significant neurologic or renal toxicity reported.

Taxol, a taxane derivative, from the bark of the western yew *Taxus brevifolia*, is a new drug that represents a new class of mitotic inhibitors that act to promote microtubular assembly and stabilize microtubules. Forastiere and colleagues reported the preliminary results of their phase II trial in recurrent or metastatic inoperable disease.[114] Of the 19 evaluable patients, two complete and seven partial responses were seen. The toxicities were manageable. Several studies are in progress or planned including a comparative study with methotrexate and a combined study with cisplatin, which is currently accruing patients. Taxol is also being studied in relapsed disease in patients previously treated with other chemotherapy.[67] Taxotere has also begun phase II trials.[115] In a preliminary report of 14 presently evaluable patients with recurrent or metastatic disease, two complete responses of 7 and greater than 4 months and three partial responses of 3, 3, and 4 months were seen. The toxicity has principally been neutropenia with 11 admissions for febrile neutropenia. The regimen has been administered on an outpatient basis and accrual is ongoing. Topotecan, a specific inhibitor of topoisomerase-1, has also entered phase II trials in recurrent head and neck cancer, and very preliminary information suggests activity worthy of additional pursuit.[116]

Folate antagonist analogues of methotrexate, 10-ethyl-10 deazaaminopterin (10-EdAM)[117, 118] and Trimethotrexate[119] have also been used in small phase II studies showing comparable responses to methotrexate when used as single agents. Epirubicin, an anthracycline derivative, has been shown to have a total response rate in previously untreated patients (neoadjuvant treatment) of 57% to 63% when combined with other agents and a total response rate in the range of 30% as a single agent.[92, 120, 121] Many other agents have been investigated with response rates typically less than 10%.[4, 122–125]

Because of the relatively poor results seen to date with conventional chemotherapy in recurrent disease, other avenues of investigation have lead to trials of various biologic agents alone or in combination with chemotherapy. Vlock and colleagues have used interferon-α alone in advanced disease with one complete response in 14 patients treated.[126] The combination of interferon-α with cisplatin and 5-fluorouracil has been previously discussed in this review. Interleukin-2 has been administered as a perilesional and intranodal injection alone and in conjunction with concurrent chemoradiotherapy.[127, 128] These represent phase I and II trials with a 66% complete response rate in the concurrent phase II trial in previously untreated patients. Other trials have combined interferon-α and interleukin-2.[129, 130] Other biologic agents and combinations, including tumor necrosis factor and interleukin-1, are undergoing phase I investigation to which patients with recurrent disease have been enrolled and results are awaited.[131]

Through the chemoprevention trials of synthetic and natural retinoids to reverse leukoplakia and reduce the incidence of second primary tumors after successful treatment of the primary, interest has been generated to treat patients with recurrent disease with retinoids.[132–135] Trials of trans-retinoic acid are currently ongoing in this patient population and results are awaited.[136]

In addition to biologics and retinoids, the delivery of chemotherapy other than intravenously has been explored. Now that technical problems of pumps and delivery have been solved, intra-arterial chemotherapy has been investigated on a limited basis.[137] Conceptually, the rationale of infusing a defined tumor supplying vasculature is appealing in a tumor type with a high frequency of local recurrence. However, there is a reluctance to subject patients to local therapies that are technically arduous when response rates have not been shown to be clearly superior to conventional intravenous administration.[138, 139] Two recent reports of small phase II trials of concurrent use of cisplatinum intra-arterially along with external beam irradiation have yielded striking response rates. In one, 13 of 13 patients who received radiation, in addition to cisplatinum, had a complete response.[140] In the other trial, cisplatinum was administered weekly intra-arterially through the tumor nutrient artery concurrently with external beam irradiation. Of the 18 presently evaluable patients, all have had a complete local response.[141] Toxicity in these trials has been acceptable. Interleukin-2 has also been tried in a dose-seeking phase I trial given intra-arterially.[142] Along these lines, investigators at the University of Pittsburgh are evaluating the response and toxicity of concurrent intravenous chemotherapy with brachytherapy in patients with previously heavily treated but locally recurrent disease.[143] Accrual to this trial is ongoing.

NEOADJUVANT CHEMOTHERAPY

Because of the overall poor results of chemotherapy in recurrent disease, the morbidities associated with surgery and radiation, and major issues of quality of life,[144, 145] there has been much work in the past decade with various integrations of chemotherapy, radiation therapy, and surgery (both conventional oncologic surgery, salvage primary surgery, and selective neck dissection).[146, 147] These can be loosely divided into neoadjuvant (induction) chemotherapy preceding definitive surgery or radiation, concurrent chemotherapy and irradiation initially evaluated in locally advanced inoperable but not metastatic disease, and adjuvant chemotherapy given typically before or after radiation but usually following surgery in high risk patients. Neoadjuvant chemotherapy was investigated extensively in the 1980s and has lead to the concept of organ preservation. This is one of the areas of intense interest for this decade.

Contrasted with the 30% total response rates in recurrent disease, multiple studies have demonstrated total response rates of 80% or more with complete response rates as high as 66% in induction or neoadjuvant trials. These dramatic differences in response rates are with the same cisplatin and infusional fluorouracil regimens with or without various modifications (i.e., interferon, leucovorum), as previously discussed.[6, 29, 56, 81, 148, 149] The neoadjuvant studies have also confirmed that locoregional control and survival are the highest in the patients who obtain complete response with the initial chemotherapy.[81, 150–153] Of those with complete clinical responses, 30% to 70% will also be found to have pathologic complete responses at the primary site at rebiopsy or on evaluation of the full surgical specimen from definitive resection.[151, 154, 155] However, the neoadjuvant trials of chemotherapy preceding locoregional treatment have not documented increased survival rates but have demonstrated either a significant reduction or a trend to reduction in distant metastases in the chemotherapy arms.[79, 156, 157] The limitations of these trials[156, 157] have been repeatedly addressed[6, 158] and essentially are that since the response rates, particularly complete response rates (3% to 19%), are lower than those presently reported in cisplatin with fluorouracil combinations, this likely influences the survival results. Even with this, however, the rate of distant metastases was lower in the chemotherapy arm. Several other randomized trials of neoadjuvant chemotherapy included patients with both resectable and unresectable cancer.[159–164] In general, the findings of these studies are similar, i.e., no survival benefit for the chemotherapy arm. The criticisms of these studies included failure to stratify for stage, suboptimal chemotherapy dosing, and differences in the numbers of patients taken to surgery in the groups.[158] The goal of the neoadjuvant studies was to improve survival, which, as mentioned, was not accomplished. However, the responsiveness to chemotherapy of previously untreated patients was demonstrated, and that the patients in the control arms did not do better because of the delays to surgery required by the neoadjuvant chemotherapy was also shown. Additionally, these studies demonstrated that previous chemotherapy did not increase the perioperative complications and also that previously administered chemotherapy did not appreciably reduce the tissue tolerance to radiation therapy.

ORGAN PRESERVATION TRIALS

In the early 1980s, the Wayne State group reported that a response to cisplatin combination predicted for further response to radiation therapy and, conversely, less than partial response to chemotherapy meant poor response to subsequent radiation therapy and poor outcome.[165, 166] This lead to their practice of offering chemotherapy initially to patients who refused surgery for operable lesions, followed by radiation in those who responded and readvising for surgery in partial responders. This same policy had also been reported by Fletcher and colleagues in a single institution phase II trial.[167]

Based on this accumulating information, the focus shifted from attempting to improve survival (which could not be shown in the neoadjuvant trial) to organ preservation. It is intuitively obvious the vital role that the organs of the head and neck play in our everyday function, namely nutrition, communication, and self-image, and thus, the necessary derangements often required by surgical procedures may have an impact on quality of life despite the remarkable advances in reconstructive surgery and rehabilitation.[144, 145]

Jacobs and colleagues reported on a pilot study in 30 patients with resectable stage III and IV disease.[150] The population of this study included those with cancer in multiple sites (oral cavity, n = 11; oropharynx, n = 7; hypopharynx, n = 6; larynx, n = 6). Patients received three courses of cisplatinum with infusional 5-fluorouracil (100 mg/m^2, day 1 and 1,000 mg/m^2 by continuous infusion, days 1 to 5 respectively) every 3 weeks. The first 8 patients received bleomycin instead of fluorouracil during the first chemotherapy cycle. The response rate to chemotherapy was 60% complete clinical response and 30% partial response at the primary site, and a 48% complete clinical response in the nodal disease and 40% partial response in the nodes. Conversely, 17% had either stable or progressive disease in either the primary, or the nodes, or both. Of the 18 patients with complete clinical response, 6 were found to have persistent disease at the primary site at rebiopsy and 2 were found to have disease in the nodal area. The 6 patients with persistent primary disease went on to conventional surgical extirpation, while the 2 with disease only at the nodal site underwent a neck dissection. Thus, 10 patients had surgery eliminated from their treatment plan and they went on to radiation therapy. All patients who either had partial response, no response, or progression after two cycles of chemotherapy, or had residual pathologic disease despite complete clinical response, had conventional extirpative surgery and radiation. Overall survival rates of the patients requiring surgery and those who did not were essentially the same but the numbers are small. Two other nonrandomized studies of organ preservation by induction chemotherapy were reported from France and Michigan.[168, 169] Both confirmed that surgery could be eliminated in some patients who show excellent response to induction chemotherapy. The first large randomized trial of organ preservation, in this case the larynx, has now been reported. This study, done by the Department of Veterans Affairs Laryngeal Cancer Study Group, was a prospectively designed, randomized comparison between neoadjuvant chemotherapy followed by radiation in responders and surgery in nonresponders versus conventional surgery and postoperative radiation in stage III and IV operable squamous cell carcinoma of the larynx.[79] Using neoadjuvant chemotherapy with standard cisplatin with fluorouracil (100 mg/m^2, day 1 and 1,000 mg/m^2 continuous infusion, days 1 to 5, respectively, repeated every 21 days for three cycles in responders), the incidence of complete response after two cycles was 31% and after three cycles was 49%. Responders went on to radiation therapy. The most significant finding in this trial was that survival with a median follow-up period of 33 months was the same in both groups and that 64% of patients assigned to neoadjuvant chemotherapy followed by radiation had the larynx preserved. Of additional interest was that distant metastases were less (11%) in the chemotherapy arm compared to the surgery plus radiation arm (17%). Also of note, over 70% of local and regional recurrences were detected in the first year after therapy and nearly all were discovered within 2 years. If there is any criticism of this study, it would be that there was no radiation only arm so that the precise role of the induction chemotherapy remains somewhat uncertain, particularly in more limited stage disease.

Norris and colleagues have reviewed their ongoing trials over the past decades.[147] Their complete response rate has risen from 26% to 57% as the use of planned primary site ablative surgery fell from 47% to 14%. Survival rates over this period did not change. They have noted some increase in local failure in the nonoperative groups but surgical salvage seems to be effective. The place of post−organ preservation management of regional disease, particularly when bulky nodal disease existed pretreatment, with various neck dissection techniques will also need to be explored.[146] Several other phase II organ sparing trials in advanced resectable disease have been reported preliminarily for sites other than the larynx.[170-175] The chemotherapy used neoadjuvantly in these nonrandomized trials is cisplatin with fluorouracil or carboplatinum with fluorouracil.

The organ preservation trials have had, as a common theme in advanced operable disease, chemotherapy followed sequentially by radiation in responders (the primary site receiving 6,500 cGy to 7,500 cGy and the nodal disease receiving doses varying from 5,000 cGy to 7,500 cGy depending on involvement). Because of the finding of different quantitative responses in the primary and nodal sites, particularly in bulky nodal disease, an evolving role for salvage neck dissection is emerging when there is a pathologic complete response in the primary site but not the neck.[146]

CONCURRENT CHEMO-RADIOTHERAPY

Concurrent chemotherapy and radiation has been used in locally advanced, usually unresectable head and neck cancer since the 1960s.[176, 177] The biologic rationale for combined radiotherapy and chemotherapy has been extensively reviewed by Fu and colleagues and Vokes and colleagues, and the reader is referred to these in-depth, excellent reviews.[178, 179] This treatment has been used in several different carcinomas (anus, pancreas, cervix, small cell lung cancer, and esophagus) besides squamous cell carcinoma of the head and neck. Since several of the drugs with activity in head and neck cancer have in common with radiation mucositis as part of their toxicity profile, this local toxicity has always been a concern in studies of concurrent chemoradiation therapy. Although toxicity can be grade 3 or 4 and require temporary feeding tubes for nutritional and fluid requirements, it has not been, in most studies, dose limiting. There is, however, important work that has been done with symptom control, and research needs to continue.[180] One very provocative report by White and colleagues deserves mention here.[181] In a nonrandomized trial looking at induction therapy with cisplatin with fluorouracil by infusion followed by surgery and radiation, some striking differences in response rates were seen. The first 19 patients in this trial received metoclopramide hydrochloride as part of their antiemetic regimen while the following 21 received droperidol. The response rate to chemotherapy for the first group was 32% and 52% in the second. The 2-year survival rates were 26% and 62%, respectively. The authors wondered if the metabisulfide previously present in commercially available metoclopramide hydrochloride preparations may have inactivated the platin species. Unexpected drug interaction should always be considered in situations where responses are unexpectedly different. In this case, whether this was in fact the cause of the response difference is speculative but is a reminder to consider all aspects of the therapeutic prescription. One of the most novel approaches to symptom control is the potential use of growth factors in an effort to ameliorate mucositis. Results of these studies are presently awaited. A full review of supportive care for mucositis is beyond the scope of this review but represents an extremely important aspect of any trial, particularly those involving concurrent therapy. Additionally, treatment schemes to reduce additive toxicity, which rapidly alternate the chemotherapy and radiation (for example, the Merlano and colleagues trial), are being reported.[182] Here, cisplatin with fluorouracil (20 mg/m^2 daily $\times$ 5 and 200 mg/m^2 daily $\times$ 5 bolus) were given usually on an outpatient basis at weeks 1, 4, 7, and 10, and radiation doses of 10 Gy/week were given at weeks 2 and 3, 5 and 6, and 8 and 9, while the radiation only arm received standard radiation without planned interruptions (10 Gy weekly to a total dose of 70 Gy). With this scheme, rates of grade 3 and 4 mucositis were essentially equivalent in the treatment groups (i.e., 19% in the combined modality group and 18% in the radiation only group). There was a total of 157 patients who were completely evaluable in this trial. Whether the absence of significantly increased mucositis has to do with the scheme of alternating treatment or the way the fluorouracil or cisplatin is delivered is unknown. Mucositis seems to be a significantly greater problem in studies where infusional fluorouracil and large bolus injections of cisplatinum are used concurrently with radiotherapy. Adelstein and colleagues reported grade 3 mucositis in 27 (49%) of the 55 patients treated with cisplatin 75 mg/m^2 day 1 followed by fluorouracil 1 g/m^2 by infusion for 4 days concurrently with radiation 30 Gy in 3 weeks.[183] This was followed by the same chemotherapy beginning day 28 without radiation. Then, after reassessment, a third course of chemotherapy was delivered, day 63 concurrently with radiation (30 Gy to 34 Gy) in 3 weeks. The average weight loss for all patients in this trial was 11.7% of body weight (mean 8.5 kg). There was one presumed fluorouracil cardiotoxic death. In the Merlano study previously discussed, only 3% of patients in the concurrent group and 1% in the radiation only group lost greater than 10% of their body weight and there were no cardiotoxic reactions reported.[182] Although it is difficult to compare these two trials of concurrent therapy, overall survival and complete response percentages seem comparable. An evaluation of response versus toxicity will await the results of prospectively randomized comparisons of specific concurrent treatment strategies.

In addition to the issues of toxicity and how they might relate to quality of life, combined toxicity raises another concern in the concurrent trials. The RTOG in a retrospective review of 426 patients found that patients with prolonged radiation treatment elapsed days, defined as 14 or more days beyond the protocol prescription, exhibited significantly poorer locoregional control and absolute survival.[184] In multivariant analysis, this was found to be an independent risk factor for control and survival. Of course, this analysis was done for radiation alone, but this does raise concerns for concurrent trials. Since mucositis is often the dose-limiting toxicity, the necessary delays in delivery of the radiation, which could be brought about by attempting to maximize the chemotherapy, might lead to an overall compromise of effectiveness of the concurrent program.

These concerns aside, benefit has been suggested by several randomized single-agent trials using fluorouracil, bleomycin, mitomycin, or cisplatin in conjunction with radiation.[185–188] Single-agent cisplatin has recently been reported in organ preservation-like trials with concurrent radiation with complete response rates in excess of 60%.[189, 190] One of these pilot trials by Gaspirini and colleagues included 5 patients with recurrent disease, but in these patients the complete response rate was only 20%.[190] The prior treatment of these patients with recurrence was not mentioned, and the number is too small for significant conclusion, but the contrast in de novo versus recurrent response to the same therapy is nonetheless striking. Carboplatin has also been reported in several phase II concurrent trials of advanced stage unresectable disease with excellent response rates in the range of 60%. Dosing varied from 70 mg/m^2 intravenously daily, days 1 to 5 and 29 to 33 of concurrent radiation;[191, 192] to 30 mg/m^2 intravenous bolus for 5 consecutive days during weeks 1, 3, 5 and 7 of concurrent radiation;[193] to a recommended dose of 100 mg/m^2 weekly during concurrent radiation.[62]

Despite the concerns of additive toxicity, several phase II trials have reported encouraging response in survival data for various combinations of chemotherapy concurrent with radiation.[102, 103, 108, 148, 194–198] Several of these phase II trials are non–cisplatin based. Trials reported by Eskandari and colleagues used concurrent weekly 5-fluorouracil (500 mg/m^2 intravenous bolus at hour 1) with leucovorin (500 mg/m^2 intravenous infusion for 2 hours) during conventional radiation (1.8 Gy/day, 5 days/week × 8 weeks).[199] Grade 3 and 4 mucositis was the dose-limiting toxicity. The complete response rate was 65% and the partial response rate was 19% in a total of 43 patients treated. At 48 months, the overall survival and disease-free survival rates were 31% and 29.5%, respectively. Another non–cisplatin combination has been explored by Vokes and colleagues using 5-fluorouracil with hydroxyurea with concurrent conventional fraction radiation.[103] This combination has also shown significant activity, and in earlier stage patients (stage II and III, as part of an organ preservation effort) showed complete response rate of 92% (23 of 24 evaluable patients) with a 2-year survival rate of 87% ± 7%.

There have been several randomized trials comparing combination chemotherapy with concurrent radiation to induction (neoadjuvant) chemotherapy with the same drugs followed by radiation sequentially. Three trials have demonstrated a disease-free and survival advantage to the concurrent treatment,[200–202] while one trial showed improved overall response in the concurrent arm but similar survival rates despite better regional control in the concurrent group.[203]

A recently reported prospectively randomized comparison between radiation alone and radiation interdigitated with chemotherapy in patients with advanced stage unresectable disease showed complete responses in 42% of the concurrent arm and 22% of the radiation arm (p = 0.037).[182] Median survival for the concurrent arm was 16.5 months and 11.7 months in the radiation only group (p < 0.05) with a 3-year survival rate of 41% and 23%, respectively. Although a significant survival benefit is present for the concurrent group over radiation only, there is still, of course, room for improvement. A smaller trial by Weissler and colleagues also showed a statistically significant disease-free survival rate for the concurrently treated patients with inoperable disease.[204]

Radiation has also been used concurrently with purified natural interferon (6 million units daily for 4 weeks, then thrice weekly for 2 months) and compared to radiation alone in a small number of patients with operable disease.[22] There was no survival benefit seen for the interferon group but there was significant toxicity (mucositis) in this group, which terminated the study.[205]

ADJUVANT CHEMOTHERAPY

The principal role of adjuvant therapy in potentially curable groups of patients is to improve the response to the primary therapeutic intervention (i.e., surgery, radiation, or both). The chemotherapy should irradicate distant micrometastatic disease and offer additive, perhaps synergistic, benefit at the locoregional site to the locoregional treatment. This concept should be tested where the adjuvant chemotherapy is likely to show its greatest benefit; this would be in patients at high risk for recurrence.[27, 30–34] Johnson and colleagues have explored adjuvant chemotherapy (methotrexate and 5-fluorouracil) given subsequent to surgery and radiation in high risk patients.[206, 207] High risk in these trials was defined as extracapsular spread in cervical nodes. In this single arm, nonrandomized trial, the 20-month disease-free survival rate was 66% compared to their historical control of surgery and radiation alone with a 38% survival rate. However, Domenge and colleagues, using combination chemotherapy (cisplatin, methotrexate, and bleomycin every 3 weeks for three cycles followed by five cycles of monthly methotrexate) following surgery and radiation in a prospective randomized trial with a total of 287 patients, were unable to demonstrate a survival benefit for the chemotherapy arm.[208] Entry criteria also required the presence of extracapsular spread. Because of the seemingly disparate results, continued evaluation of adjuvant chemotherapy is ongoing at the University of Pittsburgh and other locations, in high risk patients.

In two very large, prospectively randomized trials of adjuvant chemotherapy, both the Head and Neck Contracts Program and the Intergroup Study 0034, which included advanced but resectable squamous cell carcinoma in 462 and 448 evaluable patients, respectively, showed no difference in survival between the chemotherapy and radiation arms versus the radiation only arm.[156, 209] The incidence of distant metastases was significantly less in the chemotherapy arm of the Intergroup Study and the maintenance chemotherapy arm of the Head and Neck Contracts Program. Of note in the Intergroup Study was that when patients with close surgical margins (less than 5 mm) or in situ carcinoma at the surgical margin were analyzed separately, there was a suggestion that adjuvant chemotherapy improved survival and locoregional control. In the Head and Neck Contracts Program, Jacobs and colleagues reported on several subsets of patients that did demonstrate significantly improved survival on maintenance chemotherapy.[210] The role of adjuvant chemotherapy has yet to be proved in patients with advanced stage operable disease, but prospectively randomized comparison trials are ongoing in high risk groups.

OTHER HISTOLOGIES

Nasopharyngeal carcinoma makes up 2% of all head and neck malignancies but only 0.3% of all malignancies in the United States.[211] This tumor, however, is particularly common among the southern Chinese, and Hong Kong has the highest documented incidence in the world.[212] As a general statement, survival rates for nasopharyngeal carcinoma (NPC) progressively decline with stage when radiation alone is the treatment modality. Ho's survival experience with NPC treated with radiation alone was 84% for stage I, 67% for stage II, 40% for stage III, and 11% for stage IV.[213] Additionally, the presence of nodal disease is associated with a significantly higher rate of distant metastases.[214] Based on this information, the general approach to treatment of early stage NPC is with radiation after biopsy diagnosis and, because the survival rates are poor for advanced disease, the addition of chemotherapy in the advanced disease situation. There have been many agents and combinations used for NPC. Several recent nonrandomized trials in advanced stage disease using cisplatin with infusional 5-fluorouracil preceding radiation, carboplatin with infusional 5-fluorouracil and radiation, doxorubicin and cisplatin with or without bleomycin preceding radiation, and epirubicin with bleomycin and cisplatin preceding radiation have shown complete response rates in the 60% to 94% range and where follow-up is long enough, disease-free survival rates of 70% or more.[215–218] Al-Sarraf and colleagues treated locally advanced NPC with concurrent cisplatin, 100 mg/m^2, days 1, 21, and 42 of radiotherapy.[219] The 89% complete response rate compared favorably with the RTOG database of radiation alone. These results launched the Intergroup randomized trial of radiation with or without cisplatin plus adjuvant cisplatin with 5-fluorouracil. The International Nasopharynx Study Group has recently reported, in abstract form, preliminary results of their large (339 patients) trial of neoadjuvant chemotherapy (bleomycin, 15 mg, intravenous bolus, day 1, and 12 mg/m^2/day continuous infusion, days 1 to 5; epirubicin, 70 mg/m^2, day 1, intravenously; cisplatin, 100 mg/m^2, day 1). Cycles were repeated every 21 days times three, followed by radiotherapy (70 Gy at 2 Gy/day, 5 days/week for 7 weeks) versus radiation alone in WHO type II and III (nonkeratinizing squamous cell, undifferentiated carcinoma).[220] An initial interim analysis reveals an excess of treatment-related deaths in the chemotherapy arm (9% versus 1%) and of radiation refusal (7% versus 1%). However, there is a significant difference in disease-free survival rates favoring the chemotherapy arm (disease-free survival at 3 years 47% versus 30.5%, P < 0.02). No difference in overall survival has yet been seen. Preliminary reports of carboplatin dosing by AUC in previously untreated patients, of Ifosfamide/MESNA in a mixed population of previously treated and untreated patients, and of low-dose 5-fluorouracil continuous infusion in heavily pretreated patients have all been reported with 50%, 45%, and 30% overall response rates, respectively.[221–223] Ethesioneuroblastoma, recurrent or high risk major and minor salivary gland tumors (adenocarcinoma, adenoid cystic carcinoma, mixed malignant tumors), and chordomas have been recently reviewed by the author and the reader is referred to this review.[224]

In summary, I have attempted to review the current literature on the role of chemotherapy for the treatment of squamous cell carcinoma of the head and neck, including nasopharyngeal carcinoma. The present treatment strategies for recurrent and metastatic disease, neoadjuvant chemotherapy prior to planned surgery and as a potential organ sparing strategy, the use of concurrent chemotherapy with radiation initially in inoperable patients, some reports of this as an organ sparing strategy, and the potential risks and benefits of this strategy, and the present role, if any, for adjuvant chemotherapy have all been evaluated. Because of the limited number of patients with this disease, all patients meeting eligibility criteria for treatment on clinical trials should be enrolled and treated on these trials so that meaningful information can be gained to improve the lot of this patient population.

REFERENCES

1. Schantz SP, Harrison LB, Hong WK: Cancer of the head and neck, in DeVita VT, Hellman S, Rosenberg SA (eds): *Cancer: Principles and Practice of Oncology*, Philadelphia: J.B.Lippincott, 1993, p. 574–655.
2. Marcial VA, Pajak TF, Kramer S, et al: Radiation Therapy Oncology Group (RTOG) Studies in Head and Neck Cancer. *Semin Oncol* 15:39–60, 1988.
3. Hong WK: Adjuvant chemotherapy for resectable squamous cell carcinoma of the head and neck. Report on Intergroup Study 0034. *Int J Radiat Oncol Biol Phys* 23:885–886, 1992.
4. Armand JP, Cvitkovic E, Recondo G, et al: Salvage chemotherapy in recurrent head and neck cancer. The Institute Gustave Roussy Experience. *Am J Otolaryngol* 14:301–306, 1993.
5. Kotwall C, Sako K, Razack MS, et al: Metastatic patterns in squamous cell cancer of the head and neck. *Am J Surg* 154:439–442, 1987.
6. Clark JR, Frel E: Chemotherapy for head and neck cancer: Progress and controversy in the management of patients with no disease. *Semin Oncol* 16 (suppl 6):44–57, 1989.
7. Vikram B, Strong EW, Shah JP, et al: Failure at distant sites following multimodality treatment for advanced head and neck cancer. *Head Neck Surg* 6:730–733, 1984.
8. Vikram B, Strong EW, Shah JP: Failure at the primary site following multimodality treatment in advanced head and neck cancer. *Head Neck Surg* 6:720–723, 1984.
9. Vikram B, Strong EW, Shah JP, et al: Failure in the neck following multimodality treatment for advanced head and neck cancer. *Head Neck Surg* 6:724–729, 1984.
10. Hong WK, Lippman SM, Itri LM, et al: Prevention of secondary primary tumors with isotretinoin in squamous cell carcinoma of the head and neck. *N Engl J Med* 323:795–801, 1990.
11. Cooper JS, Pajak TF, Rubin P: Second malignancies in patients who have head and neck cancer: Incidence, effect on survival and implication based on RTOG experience. *Int J Radiat Oncol Biol Phys* 17:449–456, 1989.
12. Parker RG, Enstrom JE: Second primary cancers of the head and neck following treatment of initial primary head and neck cancers. *Int J Radiat Oncol Biol Phys* 14:561–564, 1988.
13. Slaughter DP, Southwick HW, Smejkal W: Field cancerization in oral stratified squamous epithelium. *Cancer* 6:963–968, 1953.
14. Strong MS, Incze J, Vaughan CW: Field cancerization in the aerodigestive tract—its etiology, manifestation, and significance. *J Otolaryngeal Soc* 13:1–6, 1984.
15. Vokes EE, Weichselbaum RR, Lippman SM, et al: Head and neck cancer. *N Engl J Med* 328:184–194, 1993.

16. Vokes EE (ed): *Hematology/Oncology Clinics of North America Head and Neck Cancer*. Philadelphia, W.B. Saunders, 1991.

17. Dimery IW, Hong WK: Overview of combined modality therapies for head and neck cancer. *J Natl Cancer Inst* 85:95–111, 1993.

18. Morton RP, Rugman F, Dorman EB, et al: Cisplatinum and bleomycin for advanced or recurrent squamous cell carcinoma of the head and neck: A randomized factorial phase III controlled trial. *Cancer Chemother Pharmacol* 15:283–289, 1985.

19. Brown AW, Blum J, Bulther WM, et al: Combination chemotherapy with vinblastine, bleomycin and cis-diamminechloroplatinum (II) in squamous cell carcinoma of the head and neck. *Cancer* 45:2830–2835, 1988.

20. Mercier RJ, Neal GD, Mattox DE, et al: Cisplatin and 5-fluorouracil chemotherapy in advanced or recurrent squamous cell carcinoma of the head and neck. *Cancer* 60:2609–2612, 1987.

21. Price LA, Hill BT, Calvert AH, et al: Improved results in combination chemotherapy of head and neck cancer using a kinetically based approach: A randomized study with and without Adriamycin. *Oncology* 35:26–28, 1978.

22. Kish JA, Drelichman A, Jacobs J, et al: Clinical trials of cisplatin and 5-FU infusion as initial treatment for advanced squamous cell carcinoma of the head and neck. *Cancer Treat Rep* 66:471–474, 1982.

23. Kish JA, Ensley JF, Jacobs J, et al: Randomized trial of cisplatin (CACP) and 5-fluorouracil (5-FU) infusion and CACP and 5-FU bolus for recurrent and advanced squamous cell carcinoma of the head and neck. *Cancer* 56:2740–2744, 1985.

24. Amer MH, Al-Sarraf M, Vaitkevicuis VK, et al: Factors that affect response to chemotherapy and survival of patients with advanced head and neck cancer. *Cancer* 43:2203–2206, 1979.

25. Kish JA, Weaver A, Jacobs J: Cisplatin and 5-fluorouracil infusion in patients with recurrent and disseminated epidermoid cancer of the head and neck. *Cancer* 53:1819–1824, 1984.

26. Wolf GT, Makuch RW, Baker SR: Predictive factors for tumor response to peri-operative chemotherapy in patients with squamous cell carcinoma. The Head and Neck Contracts Group. *Cancer* 54:2869–2877, 1984.

27. Leemans CR, Tuiari R, Nauta JP, et al: Regional lymph node involvement and its significance in the development of distant metastases in head and neck carcinoma. *Cancer* 71:452–456, 1993.

28. Cognetti FC, Pinnaro P, Ruggeri EM, et al: Prognostic factors for chemotherapy response and survival using combination chemotherapy as initial treatment of advanced head and neck squamous cell cancer. *J Clin Oncol* 7:829–837, 1989.

29. Dreyfuss AF, Clark JR, Wright JE, et al: Continuous infusion high-dose leucovorin with 5-fluorouracil and cisplatin for untreated stage IV carcinoma of the head and neck. *Ann Intern Med* 112:167–172, 1990.

30. Kokal WA, Gardine RL, Sheibanie K, et al: Tumor DNA content as a prognostic indicator of squamous cell carcinoma of the head and neck region. *Am J Surg* 956:276–280, 1988.

31. Schuller DE, McGuirt WF, McCabe BF, et al: The prognostic significance of metatstatic cervical lymph nodes. *Laryngoscope* 90:557–570, 1980.

32. Johnson JT, Myers EN, Bedetti CD, et al: Cervical lymph node metastases-Incidence and implications of extracapsular carcinoma. *Arch Otolaryngol Head Neck Surg* 111:534–537, 1985.

33. Snyderman NL, Johnson JT, Schramm VL, et al: Extracapsular spread of carcinoma in cervical lymph nodes: Impact upon survival in patients with carcinoma of the supraglottic larynx. *Cancer* 56:1587–1599, 1985.

34. Johnson JT, Barnes L, Myers EN, et al: The extracapsular spread of tumors in cervical node metastases. *Arch Otolaryngol Head Neck Surg* 107:725–729, 1981.

35. Spaulding MB, Vasquez J, Khan A, et al: A non-toxic adjuvant treatment for advanced head and neck cancer. *Arch Otolaryngol Head Neck Surg* 109:789–791, 1983.

36. Hill BT, Price LA, MacRae K: Importance of primary site in assessing chemotherapy response and 7-year survival data in advanced squamous cell carcinomas of the head and neck treated with initial combination chemotherapy without cisplatin. *J Clin Oncol* 4:1340–1347, 1986.

37. Bertino JR, Boston B, Capizzi RL: The role of chemotherapy in the management of cancer of the head and neck: A review. *Cancer* 36:752–758, 1975.

38. Shin DM, Lee JS, Choi G: Prognostic significance of p53 expression in head and neck squamous cell carcinoma. *Proc ASCO* 13:914, 1994.

39. Schantz SP, Savage HE, Racz T, et al: Immunologic determinants of head and neck cancer response to induction chemotherapy. *J Clin Oncol* 7:857–869, 1989.

40. Vlock DR: Immunobiologic aspects of head and neck cancer, in Vokes EE (ed): *Hematology/Oncology Clinics of North America*. Philadelphia, W.B. Saunders, 1991, pp 797–820.

41. Vogl SE, Shoenfeld DA, Kaplan PN, et al: A randomized prospective comparison of methotrexate with a combination of methotrexate, bleomycin and cisplatin in head and neck cancer. *Cancer* 56:432–442, 1985.

42. Drelichman A, Cummings G, Al-Sarraf M: A randomized trial of the combination of cisplatinum, oncovin and bleomycin (COB) versus methotrexate in head and neck cancer. *Cancer* 52:399–403, 1983.

43. DeConti RC, Schoenfeld D: A randomized prospective comparison of intermittant methotrexate, methotrexate with leucovorin and a methotrexate combination in head and neck cancer. *Cancer* 48:1061–1072, 1981.

44. Woods RL, Fox RM, Tattershall MHN, et al: Methotrexate treatment of squamous cell head and neck cancers: Dose response evaluation. *BMJ* 282:600–602, 1983.

45. Papac RJ, Jacobs EM, Foye LV, et al: Systemic therapy with amethopter in squamous carcinoma of the head and neck. *Cancer Chemother Rep* 32:47–54, 1963.

46. Wittes RE, Cvitkovic E, Shah J, et al: Cisdichlorodiammine platinum (II) in the treatment of epidermoid carcinoma of the head and neck. *Cancer Treat Rep* 61:359–366, 1977.

47. Wittes RE, Heller K, Randolph V, et al: Cisdichlorodiammine platinum (II)-based chemotherapy as initial treatment of advanced head and neck cancer. *Cancer Treat Rep* 63:1533–1538, 1979.

48. Jacobs C, Bertino JR, Goffinet DR, et al: Twenty-four hour infusion of cisplatinum in head and neck cancers. *Cancer* 42:2135–2140, 1978.

49. Veronesi A, Zagonel V, Tirelli U: High dose versus low dose cisplatin in advanced head and neck squamous carcinoma: A randomized study. *J Clin Oncol* 3:1105–1108, 1985.

50. Jacobs C, Lyman G, Velez-Garcia E, et al: A phase III randomized study comparing cisplatin and fluorouracil as single agents and in combination for advanced squamous cell carcinoma of the head and neck. *J Clin Oncol* 10:257–263, 1992.

51. Carter SK: The chemotherapy of head and neck cancer. *Semin Oncol* 4:413–424, 1977.

52. Haas DC, Coltman CA, Gottlieb JA, et al: Phase II evaluation of bleomycin. *Cancer* 38:8–12, 1976.

53. Issell BF, Borsos G, D'Aoust JC, et al: Dibromodulcitol plus bleomycin compared with bleomycin alone in head nad neck cancer. *Cancer Chemother Pharmacol* 8:171–173, 1982.

54. Al-Sarraf M: Clinical trials with fluorinated pyrimidines in patients with head and neck cancer. *Invest New Drugs* 7:71–81, 1985.

55. Tapazoglou E, Kish J, Ensley J, et al: The activity of a single agent 5-fluorouracil infusion in advanced and recurrent head and neck cancer. *Cancer* 57:1105–1109, 1986.

56. Vokes EE: Head and neck cancer, in Perry MC (ed): *Chemotherapy Source Book*. Baltimore, Williams and Wilkins, 1992, pp 918–931.

57. Eisenberger MA, Hornedo J, Silva H, et al: Carboplatin (NSC-241-240), an active platinum analog for the treatment of squamous cell carcinoma of the head and neck. *J Clin Oncol* 7:1341–1345, 1989.

58. Kaase S, Thorud E, Tausjo J, et al: Phase I/II study of carboplatin and 5-fluorouracil in patients with advanced head and neck carcinoma. *Eur J Cancer Oncol* 27:576–579, 1991.

59. Forastiere AA, Metch B, Schuller DE, et al: Randomized comparison of cisplatin plus fluorouracil and carboplatin plus fluorouracil versus methotrexate in advanced squamous cell carcinoma of the head and neck: A Southwest Oncology Group Study. *J Clin Oncol* 10:1245–1251, 1992.

60. Forastiere AA, Natale RB, Takasugi BJ, et al: A phase I/II trial of carboplatin and 5-fluorouracil combination chemotherapy in advanced carcinoma of the head and neck. *J Clin Oncol* 5:190–196, 1987.

61. Al-Sarraf M, Metch B, Kish J, et al: Platinum analog in recurrent and advanced head and neck cancer: A Southwest Oncology Group and Wayne State University study. *Cancer Treat Rep* 71:723–726, 1987.

62. Eisenberger M, Van Echo D, Aisner J: Carboplatin: The experience in head and neck cancer. *Semin Oncol* 16:34–41, 1989.

63. Aisner J, Jacobs M, Gray W, et al: Weekly carboplatin (CBP) and weekly CBP+twice weekly bleomycin (BLE) each with concurrent radiotherapy (RT) for the treatment of regionally advanced head and neck cancer. *Proc ASCO* 13:902, 1994.

64. Rowinsky EK, Cazanave LA, Donehower RC: Taxol: A novel investigational antineoplastic agent. *J Natl Cancer Inst* 82:1247–1259, 1990.

65. Rowinsky EK, Gilbert MR, McGuire WP, et al: Sequences of taxol and cisplatin. A phase I and pharmacologic study. *J Clin Oncol* 9:1692–1703, 1991.

66. Forastiere AA, Rowinsky E, Chauchy V, et al: Phase I trial of taxol and cisplatin and G-CSF in solid tumors. *Proc ASCO* 11:117, 1992.

67. Thornton D, Singh K, Putz B, et al: A phase II trial of taxol in squamous cell carcinoma of the head and neck. *Proc Am Soc Clin Oncol* 13:933, 1994.

68. Hong WK, Schaefer S, Issell B, et al: A prospective randomized trial of methotrexate versus cisplatin in the treatment of recurrent squamous cell carcinoma of the head and neck. *Cancer* 52:206–210, 1983.

69. Grose WE, Lehane DE, Dixon DO, et al: Comparison of methotrexate and cisplatin for patients with advanced squamous cell carcinoma of the head and neck region: A Southwest Oncology Group Study. *Cancer Treat Rep* 69:577–581, 1985.

70. Williams SD, Velez-Garcia E, Essessee I, et al: Chemotherapy for head and neck cancer. Comparison of cisplatin plus vinblastine plus bleomycin versus methotrexate. *Cancer* 57:18–23, 1986.

71. Campbell JB, Dorman EB, McCormick J, et al: A randomized phase III trial of cisplatinum, methotrexate, cisplatinum and methotrexate, and cisplatinum and fluorouracil in end-stage head and neck cancer. *Acta Otolaryngol (Stockh)* 103:519–528, 1987.

72. Eisenberger MA, Krasnow S, Silva H, et al: A comparison of carboplatin plus methotrexate versus methotrexate alone in patients with recurrent and metastatic head and neck cancer. *J Clin Oncol* 7:1341–1345, 1989.

73. Davis S, Kessler W: Randomized comparison of cis-diamminedichloroplatin versus cis-diamminedichloroplatinum, methotrexate, and bleomycin in recurrent squamous cell carcinoma of the head and neck. *Cancer Chemother Pharmacol* 3:57–59, 1979.

74. Jacobs C, Meyers F, Hendrickson C, et al: A randomized phase III study of cisplatin with and without methotrexate for recurrent squamous cell carcinoma of the head and neck. *Cancer* 52:1563–1569, 1983.

75. Morton RP, Stell PM: Cytotoxic chemotherapy for patients with terminal squamous carcinoma-does it influence survival? *Clin Otolaryngol* 9:175–180, 1984.

76. Clavel M, Cappelare P, Cognetti F, et al: Comparison between C (cisplatin) alone, two cisplatin containing multiple drug regimens: CABO (Cisplatin, methotrexate, bleomycin, oncovin) and CF (cisplatin-FU) in advanced head and neck carcinomas. Report on a randomized EORTC trial 24842 including 380 patients. *Cancer Chemother Pharmacol* 23(suppl 2):c73–(A292s), 1989.

77. Choksi A, Dimery I, James P, et al: 24-hour infusion cisplatin (DDP) and 5-day infusion 5-fluorouracil (5-FU) in recurrent head and neck squamous cancer (HNSC). *Proc ASCO* 5:138, 1986.

78. Rowland KM Jr, Taylor SG, Spiers AS, et al: Cisplatin and 5-FU infusion chemotherapy in advanced, recurrent cancer of the head and neck: An Eastern Oncology Group pilot study. *Cancer Treat Rep* 70:461–464, 1986.

79. Department of Veterans Affairs Laryngeal Cancer Study Group. Induction chemotherapy plus radiation compared with surgery plus radiation in patients with advanced laryngeal cancer. *N Engl J Med* 324:1685–1690, 1991.

80. Al-Sarraf M: Head and neck cancer: Chemotherapy concepts. *Semin Oncol* 15:70–85, 1988.

81. Rooney M, Kish J, Jacobs J, et al: Improved complete response rate and survival in advanced head and neck cancer after three courses induction therapy with 120 hour 5-fluorouracil infusion and cisplatin. *Cancer* 55:1123–1128, 1985.

82. Clark JR, Fallon BG, Dreyfuss AI, et al: Chemotherapy strategies in the multidisciplinary treatment of head and neck cancer. *Semin Oncol* 15 (suppl 3):36–44, 1988.

83. DiBlasio B, Barbieri W, Bozzetti A, et al: A prospective randomized trial in resectable head and neck carcinoma: Loco-regional treatment with and without neoadjuvant chemotherapy. *Proc ASCO* 13:899, 1994.

84. Sako K, Razack MS, Kalnins I: Chemotherapy for advanced and recurrent squamous cell carcinoma of the head and neck with high and low dose cisdichlorodiammine platinum. *Am J Surg* 136:529–533, 1978.

85. Merlano M, Tatarek R, Grimaldi A, et al: Phase I-II trial with cisplatin and 5FU in recurrent head and neck cancer: An effective outpatient schedule. *Cancer Treat Rep* 69:961–964, 1985.

86. Robben NC, Pippas AW, Moore JO: The syndrome of 5-fluorouracil cardiotoxicity. *Cancer* 71:493–509, 1993.

87. Burger AJ, Mannino S: 5-Fluorouracil-induced coronary vasospasm. *Am Heart J* 114:433–436, 1987.

88. Rezkalla S, Kloner RA, Ensley J, et al: Continuous ambulatory ECG monitoring during fluorouracil therapy: A prospective study. *J Clin Oncol* 7:509–514, 1989.

89. Fonseca E, Cruz JJ, Martin G, et al: Neoadjuvant chemotherapy in locally advanced head and neck cancer (HNC). *Proc ASCO* 13:917, 1994.

90. Forastiere AA, Belliveau JF, Goven PG, et al: Pharmacokinetic and toxicity evaluation of five-day continuous infusion versus intermittant bolus cis-diamminedichloroplatinum (II) in head and neck cancer patients. *Cancer Res* 48:3869–3874, 1988.

91. Ellerton JA, Borgelt B: Effectiveness of Ifosfamide-mesna (IFEX) and OVP-16 as an alternative to cisplatin (DDP) 5-FU in patients with advanced head and neck cancer. *Proc ASCO* 13:935, 1994.

92. Riverola E, Negro A, Zuslovich Z, et al: Cisplatin (DDP), epirubicin, bleomycin, methotrexate and vincristine sequential neoadjuvant chemotherapy for locally advanced squamous head and neck cancer. *Proc ASCO* 13:929, 1994.

93. Ensley J, Kish J, Tapazoglou E, et al: An intensive, five course, alternating combination chemotherapy induction regimen used in patients with advanced unresectable head and neck cancer. *J Clin Oncol* 6:1147–1153, 1988.

94. Ensley J, Kish J, Tapazoglou E, et al: Continued intensification of an alternating regimen in patients with advanced, untreated squamous cancers of the head and neck. *Proc ASCO* 7:154, 1988.

95. Lopez A, Bruuet J, DeAndres, et al: Randomized trial of neoadjuvant cisplatin and fluorouracil (CF) versus carboplatin and fluorouracil (CBDCA-F) in patients with stage IV-Mo head and neck cancer. *Proc ASCO* 13:907, 1994.

96. Sauti DV, McHenry CS, Sommer H: Mechanism of interaction of thymidylate synthetase with 5-fluoro-deoxyuridylate. *Biochemistry* 13:471–481, 1974.

97. Danenberg PV, Langenbach RJ, Heidelberger C: Structures of irreversible complexes of thymidylate syntetase and fluorinated pyrimidine nuceotides. *Biochemistry* 13:926–933, 1974.

98. Lockshin A, Danenberg PV: Biochemical factors affecting the tightness of 5-Fluorodeoxyuridylate binding of human thymidylate synthetase. *Biochem Pharmacol* 30:247–257, 1980.

99. Vokes EE, Choi KE, Schilsky RL, et al: Cisplatin, fluorouracil and high-dose leucovorin for recurrent or metastatic head and neck cancer. *J Clin Oncol* 6:618–626, 1988.

100. Vokes EE, Schilsky RL, Weichselbaum RR, et al: Induction chemotherapy with cisplatin, fluorouracil, and high-dose leucovorin for locally advanced head and neck cancer: A clinical and pharmacologic analysis. *J Clin Oncol* 8:241–247, 1990.

101. Lehmann OA, Santos RL, Butagelj E, et al: Cisplatin and fluorouracil (CF) versus cisplatin, fluorouracil and leucovorin (CFL) in advanced head and neck cancer. *Proc ASCO* 13:927, 1994.

102. Vokes EE, Panje WR, Schilsky RL, et al: Hydroxyurea, 5-fluorouracil and concommitant radiotherapy in poor prognosis head and neck cancer. A phase I-II study. *J Clin Oncol* 7:761–768, 1989.

103. Vokes EE, Haraf DJ, Mick R, et al: Concommitant chemoradiotherapy for intermediate stage head and neck cancer (HNC). *Proc ASCO* 13:909, 1994.

104. Gandia D, Wibault P, Guillot T, et al: Simultaneous chemoradiotherapy as salvage treatment in locoregional recurrences of squamous head and neck cancer. *Head Neck* 15:8–15, 1993.

105. Weppelmann B, Wheeler RH, Peters GE, et al: Treatment of recurrent head and neck cancer with 5-fluorouracil, hydroxyurea and irradiation. *Int J Radiat Oncol Biol Phys* 22:1051–1056, 1992.

106. Wadler S, Schwartz EL: Antineoplastic activity of the combination of inter-

feron and cytotoxic agents against experimental and human malignancies: A review. *Cancer Res* 50:3473–3486, 1990.

107. Wadler S, Schwartz EL, Goldman M, et al: Fluorouracil and recombinant Alpha-2a-Interferon. An active regimen against advanced colorectal carcinoma. *J Clin Oncol* 7:1769–1775, 1989.

108. Kies M, Haraf D, Mick R, et al: Cisplatin, 5FU, Leucovorin and Interferon alpha-2B (PFL-alpha) followed by concurrent 5FU-hydroxyurea (HU) and radiation (FHX) for stage IV squamous cell cancer of the head and neck. *Proc ASCO* 13:913, 1994.

109. Arquette MA, Mortimer JE, Loehrer PJ, et al: A phase II Hoosier Oncology Group Trial of interferon alpha-2B (IFN) added to cisplatin (CDDP) and 5-fluorouracil (FU) in recurrant or metastatic head and neck cancer. *Proc ASCO* 13:901, 1994.

110. Cervellino JC, Araujo CE, Pirisi C, et al: Ifosfamide and mesna for the treatment of advanced squamous cell head and neck cancer. A Getlac study. *Oncology* 48:89–92, 1991.

111. Domenge C, Schwaab G, Marandas P, et al: Phase II feasability study of Ifosfamide/mesna and methotrexate in recurernt advanced squamous cell head and neck cancer. *Proc ASCO* 13:944, 1994.

112. Gupta V, Arena S, Hilal E, et al: High response rate to cisplatin and Ifosfamide/mesna in head and neck cancer. *Proc ASCO* 13:936, 1994.

113. Buesa JM, Fernandez R, Esteban E: A phase II trial of ifosphamide in recurrent and metastatic head and neck cancer. *Ann Oncol* 2:151–152, 1991.

114. Forastiere AA: Use of Paclitaxel (Taxol) in squamous cell carcinoma of the head and neck. *Semin Oncol* 20 (suppl 3):56–60, 1993.

115. Dreyfuss A, Clark J, Norris C: Taxotere (TXTR) for advanced incurable squamous cell carcinoma of the head and neck. *Proc ASCO* 13:931, 1994.

116. Robert F, Wheeler RA, McHenry DC, et al: Phase II study of topotecan in advanced head and neck cancer. Identification of an active new agent. *Proc ASCO* 13:905, 1994.

117. Green MD, Sherman P, Zalcberg J: Phase II study of 10-EdAM in patients with squamous cell carcinoma of the head and neck, previously untreated with chemotherapy. *Invest New Drugs* 10:31–34, 1992.

118. Schornagle J, Cappalare J, Verwey F, et al: A randomized phase II study of 10-ethyl-10-deazo-aminopterin (10-EdAM) and methotrexate in advanced head and neck squamous cell cancer. *Proc ASCO* 8:175, 1989.

119. Robert F: Trimethotrexate as a single agent in patients with advanced head and neck cancer. *Sem Oncol* 15 (suppl 2):22–26, 1988.

120. Magee MJ, Henand J, Bosl GJ, et al: Phase II trial of 4-epi-doxorubicin in advanced carcinoma of head and neck origin. *Cancer Treat Rep* 69:125, 1985.

121. Maipang T, Wataraarepornchai S, Panjapiyakul C, et al: Cisplatinum-epirubicin chemotherapy for advanced unresectable squamous cell carcinoma of the head and neck. *Head Neck* 15:109–114, 1993.

122. Kaplan BH, Vogl SE, Cinberg J, et al: Phase II trial of vindesine in squamous cancer of the head and neck. *Proc ASCO* 3:199, 1983.

123. Vogl SE, Ryan L, Wernz J, et al: Ineffective agents in the chemotherapy of head and neck cancer (HNCA), mitoxanthrone (DHAD), dibromodulcitol (DBD), and vinblastine (VLB). *Proc AACR* 26:171, 1985.

124. Leaf A, Schwartz E, Ritch P: A phase II study of Amonafide (AM) in carcinoma of the head and neck. (CHN). *Proc ASCO* 13:924, 1994.

125. Testolin A, Redcher G, Pozza F, et al: Vinorelbine (VNB) in pre-treated advanced head and neck squamous cell carcinoma: A phase II study. *Proc ASCO* 13:938, 1994.

126. Vlock DR, Johnson JT, Myers E, et al: Preliminary trial of non-recombinant interferon alpha in recurrent squamous cell carcinoma of the head and neck. *Head Neck* 13:15–21, 1991.

127. Selvaggi KJ, Vlock DR, Johnson JT, et al: Phase Ib trial of peritumoral and intranodal injections of IL-2 in patients with advanced squamous cell carcinoma of the head and neck. *Proc ASCO* 9:690, 1990.

128. Crispino S, Paolorossi F, Colombo A, et al: Concommitant radiotherapy (RT) and carboplatinum (C)—5FU (F) plus interleukin-2 (IL-2) in locally advanced N2-N3 head and neck squamous cell carcinoma. *Proc ASCO* 13:898, 1994.

129. Urba SG, Forastiere AA, Wolfe GT, et al: Intensive recombinant interleukin-2 and alpha interferon therapy in patients with advanced head and neck squamous carcinoma. *Cancer* 71:2326–2331, 1993.

130. Schantz SP, Dimery I, Lippman SM, et al: A phase II study of interleukin-2 and interferon-alpha in head and neck cancer. *Invest New Drugs* 10:217–223, 1992.

131. Tamura T, Sasaki Y, Shinkai T, et al: Phase I study of combination therapy with interleukin-2 and B-Interferon in patients with advanced malignancy. *Cancer Res* 49:730–735, 1989.

132. Meysken FL Jr: Coming of age-The chemoprevention of cancer. *New Engl J Med* 323:825–827, 1990.

133. Smith MA, Parkinson DR, Cheson BD, et al: Retinoids in cancer therapy. *J Clin Oncol* 10:839–864, 1992.

134. Hong WK, Endicott J, Itri LM, et al: 13-cis-retinoic acid in the treatment of oral leukoplakia. *N Engl J Med* 315:1501–1505, 1986.

135. Hong WK, Lippman SM, Itri LM, et al: Prevention of second primary tumors with isotretinoin in squamous cell carcinoma of the head and neck. *N Engl J Med* 323:795–801, 1990.

136. Smith DC, Jacob HE, Branch RA, et al: A phase II trial of All-Trans-Retinoic Acid (ATRA) in advanced squamous cell carcinoma of the head and neck. *Proc ASCO* 13:930, 1994.

137. Nervi C, Arcangeli G, Casale C, et al: A re-appraisal of intra-arterial chemotherapy. Results obtained in 145 patients with head and neck cancer treated during 1963–1966 with intra-arterial chemotherapy followed by radical radiotherapy. *Cancer* 26:577–582, 1970.

138. Baker SR, Forastiere AA, Wheeler R, et al: Intra-arterial chemotherapy for head and neck cancer. An update on the totally implantable infusion pump. *Arch Otolaryngol Head Neck Surg* 113:1183–1190, 1987.

139. Forastiere AA, Baker SR, Wheeler R, et al: Intra-arterial cisplatin and FUDR in advanced malignancies confined to the head and neck. *J Clin Oncol* 5:1601–1606, 1987.

140. Los G, Vicario D, Barton RM, et al: Selective intra-arterial infusion of high dose cisplatin in advanced head and neck cancer patients results in high tumor platinum concentrations and cisplatin DNA adduct function. *Proc ASCO* 13:908, 1994.

141. Vicario D, Robbins KT, Storniolo AM, et al: Phase II study of highly selective supradose intra-arterial cisplatin with concurrent radiotherapy in advanced upper aerodigestive tract carcinoma. *Proc ASCO* 13:911, 1994.

142. Gore ME, Riches P, MacLennan K, et al: Phase I study of intra-arterial interleukin-2 in squamous cell carcinoma of the head and neck. *Br J Cancer* 66:405–407, 1992.

143. Jacob HE, Johnson JT, Cano E: Personal communication, 1994.

144. McNeil BJ, Weichselbaum R, Pauker SG: Speech and survival trade offs between quality and quantity of life in laryngeal cancer. *N Engl J Med* 305:982–987, 1981.

145. List M, Ritter-Sterr C, Baker T, et al: A longitudinal assessment of quality of life in laryngeal cancer patients. *Proc ASCO* 13:916, 1994.

146. Wolf GT, Fisher SG: Effectiveness of salvage neck dissection for advanced regional metastases when induction chemotherapy and radiation are used for organ presentation. *Laryngoscope* 102:934–939, 1992.

147. Norris CM Jr, Busse PM, Clark JR: Evolving role of surgery after induction chemotherapy and primary site radiation in head and neck cancer. *Semin Surg Oncol* 9:3–13, 1993.

148. Vokes EE, Weichselbaum RR, Mick R, et al: Favorable long term survival following induction chemotherapy with cisplatin, fluorouracil, and leucovorin and concommitant chemoradiotherapy for locally advanced head and neck cancer. *J Natl Cancer Inst* 84:877–882, 1992.

149. Vokes EE, Mick R, Lester EP, et al: Cisplatin and fluorouracil chemotherapy does not yield long term benefit in locally advanced head and neck cancer: Results from a single institution. *J Clin Oncol* 9:1376–1384, 1992.

150. Jacobs C, Goffinet DR, Goffinet L, et al: Chemotherapy as a substitute for surgery in the treatment of advanced resectable head and neck cancer. A report from the Northern California Oncology Group. *Cancer* 60:1178–1183, 1987.

151. Ervin TJ, Clark JR, Weichselbaum RR, et al: An analysis of induction and adjuvant chemotherapy in the multidisciplinary treatment of squamous cell carcinoma of the head and neck. *J Clin Oncol* 5:10–20, 1987.

152. Kies MS, Gordon LI, Hauck WW, et al: Analysis of complete responders after initial treatment with chemotherapy in head and neck cancer. *Otolaryngol Head Neck Surg* 93:199–205, 1985.

153. Vikram B, Chadha M, Yu L, et al: Production of tumor control in hypopharynx (HP) cancer after alternation chemoradiotherapy. *Proc ASCO* 13:919, 1994.

154. Spaulding MB, Kahn A, Delos Santos R, et al: Adjuvant chemotherapy in advanced head and neck cancer. *Am J Surg* 144:432–443, 1982.

155. Al-Kourainy K, Kish J, Ensley J, et al: Achievement of superior survival for histologically negative versus histologically positive clinically complete responders to cisplatin combination chemotherapy in patients with locally advanced head and neck cancer. *Cancer* 59:233–238, 1987.

156. Head and Neck Contracts Program. Adjuvant chemotherapy in advanced head and neck squamous carcinoma. *Cancer* 60:301–311, 1987.

157. Schuller DE, Metch B, Maltox D, et al: Prospective chemotherapy in advanced resectable head and neck cancer. Final report of the Southwest Oncology Group. *Laryngoscope* 98:1205–1211, 1988.

158. Forastiere AA: Randomized trials of induction chemotherapy: A critical review, in Vokes EE (ed): *Hematology/Oncology Clinics of North America. Head and Neck Cancer.* Philadelphia, WB Saunders, 1991, pp 725–736.

159. Carugati A, Pradier R, de la Torre A: Combination chemotherapy pre radical treatment for head and neck squamous cell carcinoma. *Proc ASCO* 7:589, 1988.

160. Kun LE, Toohill RJ, Holoye PY, et al: A randomized study of adjuvant chemotherapy for cancer of the upper aerodigestive tract. *Int J Radiat Oncol Biol Phys* 12:173–178, 1986.

161. Martin M, Mazeron JJ, Brun B, et al: Neoadjuvant polychemotherapy of head and neck cancer: Results of a randomized study. *Proc ASCO* 7:590, 1988.

162. Paccagnella A, Cavaniglia G, Zorat PL, et al: Chemotherapy before locoregional treatment in stage III and IV head and neck cancer: Intermediate results of an ongoing randomized phase III trial. AGSTTC study. *Proc ASCO* 9:173, 1990.

163. Stell PM, Balby JE, Strickland R, et al: Sequential chemotherapy and radio-therapy in advanced head and neck cancer. *Clin Radiol* 34:463–467, 1983.
164. Toohill RJ, Anderson T, Byhardt RW, et al: Cisplatin and fluorouracil as neo-adjuvant therapy in head and neck cancer: A preliminary report. *Arch Oto-laryngol Head Neck Surg* 113:758–761, 1987.
165. Ensley J, Jacobs J, Weaver A, et al: The correlation between response to cis-platinum combination chemotherapy and subsequent radiotherapy in pre-viously untreated patients with advanced squamous cell cancer of the head and neck. *Cancer* 54:811–814, 1984.
166. Hong WK, O'Donoghue GM, Sheetz S, et al: Sequential response patterns to chemotherapy and radiotherapy in head and neck cancer: Potential impact to treatment in advanced laryngeal cancer. *Prog Clin Biol Res* 201:191–197, 1985.
167. Fletcher GH, Jesse RH: The place of irradiation in the management of the primary lesion in head and neck cancer. *Cancer* 39:862–867, 1977.
168. Demard F, Chauvel P, Santini J, et al: Response to chemotherapy as justifi-cation for modification of the therapeutic strategy for pharyngolaryngeal car-cinomas. *Head Neck* 12:225–231, 1990.
169. Urba S, Forastiere AA, Wolfe GT, et al: Neoadjuvant chemotherapy with high dose continuous infusion cisplatin, 5 fluorouracil and mitoguanzone for head and neck cancer. *Proc ASCO* 8:172, 1989.
170. Pfister DG, Harrison L, Strong EW, et al: Organ/function preservation in ad-vanced oropharynx cancer (OPC): Results with induction chemotherapy and radiation. *Proc ASCO* 11:776, 1992.
171. Lefebvre JL, Sahmcoud T: Larynx preservation in hypopharyngeal squamous cell carcinoma: Preliminary results of a randomized study (EORTC 24891). *Proc ASCO* 133:912, 1994.
172. Martin M, Gehanno P, Depondt J, et al: A phase III study: Induction carbo-platin and 5-fluorouracil before locoregional treatment versus locoregional treatment alone in head and neck carcinomas. *Proc ASCO* 13:906, 1994.
173. Pinto HA, Goffinet DR, Fee WE: Induction chemotherapy followed by simul-taneous chemoradiotherapy (CRT) for organ preservation in advanced re-sectable head and neck cancer. *Proc ASCO* 13:903, 1994.
174. Urba S, McLaughlin P, Wolfe GT, et al: Induction chemotherapy (CT) with carboplatin (CBDCA) and 5-fluorouracil (5FU) for organ preservation in pa-tients with advanced head and neck cancer. *Proc ASCO* 13:910, 1994.
175. Dougherty D, Steinbrenner L, Garrabrant C, et al: A non-toxic, effective regi-men for induction therapy and organ preservation in advanced head and neck cancer. *Proc ASCO* 13:942, 1994.
176. Fu KK: Concurrent radiotherapy and chemotherapy, in Wittes RE (ed): *Head and Neck Cancer*. New York, Wiley, 1985, pp 221–248.
177. Awan AM, Vokes EE, Weichselbaum RR: Advances in radiation oncology in the treatment of head and neck tumors. *Adv Otolaryngol Head Neck Surg* 3:257–288, 1989.
178. Fu KK, Phillips TL: Biologic rationale of combined radiotherapy and che-motherapy, in Vokes EE (ed): *Hematology/Oncology Clinics of North America. Head and Neck Cancer*. Philadelphia, WB Saunders, 1991, pp 737–751.
179. Vokes EE, Weichselbaum RR: Concommitant chemradiotherapy: Rationale and clinical experience in patients with solid tumors. *J Clin Oncol* 8:911–934, 1990.
180. Johnson JT, Ferretti GA, Nethery WJ, et al: Oral pilocarpine for post irradia-tion xerostomia in patients with head and neck cancer. *N Engl J Med* 329:390–395, 1993.

181. White RM, Myers EM, Ashayeri E: Induction chemotherapy for advanced head and neck cancer: Modification of response to chemotherapy by anti-emetics. *J Clin Oncol* 12:45–55, 1992.

182. Merlano M, Vitale V, Rosso R, et al: Treatment of advanced squamous cell carcinoma of the head and neck with alternating chemotherapy and radio-therapy. *N Engl J Med* 327:1115–1121, 1992.

183. Adelstein DJ, Kalish LA, Adams GL, et al: Concurrent radiation therapy and chemotherapy for locally unresectable squamous cell head and neck can-cer: An Eastern Cooperative Oncology Group pilot study. *J Clin Oncol* 11:2136–2142, 1993.

184. Pajak TF, Laramore GE, Marcial VA, et al: Elapsed treatment days—A criti-cal item for radiotherapy quality control review in head and neck trials: RTOG report. *Int J Radiat Oncol Biol Phys* 20:13–20, 1991.

185. Lo TCM, Wiley AL Jr, Ansfield FJ: Combined radiation therapy and 5-fluorouracil for advanced squamous cell carcinoma of the oral cavity and oropharynx: A randomized study. *Am J Roentgenol* 126:229–235, 1976.

186. Fu KK, Phillips TL, Silverberg IJ, et al: Combined radiotherapy and chemo-therapy with bleomycin and methotrexate for advanced inoperable head and neck cancer: Update of a Norhtern California Oncology Group randomized trial. *J Clin Oncol* 5:1410–1418, 1987.

187. Weissberg JB, Sun YH, Papac RJ, et al: Randomized clinical trial of mitomycin-C as an adjuvant to radiotherapy in head and neck cancer. *Int J Radiat Oncol Biol Phys* 17:3–9, 1989.

188. Bachaud JM, Daird JM, Boussin G, et al: Combined post operative radio-therapy and weekly cisplatin infusion for locally advanced squamous cell carcinoma of the head and neck: Preliminary report of a randomized trial. *Int J Radiat Oncol Biol Phys* 20:243–246, 1991.

189. Fontanesi J, Beckford NS, Lester EP, et al: Concomitant cisplatin and hy-perfractionated external beam irradiation for advanced malignancy of the head and neck. *Am J Surg* 162:393–396, 1991.

190. Gasperini G, Recher G, Testolin A, et al: Synchronous radiotherapy and che-motherapy with cisplatin in the management of locally advanced or recur-rent head and neck cancer. *J Clin Oncol* 15:242–249, 1992.

191. Zamboglou N, Achterrath W, Schnabel T, et al: Simultaneous radiotherapy and chemotherapy with carboplatin in inoperable squamous cell carcinoma of the head and neck: A phase II study. *Cancer Invest* 10:349–355, 1992.

192. Nabholtz JM, Rapp E, Jha N, et al: Neoadjuvant chemotherapy with carbo-platin and continuous infusion 5-fluorouracil followed by concurrent car-boplatin and radiotherapy in advanced unresectable stage III and IV head and neck cancer: Preliminary results of a phase II pilot study. *Proc ASCO* 13:934, 1994.

193. Orecchia R, Urgesi A, Sacco M, et al: Daily low-dose carboplatin and stan-dard radiotherapy in unresectable head nad neck and lung cancers: A pilot study. *Tumori* 77:423–425, 1991.

194. Tomio L, Zorat PL, Peccagnella A, et al: A pilot study of concomitant radia-tion and chemotherapy in patients with locally advanced head and neck cancer. *Am J Clin Oncol* 16:264–267, 1993.

195. Adelstein DJ, Sharan VM, Earle AS, et al: Long term results after chemora-diotherapy for locally confined squamous cell head and neck cancer. *Am J Clin Oncol* 13:440–447, 1990.

196. Taylor SG IV, Murthy AK, Caldarelli DD, et al: Combined simultaneous cis-platin/fluorouracil chemotherapy and split course radiation in head and neck cancer. *J Clin Oncol* 7:846–856, 1989.

197. Wendt TG, Hartenstein RC, Wustrow TPU, et al: Cisplatin, fluorouracil with

leucovorin calcium enhancement, and synchronous accelerated radiotherapy in the management of locally advanced head and neck cancer: A phase II trial. *J Clin Oncol* 7:471–476, 1989.

198. Abitbol AA, Schwade JG, Lewin AA, et al: Hyperfractionated radiation therapy and concurrent 5-fluorouracil, cisplatin and mitomycin-C in head and neck carcinoma. A pilot study. *J Clin Oncol* 15:250–255, 1992.

199. Eskandari J, DeMuizon H, Bonnet D, et al: Advanced head and neck carcinomas. Results of combined radiotherapy and weekly concomitant 5-fluorouracil-Leucovorin modulation. *Proc ASCO* 13:896, 1994.

200. Merlano M, Corvo R, Margarino G, et al: Combined chemotherapy and radiation therapy in advanced inoperable squamous cell carcinoma of the head and neck: The final report of a randomized trial. *Cancer* 67:915–921, 1991.

201. A randomized trial of combined multidrug chemotherapy and radiotherapy in advanced squamous cell carcinoma of the head and neck: An interim reprot from the SECOG participants. *Eur J Surg Oncol* 12:289–295, 1986.

202. Adelstein DJ, Sharan VM, Earle AS: Simultaneous versus sequential combined technique therapy for squamous cell head and neck cancer. *Cancer* 65:1685–1691, 1990.

203. Taylor SG IV, Murthy AK, Vannetzel JM, et al: Randomized comparison of neoadjuvant cisplatin and fluorouracil infusion followed by radiation versus concomitant treatment in advanced head and neck cancer. *J Clin Oncol* 12:385–395, 1994.

204. Weissler MC, Melin S, Sailer SL, et al: Simultaneous chemoradiation in the treatment of advanced head and neck cancer. *Arch Otolaryngol Head Neck Surg* 118:806–810, 1992.

205. Valavaara R, Kortekangas AE, Nordman E, et al: Interferon combined with irradiation in the treatment of operable head and neck carcinoma. *Acta Oncol* 31:429–431, 1992.

206. Johnson JT, Myers EN, Srodes CH, et al: Maintenance chemotherapy for high risk patients. *Arch Otolaryngol Head Neck Surg* 111:727–729, 1985.

207. Johnson JT, Myers EN, Schramm VL, et al: Adjuvant chemotherapy for high risk squamous cell carcinoma of the head and neck. *J Clin Oncol* 5:456–458, 1987.

208. Domenge C, Marandas P, Vignoud J, et al: Post surgical adjuvant chemotherapy in extracapsular spread invaded lymph nodes of epidermoid carcinoma of the head and neck. A randomzied multicentric trial. *Proc of the 2nd International Conf on Head and Neck Cancer* 108:74, 1988.

209. Laramore GE, Scott CB, Al-Sarraf M, et al: Adjuvant chemotherapy for resectable squamous cell carcinomas of the head and neck: Report on Intergroup Study 0034. *Int J Radiat Oncol Biol Phys* 23:705–713, 1992.

210. Jacobs C, Makuch R: Efficacy of adjuvant chemotherapy for patients with resectable head and neck cancer: A subset analysis of the head and neck contracts program. *J Clin Oncol* 8:838–847, 1990.

211. Hara HJ: Malignant tumors of the nasopharynx. *J Otolaryngeal Soc* 3:187–198, 1971.

212. Waterhouse J, Muir C, Shanmugaratnam K, et al: Cancer incidence in five continents. *Int Agency Res Cancer* 4:700–701, 1982.

213. Ho JHC: An epidemiologic and clinical study of nasopharyngeal carcinoma. *Radiat Oncol Biol Phys* 4:183–197, 1978.

214. Chatani M, Teshima T, Inoue T, et al: Radiation therapy for nasopharyngeal carcinoma: Retrospective review of 105 patients based on a survey of Kansai Cancer Therapist Group. *Cancer* 57:2267–2271, 1986.

215. Dimery IW, Goepfert H, Peters LJ, et al: Survival update of advanced naso-

pharyngeal carcinoma (NPC) treated with neoadjuvant chemotherapy. *Proc ASCO* 10:197, 1991.

216. Leung WT, Shui W, Tac M, et al: Phase II study of carboplatin and 5FU combination chemotherapy in treatment of advanced NPC. *Proc ASCO* 10:199, 1991.

217. Boussen H, Benna F, Jallouli M, et al: Primary chemotherapy with ADR-BLE-CDDP versus ADR-PLAT before radiotherapy in indifferentiated nasopharyngeal carcinoma. Two year analysis and natural history after CT. *Proc ASCO* 10:203, 1991.

218. Bachouchi M, Lianes P, Armand JP, et al: Two years follow-up on bleomycin, epirubicin, cisplatin in locally advanced undifferentiated carcinoma nasopharyngeal type (UCNT). *Proc ASCO* 10:201, 1991.

219. Al-Sarraf M, Pajak RF, Cooper JS, et al: Chemoradiotherapy in patients with locally advanced nasopharyngeal carcinoma: A Radiation Therapy Oncology Group study. *J Clin Oncol* 8:1342–1351, 1990.

220. Cvitkovic E: For the Int. Nasopharynx Study Group. Instit. G-Roussy-La Grange-Savigny le Temple (France) neoadjuvant chemotherapy with epirubicin, cisplatin, bleomycin in undifferentiated nasopharyngeal cancer. Preliminary results of an international phase III trial. *Proc ASCO* 13:915, 1994.

221. Chan WK, Chi KH, Lin TH, et al: Carboplatin in nasopharyngeal carcinoma. A phase II study. *Proc ASCO* 13:922, 1994.

222. Liu JM, Chan WK, Chi KH, et al: Preliminary report of a phase II trial of Ifosfamide in patients with advanced stage nasopharyngeal carcinoma in Taiwan. *Proc ASCO* 13:923, 1994.

223. Fandi A, Taamma A, Bachouchi M, et al: Palliative treatment by low dose 5 fluorouracil continuous infusion in recurrent and/or metastatic undifferentiated nasopharyngeal carcinoma type (UNCT). *Proc ASCO* 13:946, 1994.

224. Jacob HE: Chemotherapy for cranial base tumors. *J Neurooncol* 20:327–335, 1994.

Recent Advances in the Treatment of Neurofibromatosis Type II

Robert J. S. Briggs, M.D., F.R.A.C.S.
Assistant Otolaryngologist, Royal Melbourne Hospital, Senior Lecturer
Melbourne University, Department of Otolaryngology, Melbourne, Australia

Emil A. Popovic, M.B., B.S., F.R.A.C.S.
Assistant Neurosurgeon, Department of Neurosurgery, Clinical Neuroscience
Centre, Royal Melbourne Hospital Melbourne, Australia

Derald E. Brackmann, M.D.
Clinical Professor of Otolaryngology, University of Southern California, House
Ear Clinic, House Ear Institute, Los Angeles, California

Neurofibromatosis type II (NF2) is an autosomal dominant condition, the hallmark of which is the occurrence of bilateral acoustic neuromas (vestibular schwannomas). Recent developments in understanding the genetic characteristics of NF2 include identification of the responsible tumor suppressor gene and recognition of the variable clinical manifestations. Previously, delayed diagnosis, acoustic neuroma growth, or surgical removal usually resulted in eventual total hearing loss. Early diagnosis is now facilitated by use of gadolinium enhanced magnetic resonance imaging and appropriate family screening, including DNA analysis. Early diagnosis, when the tumors are smaller, together with refinements in hearing preservation surgery, has improved our ability to prevent total hearing loss by complete surgical tumor removal. Hearing restoration is now a realistic goal in patients with NF2. Development of the auditory brain stem implant (ABI) now allows restoration of some auditory function at the time of tumor removal in those patients with large acoustic neuromas or no useful hearing.

CLINICAL AND GENETIC CHARACTERISTICS

Neurofibromatosis encompasses a heterogeneous group of neurologic disorders, the most frequent of which is neurofibromatosis type 1 (von Recklinghausen's disease, NF1). The occurrence of bilateral vestibular schwannomas is now well recognized as being pathognomonic for NF2. Formerly called central neurofibromatosis or bilateral acoustic neurofibromatosis, NF2 is a distinctly different disorder to NF1. NF1 patients tend to develop cranial tumors and dysplasias of astrocytic and neuronal origin, e.g., astrocytoma, glioma, neurofibroma, hamartoma, and het-

Advances in Otolaryngology—Head and Neck Surgery®, vol. 9
© 1995, Mosby–Year Book, Inc.

erotopia, whereas patients with NF2 develop tumors of the neuronal lining, such as schwannomas, meningioma, and ependymoma. Confirmation that these are indeed different disorders came in 1987 when genetic linkage analysis localised the NF1 gene to chromosome 17 and the NF2 gene to chromosome 22.[1-3] At least two other forms of NF have been proposed: segmental NF in which cafe au lait spots and dermal neurofibromas are confined to one or several adjacent dermatomes,[4] and multiple cafe au lait spots inherited as an autosomal dominant trait but occurring in isolation.[5]

The clinical diagnosis of NF2 has recently been redefined by the U.S. National Institutes of Health Consensus Development Conference.[6] The clinical criteria for diagnosis are the presence of bilateral vestibular schwannomas, as in the typical clinical case, or, a first-degree relative of a patient with NF2 who has one of the following pathologies: schwannoma, neurofibroma, glioma, meningioma, or posterior capsular cataract or lens opacity at a young age.

Acoustic neuromas occur most commonly as sporadic tumors that are unilateral. Affected individuals have no family history, no other tumors, and generally are over 40 years of age at diagnosis. In NF2, the tumors are bilateral; affected individuals frequently have relatives with NF2 and are often diagnosed with the tumors as adolescents or young adults, and may develop other central nervous system tumors.

All cases of vestibular schwannomas, both sporadic and familial, are thought to result from the functional loss of a tumor suppressor gene that has been localised to the long arm of chromosome 22 and which has recently been cloned.[7, 8] Numerous tumors are now known to result from the loss of function of tumor suppressor genes which, in general, code for a protein involved in one of the pathways that control the regulation of cell proliferation and/or differentiation. The most widely recognised tumor suppressor gene is p53 which is localized to the short arm of chromosome 17 and has been found to be mutated or absent in a wide range of human cancers including lung, breast, colon, sarcomas, leukemias, and gliomas.[9, 10] The p53 gene codes for a protein that controls the passage of proliferating cells through the normal cell cycles and prevents potentially dangerous DNA mutations from being passed on to subsequent generations. If certain DNA defects are detected, the cell cycle is arrested by p53 and the defect is either repaired or the cell undergoes destruction in a process called apoptosis. For a tumor suppressor gene to contribute towards tumorigenesis both of its alleles must be inactivated and therefore mutations behave as a genetically recessive trait. Patients with NF2 carry a germline mutation of one of the two NF2 alleles; therefore, all of the somatic cells have inherited this mutation from gametogenesis. An NF2 related tumor will only develop if the normal NF2 allele is inactivated, causing a failure of production of all functional NF2 protein in that cell. Because of the very high penetrance of NF2, the incidence of inactivation of a normal NF2 allele must be very high, and this explains the apparent paradox of the phenotypic picture of a dominantly-inherited disease, which results from a recessive mutation at the genetic level. In sporadic vestibular schwannomas mutations of both NF2 alleles have occurred as two spontaneous rare events in a single Schwann cell.

The NF2 gene has been isolated almost simultaneously by two separate laboratory groups.[7, 8] The gene is located on the long arm of chromosome 22, in the 22q12 region (Fig 1) and codes for an approximately 590 amino acid protein which has been called merlin[7] and schwannomin[8] by the respective groups. Schwannomin has become the popular term for the NF2 protein. It seems that the NF2 gene is a novel tumor suppressor gene because its product is a protein that appears to be involved with the integrity and function of cellular membranes and the cytoskeleton, a role not previously described with respect to tumor suppressor gene products. Schwannomin has a striking homology (of the order of 50%) to at least three cytoskeleton associated proteins: moesin, ezrin and radixin, hence the original name merlin (moesin-ezrin-radixin-like-protein). Schwannomin may therefore be involved in stable cell-cell and cell-matrix interactions and its absence may potentially lead to cell migration, changes in cell shape, or loss of contact inhibition.[8] Loss of the NF2 gene may be important in the development of sporadic meningiomas[11] although a recent study has provided evidence that familial meningioma results from a mutated chromosome 22 gene distinct from NF2.[12] It appears that the development of meningiomas may result from mutation of one of possibly two different genes along chromosome 22[13] although there is still an ongoing debate as to the existence of a defective non-NF2 gene on chromosome 22 that may be responsible for meningioma.[14]

The clinical separation of NF1 and NF2 is substantiated by the presence of the NF1 gene on the long arm of chromosome 17.[15] The NF1 gene is also a tumor suppressor gene and codes for a protein called neurofi-

REGIONS

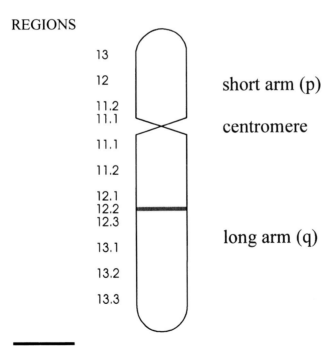

FIGURE 1.

Schematic representation of chromosome 22. The NF2 gene is represented by the shaded area on the long arm of chromosome 22.

bromin.[16] Neurofibromin has a GTPase-activating activity that catalyzes the inactivation of the protein p21-ras and functions to down-regulate one step in an important cytoplasmic pathway involved in the control of cell proliferation.[17]

The primary mutation in NF2 is inherited in the germline, with about one-half of all cases of NF2 representing a new mutation. Prevalence studies in the United Kingdom have documented the incidence of NF2 as high as 1 in 33,000 to 40,000 live births.[18] Inheritance is autosomal dominant and so each offspring of an affected individual has a 50% chance of being a carrier. The NF2 gene is highly penetrant, with gene carriers having a 95% chance of developing bilateral vestibular schwannomas. A significant maternal gene effect has been demonstrated with onset of symptoms or diagnosis occurring approximately 5 years earlier (average 18 years) in maternally than in paternally inherited cases.[18, 19] The age of onset is variable, however, with tumors presenting as late as the seventh decade of life or as early as the first 12 months. Approximately one-half of NF2 patients are symptomatic by 30 years of age and 90% of carriers will be affected by age 50.[20] Clinical presentation is also heterogeneous.[21, 22] Some families are characterized by a relatively benign form in which vestibular schwannomas are the only usual features. In these cases age of onset is later, usually after 25 years, and tumor progression may be very slow without significant hearing loss occurring. Other families have a severe form with early onset, usually less than 15 years, of rapidly progressive and multiple intracranial and spinal tumors. The peripheral features are more pronounced in these severe cases.

In addition to vestibular schwannomas, a variety of central nervous system, ophthalmologic, and dermatologic manifestations are seen with NF2. Schwannomas of other cranial nerves and spinal nerve roots occur as well as meningiomas and spinal cord ependymonas. Juvenile posterior subcapsular cataracts are common, and less frequently, iris Lish nodules are observed. Dermatologic manifestations are less common in NF2, skin tumors are predominantly schwannomas, and variable skin hyperpigmentation may occur.

DIAGNOSTIC ADVANCES

The diagnostic criteria for NF2 were defined at the National Institutes of Health consensus development conference on neurofibromatosis in 1987 and revised in 1991.[6, 23] The criteria for NF2 are met if a person has either of the following: bilateral VIII masses seen with appropriate imaging techniques (eg, computed tomography [CT] or magnetic resonance imaging [MRI]), or a first-degree relative (parent or sibling) with NF2 and either a unilateral VIII nerve mass or one of either neurofibroma, meningioma, glioma, schwannoma, or juvenile posterior subcapsular lenticular opacity.

MAGNETIC RESONANCE IMAGING

The most significant development in the diagnosis of NF2 was the introduction in 1988 of the contrast agent gadolinium DTPA (Gadopentetic acid, Magnevist, Burlix Laboratories, Inc., Wayne, NJ) for magnetic resonance imaging. Gadolinium enhanced MRI is currently the most sensitive imaging method for the detection of vestibular schwannomas (Fig 2). Gadolinium provides an indicator of disruption of the blood brain barrier and schwannomas as small as 2 mm are detectable. For this reason, on the basis of imaging, the exclusion of bilateral vestibular schwannomas can now only be made after gadolinium enhanced MRI with 1.5 mm overlapping, 3.0 mm thick cuts through the posterior fossa. Computed tomographic scan with intravenous contrast can be used to demonstrate larger tumors; however, resolution is considerably inferior to MRI. Intracannalicular tumors will generally not be demonstrated on CT scan unless subarachnoid air contrast is utilized. Some patients will not tolerate MRI due to claustrophobia and in this case CT scanning may be necessary. Gadolinium is also considerably safer than iodinated contrast media; however, anaphylactoid reactions have been reported and so it is not entirely without risk.[24, 25]

All individuals diagnosed with NF2 should undergo MRI of the total neuraxis with and without gadolinium contrast in order to document spinal nerve root schwannomas or spinal cord ependymonas. Individuals without spinal lesions tend to have a more benign form of the disorder and have a longer life expectancy. Magnetic resonance imaging now allows for the spinal tumors to be diagnosed and monitored noninvasively with similar sensitivity to myelography and follow up CT scanning. (Fig 3)

DNA ANALYSIS

The most recent development in diagnosis of NF2 is the use of DNA analysis to directly identify the NF2 gene mutation.[26] Until 1993 genetic

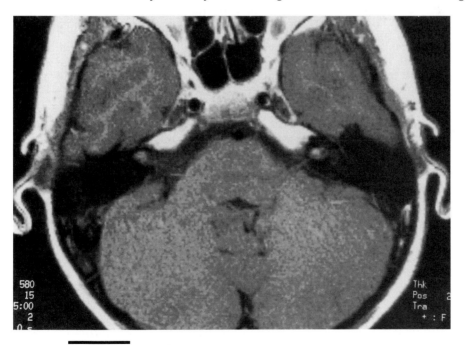

FIGURE 2.
Gadolinium enhanced MRI scan demonstrating bilateral small vestibular schwannomas.

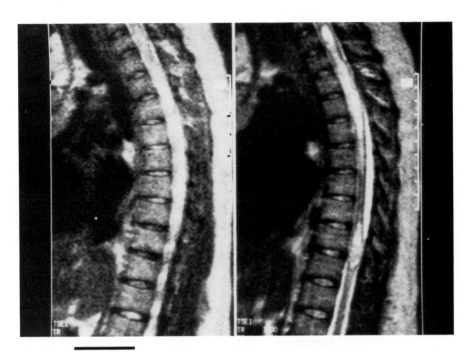

FIGURE 3.
Magnetic resonance scan demonstrating spinal cord ependymomas.

screening for relatives of an NF2 patient was time consuming and neces-sitated genetic linkage analysis. This requires two previous affected gen-erations. Linkage analysis screens blood lymphocyte DNA for identifiable genetic loci that associate closely with the mutant NF2 gene along chro-mosome 22 but only provides probability odds of a relative harboring NF2.[27] With the isolation of the NF2 gene, members of NF2 families can now be directly tested for mutations and unaffected individuals can be spared repeated medical evaluation.[6] Unfortunately, these new direct screening tests are also currently very time consuming, costly, and are only available in a few limited facilities that can screen for only a lim-ited number of all the possible NF2 mutations. The current difficulties of performing a full mutation screen in each at-risk individual suggest that screening for the NF2 gene will not be immediately available in most DNA diagnostic laboratories.[26] Tumors of NF2 patients can be stored in liquid nitrogen for future analysis against relatives' DNA, but until direct ge-netic screening becomes generally available the traditional clinical follow-up will remain the standard management of affected individuals and their families.

Any young patient (less than 40 years of age) with a unilateral ves-tibular schwannoma should be suspected of having NF2. Magnetic reso-nance imaging with gadolinium enhancement is particularly important in such patients as there have been numerous cases where CT imaging failed to demonstrate the contralateral tumor. When NF2 is suspected the full battery of audiologic tests including acoustic reflex studies and audi-tory brain stem response testing should be performed, although these also may be normal even in the presence of small tumors. Clinical examination should include complete ophthalmologic and dermatologic assessment.

HEARING PRESERVATION TUMOR REMOVAL—REFINEMENT OF TECHNIQUES

The results of hearing preservation acoustic neuroma removal in NF2 patients have been worse than in patients with unilateral tumors.[28-30] It is now accepted that the vestibular schwannomas in NF2 tumors are histologically the same as sporadic tumors. This has been confirmed by recent genetic studies. The apparent greater invasiveness in NF2 tumors, as demonstrated in the histologic study by Linthicum,[31] may represent a polyclonal origin within the vestibular nerve, rather than a difference in growth pattern and histology. The poorer hearing preservation results may be secondary to larger tumor size and possibly this polyclonal origin. Doyle and Shelton[32] have reviewed the experience at the House Ear Clinic with middle fossa craniotomy tumor removal and reported a 67% hearing preservation rate for NF2 patients. Only 38%, however, had serviceable hearing.

With increased use of the middle fossa approach and several technical modifications, the rate of hearing preservation has improved. Changes in technique include wider medial bone removal, medial to lateral dissection of tumor and preservation of nontumor neural elements. Most recently, Brackmann et al. reported that 71% of a series of 24 consecutive patients had hearing preserved at or near preoperative levels.[33] Although only two of this series were NF2 patients (both had their hearing preserved), we believe such improved results will also be likely in patients with NF2 particularly if their tumors are diagnosed while still intracannalicular.

CRITERIA FOR HEARING PRESERVATION

Serviceable contralateral hearing must be present if tumor removal for hearing preservation is to be attempted. The potential for successful hearing preservation is limited by a number of factors, primarily tumor size. The inverse relationship between tumor size and the rate of hearing preservation is now generally accepted. In reported series of unilateral tumors, the upper limit of tumor size for middle fossa hearing preservation has generally been sited as 1.5 cm and 1.5 to 2 cm for retrosigmoid-suboccipital removal.[34-39] Only exceptional cases of hearing preservation in tumors 3 cm and larger have been reported. Gardner and Robertson estimated an overall 33% hearing preservation rate for a total of 394 unilateral tumors removed by either middle fossa or retrosigmoid procedures in their literature review.[40]

As noted, the overall hearing preservation rate for bilateral tumors is even lower. For tumors 2 cm or larger in greatest diameter the chance of preserving serviceable hearing is too small to justify surgical removal until other factors necessitate it. As demonstrated for patients with unilateral tumors, a comprehensive audiologic evaluation can be helpful in the assessment of likely hearing preservation. The preoperative hearing level provides some indication of the degree of involvement of the cochlear nerve and cochlear blood supply by the tumor and the greater the involvement, the greater likelihood of further hearing loss with surgery.[41] Assessment of VIII nerve integrity by audiologic parameters such as audiogram, speech discrimination score, auditory brain stem response (ABR), and electronystamography has been shown to have predictive value for successful hearing preservation. Hypoactive caloric response on electronystamography, indicating superior vestibular nerve involvement and an auditory brain stem response interaural wave V latency difference of less than 0.4 ms are positive prognostic indicators.[42] For unilateral tumors, poor prognostic indicators such as speech reception threshold (SRT) greater than 50 dB and speech discrimination score (SDS) less than 50% indicate that attempted hearing preservation is pointless in the setting of a normal contralateral ear. For NF2 patients, any preserved hearing is potentially useful; thus, provided tumor size is favorable, less conservative audiologic criteria than the 50-50 rule (SRT and SDS) may be used when attempted hearing preservation is considered.

SURGICAL APPROACH

The choice of surgical approach for hearing preservation tumor removal is determined by the tumor site and size. We prefer the *middle cranial fossa approach* because exposure of the full length of the internal auditory canal (IAC) is possible. Increased physician awareness, use of gadolinium enhanced MR imaging, and appropriate screening of NF2 families is resulting in the early diagnosis of intracannalicular tumors. The middle cranial fossa approach is ideal for these small intracannalicular tumors and those that extend less than 1.0 cm beyond the porous acousticus into the cerebellopontine angle (CPA).

The *retrosigmoid-suboccipital approach* provides greater access to the CPA than does the middle cranial approach; however, the posterior semicircular canal and vestibule limit access to the lateral fundus of the IAC. If hearing is to be preserved, the labyrinth must not be entered and so dissection of the IAC fundus must be accomplished blindly with the possibility of subtotal tumor removal and tumor recurrence. The retrosigmoid approach is ideally suitable for tumors that are more medially situated with up to 2 cm of CPA extension but without involvement of the IAC fundus, as shown on MRI. Unfortunately, among NF2 patients, few tumors fall into this category. Usually the tumor fills the fundus of the internal auditory canal.

Deterioration in hearing level over time has been documented after removal of unilateral tumors. This may present a significant problem in the case of initially successful NF2 tumor removal. Also, as noted above, successful hearing preservation requires preservation of the cochlear nerve and blood supply. This is achieved by preserving nontumor neural elements that often include remnants of the vestibular nerve. In view of the potential for polyclonal origin of vestibular schwannomas in NF2, it seems likely that second tumors may develop at some time subsequent to hearing preservation tumor removal. Long-term follow-up of all patients who have had attempted hearing preservation procedures is necessary in order to assess whether this is the case.

HEARING RESTORATION—AUDITORY BRAIN STEM IMPLANT

Another exciting advance in the management of NF2 is the success of the auditory brain stem implant. Development of the ABI has progressed to the stage of a multicenter international clinical trial. The first cochlear nucleus implant was performed in 1979 by Drs. William House and William Hitselberger.[43] They implanted a pair of electrodes into the cochlear nucleus of a human volunteer with NF2 during the surgical procedure to remove the second side acoustic neuroma. Since then, a total of 35 patients have been implanted with a variety of prototype devices. Stimulation of the electrodes has produced auditory sensation in most patients, with results similar to a single channel cochlear implant.[44] Currently, a multielectrode prosthesis connected to a subcutaneous electromagnetic receiver (similar to the cochlear corporation multichannel cochlear implant) is implanted (Fig 4). The electrode array is placed over the surface of the cochlear nucleus within the lateral recess of the fourth ventricle (Figs 5 and 6).[45] Stimulation is through a transcutaneous coil system with a variety of speech processing strategies available depending on the results of electrode mapping.

The ABI is designed for those patients with loss of cochlear nerve function secondary to resection of bilateral vestibular schwannomas. Currently the ABI has only been approved for implantation at the time of tumor removal. A translabyrinthine approach is utilized for tumor removal so as to allow the most lateral access to the anteriorly facing lateral recess. After tumor removal has been completed, the foramen of Luschka and lateral recess of the fourth ventricle identified by anatomic landmarks, such as the stump of the cochleovestibular nerve, choroid plexus, and taenia. The electrode array is then inserted fully within the lateral

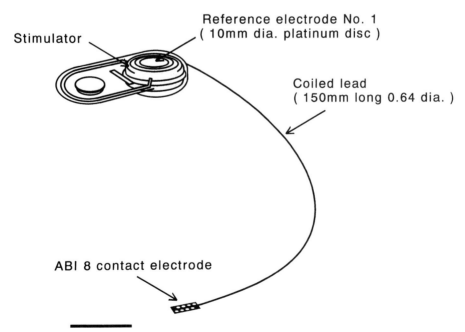

FIGURE 4.

Schematic representation of the multielectrode auditory brain stem implant.

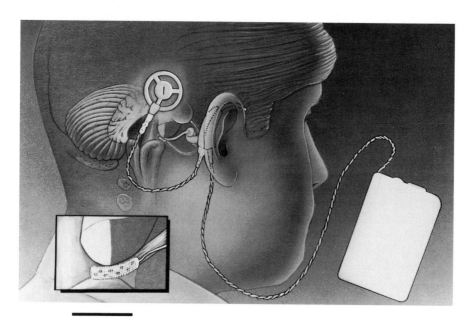

FIGURE 5.
Schematic representation of the auditory brain stem implant with speech processor and transcutaneous coil transducer. Insert shows multielectrode array within lateral recess of fourth ventricle.

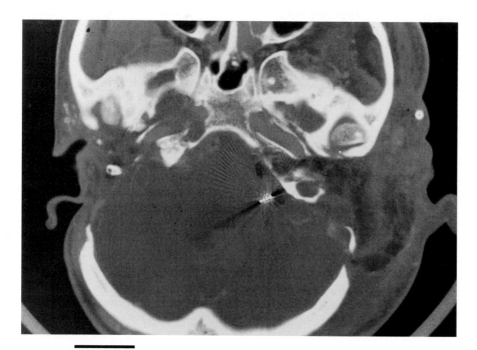

FIGURE 6.
Computed tomographic scan demonstrating the brain stem implant electrode array within the lateral recess of fourth ventricle.

recess with the electrodes facing superiorly to contact the cochlear nuclei. After placement of the electrode array, intraoperative electrophysiologic monitoring by electrically evoked auditory brain stem responses is performed to ensure that the electrodes do activate the auditory system and to assess for activation of nonauditory brain stem structures (V, VII, IX, X) and vital sign changes.[45]

Most implanted patients receive auditory stimulation without significant nonauditory side effects. They are able to utilize the auditory sensation to supplement lip reading and recognize simple temporal sequences. All 11 patients with the Cochlear Corporation multichannel ABI have superior speech recognition performance compared to those with the previous single channel implant. The current criteria for ABI patient selection are listed in Table 1.

The multielectrode ABI developed by the House Ear Institute and Cochlear Corporation has eight active electrodes. In Europe a 22 electrode ABI has been developed and was first implanted in 1992. The patient had total hearing loss following gamma knife irradiation for NF2 and with electrical stimulation regained sound perception sufficient to supplement lip reading.[46]

COCHLEAR IMPLANT

In some NF2 patients a multichannel cochlear implant may be used to partially restore hearing as reported by Hoffman et al.[47] Suitable patients are those with nonaidable hearing who have an intact cochlear nerve following tumor removal. In general, such patients will be those who have undergone removal of a small tumor with unsuccessful attempted hearing preservation. In such cases the cochlear nerve is often preserved intact and the hearing loss is presumed secondary to disturbance of the cochlear blood supply. Preservation of a functional cochlear nerve is unlikely in cases where tumor removal is necessitated by tumor size, particularly as every attempt at total tumor removal should be made. In the occasional small tumor with total hearing loss, preservation of the cochlear nerve may be attempted during tumor removal with the view to subsequent cochlear implantation. Zwolan et al.[48] have even demonstrated that the labyrinthectomy performed as part of the translabyrinthine approach may not prevent successful cochlear implantation. Successful promontory or round window stimulation provides an indication of viable spiral ganglion cells and functional cochlear nerve. It is not,

---

TABLE 1.
Criteria for Auditory Brain Stem Implant

Evidence of bilateral VIII nerve tumors
Competency in the English language
Age of 15 years or older
Psychological suitability
Willingness to comply with research follow-up protocol
Realistic expectations

however, prerequisite for implantation. Electrically evoked ABR is becoming increasingly feasible and hopefully will provide a sensitive method of selecting patients who will benefit from cochlear implantation. Intracochlear electrically evoked ABR, as described by Montandon et al,[49] may be the only way of demonstrating those patients who will not benefit from cochlear implantation.

FAMILY SCREENING—PATIENT EDUCATION

In view of the autosomal dominant inheritance of NF2 and the devastating consequences of the condition, it is essential that every patient is appropriately educated and their family screened to identify other affected or at-risk individuals. It is the responsibility of the physician to commence patient education by fully informing the individual and their family of the nature of NF2 and the genetic implications.[50] Genetic counseling should be made available and the geneticist should become involved in family screening. Patients should be referred to organisations such as the California NF2 research group, which can provide multidisciplinary care and counseling for NF2 patients and their families.

Diagnostic screening must be offered and should be encouraged for all at-risk first-degree relatives of patients with NF2. Those at-risk relatives who already have manifestations of NF2 can usually be identified by routine clinical and audiologic testing. Careful dilated ophthalmic examination is required to identify posterior capsular lens opacities. Alterations in pure tone hearing thresholds, speech discrimination, acoustic reflex thresholds, and ABR wave-forms or latencies indicate the necessity for MRI. It is now well recognized, however, that tumors may be present with normal audiologic parameters; thus, ideally all at-risk first-degree relatives should have gadolinium enhanced MRI performed to exclude asymptomatic lesions.

As discussed above, where families have two or more affected generations, genetic linkage DNA analysis using chromosome markers located close to the NF2 gene on chromosome 22 can be used to identify asymptomatic gene carriers.[27] Such early diagnosis will allow close follow-up examination and hopefully hearing preservation tumor removal prior to significant hearing impairment. It is recommended that at-risk individuals should have repeat MRI scans every 3 years, at least until the age of 50 when the risk of manifesting NF2 is greatly diminished, although not eliminated.

As well as education about the nature of their condition, all NF2 patients and families should commence appropriate rehabilitation. This should be in the anticipation of eventual profound or total hearing loss. Instruction in speech reading, signing, and use of the telephone typewriter (TTY) should be undertaken, preferably before significant hearing loss occurs.

TREATMENT STRATEGIES

Management of the individual NF2 patient requires a comprehensive multidisciplinary approach. Treatment strategies are determined by the patient's age, sex, the size and growth rate of the vestibular schwannomas, and level, quality, and rate of change of hearing in each ear. The presence of other intracranial or spinal tumors and any associated neurologic deficit is also considered. Also social, psychological, and occupational circumstances need to be considered in deciding which of the following treatment options to recommend.

OBSERVATION WITHOUT SURGICAL INTERVENTION

The presence of vestibular schwannomas alone is not indication for surgical removal. Tumor size and hearing level may remain stable for many years, and observation without surgical intervention should be the initial approach in many neurologically stable cases. Observation is recommended when a tumor is present in an only hearing ear, even if the tumor is small, or when there is bilateral hearing but tumors that are too large for likely hearing preservation removal. The patient must be neurologically stable, however, and there must be no risk from tumor size, i.e., brain stem compression or hydrocephalus. Close follow-up is essential and should be initially at 6 months and then annually. Magnetic resonance imaging is repeated to document tumor growth or development of obstructive hydrocephalus. Clinical examination and audiometry is performed to document any change in hearing level and identify impending problems such as involvement of other cranial nerves or raised intracranial pressure. The patient is encouraged to notify the otologist immediately in the case of any fluctuation of hearing or onset of other symptoms. Surgical intervention is considered if further hearing loss occurs or when the tumor reaches sufficient size (approximately 3 cm) to produce symptoms.

HEARING PRESERVATION SURGERY—TOTAL TUMOR REMOVAL

Hearing preservation removal of vestibular schwannomas is a reasonable goal in selected NF2 patients and should be considered when there is bilateral serviceable hearing and small tumors. Total tumor removal with attempted hearing preservation through a middle cranial fossa approach is recommended for patients in whom one, or preferably both, of their tumors fulfill the above criteria for likely successful hearing preservation. Even with small tumors, there is usually some asymmetry, if only slight, in tumor size and hearing levels. Our policy has been to recommend surgical removal on the side with the larger tumor and/or greater hearing impairment. This retains the better hearing which should last the longest, should hearing be lost at the time of tumor removal. This approach is in contrast to that advocated by Glasscock et al,[51] who recommend removal of the smaller tumor on the side with better hearing on the basis that it is the best opportunity to save hearing.

In choosing the tumor to be initially treated, the relative chances of hearing preservation must be carefully assessed. Factors such as a large discrepancy in tumor size suggest the need to treat the smaller tumor in order to enhance the likelihood of hearing preservation. Hearing in the contralateral ear must at least be serviceable even if the tumor is too large for a likely hearing preservation removal. If hearing is successfully preserved at a serviceable level, removal of the contralateral tumor (if suitable) is recommended after 6 months. At least this delay is necessary to demonstrate that the hearing is stable in the operated ear. If the initial tumor removal results in hearing loss, the contralateral tumor is observed and hearing preservation surgery is not attempted.

Occasionally there will be a tumor suitable for attempted hearing preservation removal in an only hearing ear, possibly following failed contralateral hearing preservation tumor removal. As noted above, we recommend observation in this circumstance. Some patients, however, may request surgery despite the chance of total hearing loss, understanding that this provides the only chance for permanent hearing preservation.

INTERNAL AUDITORY CANAL DECOMPRESSION WITHOUT TUMOR REMOVAL—MIDDLE FOSSA APPROACH

Where there is progressive hearing loss in the situation of unilateral hearing or tumors too large for likely hearing preservation tumor removal, decompression of the tumor within the IAC, without tumor removal, can be performed in the hope of stabilizing or even improving hearing. Such IAC decompression has been performed through a middle fossa craniotomy approach.

If progression or fluctuation of hearing impairment occurs in a patient being observed, then decompression of the tumor within the IAC is recommended. A middle fossa craniotomy is utilized and bone is widely removed medial to the cochlea and superior semicircular canal to decompress the IAC. The dura of the IAC and the porous acousticus is incised along its posterior border and reflected to allow maximal tumor decompression. Intraoperative monitoring with ABR and facial electromyogram is used routinely. The tumor is not debulked as this significantly increases the risk of further hearing loss. Since the report by Gadre et al,[52] middle fossa decompression has been performed in a further seven patients.

PARTIAL TUMOR REMOVAL—RETROSIGMOID APPROACH

The only circumstance in which partial tumor removal should be considered is when a patient has good unilateral hearing and a tumor that is symptomatic due to large size. In this circumstance, debulking of the tumor through a retrosigmoid craniotomy may be performed in the hope of reducing the risk and relieving symptoms due to pressure, while retaining serviceable hearing. A cuff of tumor capsule is left in an attempt to protect the seventh and eighth nerves and cochlear blood supply. This is only a temporizing measure and unfortunately in our experience, partial tumor removal in NF2 patients has usually resulted in significant hearing impairment. Also, rapid tumor regrowth usually occurs, presumably due to the preserved vascular supply to the tumor capsule.

NON–HEARING PRESERVATION—TRANSLABYRINTHINE TOTAL TUMOR REMOVAL

Where hearing preservation is no longer possible, due to tumor size or previous hearing loss, total tumor removal with facial nerve preservation is the goal. Sacrifice of residual hearing may be necessary if a large tumor is producing symptomatic brain stem compression. We have favored the translabyrinthine approach as this allows safe tumor removal with maximal preservation of facial nerve function.

The translabyrinthine approach is recommended for tumors of any size in an ear without useful hearing or for large tumors producing symptomatic brain stem compression, even if there is residual hearing. As noted by Linthicum, NF2 tumors are often of considerable size before hearing impairment occurs and diagnosis is made.[31] For large tumors in particular, the translabyrinthine approach allows safe tumor removal with minimal cerebellar retraction and maximal preservation of facial nerve function.[53]

HEARING RESTORATION—AUDITORY BRAIN STEM IMPLANT

Perhaps the greatest advantage of the translabyrinthine approach is that it allows direct access to the lateral recess of the fourth ventricle for placement of the ABI electrode array. Patients with NF2 who fulfill the above criteria for translabyrinthine tumor removal should be considered for hearing restoration by auditory brain stem implantation, even if hearing remains serviceable in the contralateral ear.

OTHER ISSUES IN THE MANAGEMENT OF PATIENTS WITH NF2

STEREOTACTIC RADIATION THERAPY

Stereotactic radiation therapy was initially thought to be an answer to the dilemma of how to manage bilateral acoustic neuromas. Patients with NF2 have frequently been submitted for radiosurgery to the second side tumor. Unfortunately, this often results in progression of their hearing impairment and does not guarantee control of tumor growth. While studies with long-term follow-up are not yet available, reported hearing results have been worse than those for microsurgical removal of small tumors. Only 38% report having useful hearing preserved after 12 months; in addition, facial nerve dysfunction occurred in 34% of patients.[54] For large tumors, there is increased risk of radiation necrosis of the adjacent brain stem and cerebellum. In our experience, radiation induced fibrosis has complicated tumor removal when surgery became necessary due to continued growth, and in one case the fibrosis and anatomical distortion following radiation prevented successful placement of an ABI.[55] Stereotactic radiotherapy should be considered only in patients who are poor surgical risks or refuse surgery.

MANAGEMENT OF NONAUDITORY MANIFESTATIONS OF NF2

Advances in the management of NF2 related tumors have been the same as those for sporadic neurologic tumors and particularly relate to improvements in the diagnosis (especially MRI). Technical advances with the use of laser, computer-assisted stereotactic localization and resection, angiography and tumor embolization, ultrasonic tumor removal, stereotactic radiosurgery,[56] and intraoperative monitoring, such as somatosensory, brain stem, cranial nerve and motor evoked potentials all hopefully contribute to reduced morbidity rates and improved outcome. A discussion of the surgical management of the nonvestibular cranial nerve and spinal nerve root schwannomas, meningiomas, or spinal cord ependymomas is beyond the scope of this chapter. In general, such lesions are observed until the risk from size or development of symptoms necessitates removal.

Occular abnormalities are important both in the diagnosis and management of the patient with NF2. Posterior subcapsular and/or capsular cataracts are found in up to 80% of affected individuals and are particularly diagnostic when they occur at an early age. The lens opacification may progress with age and prompt surgical removal of the cataract must be considered, particularly in patients who may already be limited by hearing loss.

FUTURE POSSIBILITIES

A variety of possibilities exist for future control of tumor growth. Angiogenic growth factor inhibition has shown, in vitro, to suppress growth of human nerve sheath tumors.[57] Cloning of the NF2 gene product may provide a tumor suppressor factor that can be administered locally or systemically to suppress vestibular schwannoma growth rate. Somatic gene therapy may eventually be possible with replacement of the inactivated NF2 gene in order to prevent tumorigenesis.

SUMMARY

The importance of early diagnosis of NF2 is paramount for both the individual and family. Recent advances including identification of the NF2 gene and recognition of the variable clinical manifestations, as well as the use of gadolinium enhanced MRI have made the early diagnosis of small tumors more frequent. Total surgical tumor removal with hearing preservation is, therefore, more feasible and should be considered in appropriate patients. For those patients with NF2 with large tumors or more profound hearing loss, development of the ABI has made the restoration of useful auditory function a realistic goal at the time of tumor removal. These developments, combined with the rarity and severity of NF2, have stimulated calls for the establishment of a register of patients and families and management by a few supraregional centers.[58]

REFERENCES

1. Rouleau GA, Wertelecki W, Haines JL, et al: Genetic linkage of bilateral acoustic neurofibromatosis to a DNA marker on chromosome 22. *Nature* 329:246–248, 1987.
2. Barker D, Wright E, Nguyen L, et al: Gene for von Recklinghausen neurofibromatosis is in the pericentromeric region of chromosome 17. *Science* 236:1100–1102, 1987.
3. Seizinger BR, Rouleau GA, Ozelius LJ, et al: Genetic linkage of von Recklinghausen neurofibromatosis to the nerve growth factor receptor gene. *Cell* 49:589–594, 1987.
4. Miller RM, Sparkes RS: Segmental neurofibromatosis. *Arch Dermatol* 113:837–838, 1977.

5. Riccardi VM: Neurofibromatosis: Clinical heterogeneity. *Curr Prob Cancer* VII:1–24, 1982.

6. National Institutes of Health Consensus Development Conference Statement on Acoustic Neuroma, December 11–13, 1991. *Arch Neurol* 51:201–207, 1994.

7. Trofatter JA, MacCollin MM, Rutter JL, et al: A novel moesin-, ezrin-, radixin-like gene is candidate for the neurofibromatosis 2 tumor suppressor. *Cell* 72:791–800, 1993.

8. Rouleau GA, Merel P, Lutchman M, et al: Alteration in a new gene encoding a putative membrane-organizing protein causes neuro-fibromatosis type 2. *Nature* 363:515–521, 1993.

9. Donehower LA, Bradley A: The tumor suppressor p53. *Biochim Biophys Acta* 1155:181–205, 1993.

10. Levine AJ: The tumor suppressor genes. *Annu Rev Biochem* 62:623–651, 1993.

11. Seizinger BR, de la Monte S, Atkins L, et al: Molecular genetic approach to human meningioma: loss of genes on chromosome 22. *Proc Natl Acad Sci USA* 84:5419–5423, 1987.

12. Pulst S-M, Rouleau GA, Marineau C, et al: Familial meningioma is not allelic to neurofibromatosis 2. *Neurology* 43:2096–2098, 1993.

13. Murphy M, Pyket MJ, Harnish P, et al: Identification and characterization of genes differentially expressed in meningiomas. *Cell Growth Differ* 4:715–722, 1993.

14. Sanson M, Marineau C, Desmaze C, et al: Germline deletion in a neurofibromatosis type 2 kindred inactivates the NF2 gene and a candidate meningioma locus. *Hum Mol Genet* 2:1215–1220, 1993.

15. Barker D, Wright E, Nguyen K, et al: Gene for von Recklinghausen neurofibromatosis is in the pericentromeric region of chromosome 17. *Science* 236:1100–1102, 1987.

16. Xu G, O'Connell P, Viskochil D, et al: The neurofibromatosis type 1 gene encodes a protein related to GAP. *Cell* 62:599–608, 1980.

17. Gutman DH, Collins F: The neurofibromatosis type gene and its protein product, neurofibromin. *Neuron* 10:335–343, 1993.

18. Evans DGR, Huson SM, Donnai D, et al: A genetic study of type 2 neurofibromatosis in the United Kingdom 1. Prevalence, mutation rate, fitness, and confirmation of maternal transmission effect on severity. *J Med Genet* 29:841–846, 1992.

19. Kanter W, Eldridge R: Evidence of a maternal effect in central neurofibromatosis. *Lancet* 2:903, 1978.

20. Wertelecki W, Rouleau GA, Superneau DW, et al: Neurofibromatosis 2: Clinical and DNA linkage studies of a large kindred. *N Engl J Med* 318:684–688, 1988.

21. Evans DGR, Huson SM, Neary W, et al: A clinical study of neurofibromatosis. *Q J Med* 304:603–618, 1992.

22. Eldridge R, Parry DM, Kaiser-Kupfer MI: Neurofibromatosis 2: Clinical heterogeneity and natural history in 39 individuals in 9 families and 16 sporadic cases. *Am J Hum Genet* 49:133(A676), 1991.

23. Neurofibromatosis Conference Statement. National Institutes of Health Consensus Development Conference. *Arch Neurol* 45:575–578, 1988.

24. Lufkin RB: Severe anaphylactoid reaction to Gd-DTPA. *Radiology* 176:879, 1990.

25. Weiss KL, Jhaveri HS: Severe anaphylactoid reaction after IV Gd DTPA. Society of Magnetic Resonance Imaging, Abstracts, 8th Annual meeting Washington, D.C. 1990.

26. MacCollin M, Mohney T, Trofatter J, et al: DNA diagnosis of neurofibromatosis 2. *JAMA* 270:2316–2320, 1993.

27. Ruttledge MH, Narod SA, Dumanski JP, et al: Presymptomatic diagnosis of neurofibromatosis 2 with chromosome 22 markers. *Neurology* 43:753–1760, 1993.

28. Hughes GB, Sismanis A, Glasscock ME III, et al: Management of bilateral acoustic tumors. *Laryngoscope* 92:1351–1359, 1982.

29. Montgomery WW: Bilateral acoustic neuromas. *Ann Otol Rhinol Laryngol* 87:135–137, 1978.

30. Sterkers JM: Removal of bilateral acoustic neuromas with preservation of hearing. A comparison of the retrosigmoid and translabyrinthine approach, in Silverstein H, Norrel H (eds): *Neurological Surgery of the Ear*, vol 2. Birmingham, AL: Aesculapius Publishing, 1979, pp 269–277.

31. Linthicum FH: Unusual audiometric and histologic findings in bilateral acoustic neuromas. *Ann Otol* 81:433–437, 1972.

32. Doyle KJ, Shelton C: Hearing preservation in bilateral acoustic neuroma surgery. *Am J Otol* 14:562–565, 1993.

33. Brackmann DE, House JR, Hitselberger WE: Technical modifications to the middle cranial fossa approach in removal of acoustic neuromas. *Am J Otol*, 15:614–619, 1994.

34. Gantz BJ, Parnes LS, Harker LA, et al: Middle cranial fossa acoustic neuroma exicision: Results and complications. *Ann Otol Rhinol Laryngol* 95:454–459, 1986.

35. Wade PJ, House W: Hearing preservation in patients with acoustic neuromas via the middle fossa approach. *Otolaryngol Head Neck Surg* 92:184–193, 1984.

36. Glasscock ME, Hays JW, Josey AF, et al: Middle fossa approach for acoustic tumor removal and preservation of hearing, in Brackmann DE (ed): *Neurological Surgery of the Ear and Skull Base*. New York, Raven Press, 1982, pp 223–226.

37. Smith MFW: Conservation of hearing in acoustic schwannoma surgery. *Am J Otol* 99:405–408, 1985.

38. Cohen NL, Hammerrschlag P, Berg H, et al: Acoustic neuroma surgery: An eclectic approach with emphasis on preservation of hearing. The New York-Bellevue experience. *Ann Otol Rhinol Laryngol* 95:21–27, 1986.

39. Silverstein H, McDaniel A, Norrel H, et al: Hearing preservation after acoustic neuroma surgery with intraoperative direct eighth cranial nerve monitoring: A classification of results. *Otolaryngol Head Neck Surg* 95:285–291, 1986.

40. Gardner G, Robertson JH: Hearing preservation in unilateral acoustic neuroma surgery. *Ann Otol Rhinol Laryngol* 97:55–66, 1988.

41. Josey AF, Glasscock ME III, Jackson CG: Preservation of hearing in acoustic tumor surgery: Audiologic indicators. *Ann Otol Rhinol Laryngol* 97:626–630, 1988.

42. Shelton C, Brackmann DE, House WF: Acoustic tumor surgery: Prognostic factors in hearing conservation. *Arch Otolarygnol Head Neck Surg* 115:1213–1216, 1989.

43. Edgerton BJ, House WF, Hitselberger WE: Hearing by cochlear nucleus stimulation in humans. *Ann Otol Rhinol Laryngol Suppl* 91:117–124, 1982.

44. Shannon RV, Fayad J, Moore J, et al: Auditory brainstem implant: II Postsurgical issues and performance. *Otolaryngol Head Neck Surg* 108:634–642, 1993.

45. Brackmann DE, Hitselberger WE, Nelson RA, et al: Auditory brainstem implant: II Postsurgical issues in surgical implantation. *Otolaryngol Head Neck Surg* 108:624–633, 1993.

46. Laszig R, Kuzma J, Siefert V, et al: The Hannover auditory brainstem implant: A multiple electrode prosthesis. *Eur Arch Otorhinolaryngol* 248:420–421, 1991.

47. Hoffman RA, Kohan D, Cohen NL: Cochlear implants in the management of bilateral acoustic neuromas. *Am J Otol* 13:525–529, 1992.

48. Zwolan TA, Shepherd NT, Niparko JK: Labyrinthectomy with cochlear implantation. *Am J Otol* 14:220–223, 1993.

49. Montandon P, Kasper A, Pelizzone M: Exploratory cochleotomy. *ORL J Otorhinolaryngol Relat Spec* 54:295–298, 1992.

50. Evans DGR, Huson SM, Neary W, et al: A genetic study of type 2 neurofibromatosis in the United Kingdom: II guidlines for genetic counselling. *J Med Genet* 29:847–852, 1992.

51. Glasscock ME III, Hart MJ, Vrabec JT: Management of bilateral acoustic neuroma. *Otolaryngol Clin North Am* 25:449–469, 1992.

52. Gadre AK, Kwartler JA, Brackmann DE, et al: Middle fossa decompression of the internal auditory canal in acoustic neuroma surgery: A therapeutic alternative. *Laryngoscope.* 100:948–952, 1990.

53. Briggs RJS, Luxford WM, Atkins JS, et al: Translabyrinthine removal of large ($\geq$ 4cm) acoustic neuromas. *Neurosurgery* 34:785–792, 1994.

54. Lunsford LD, Linskey ME: Stereotactic radiosurgery in the treatment of patients with acoustic tumors. *Otolaryngol Clin North Am* 25:471–491, 1992.

55. Slattery WH, Brackmann DE: Results of surgery following stereotactic irradiation for acoustic neuromas. *Am J Otol,* accepted 1994.

56. Kelly PJ, Goerss SJ, Kall BA: Evolution of contemporary instrumentation for computer assisted stereotactic surgery. *Surg Neurol* 30:204–215, 1988.

57. Takamiya Y, Friedlander RM, Brem H: Inhibition of angiogenesis and growth of human nerve-sheath tumors by AGM-1470. *J Neurosurg* 78:470–476, 1993.

58. Evans DGR, Ramsden R, Huson SM, et al: Type 2 neurofibromatosis: The need for supraregional care? *J Laryngol Otol* 107:401–406, 1993.

Nasopharyngeal Carcinoma*

Silloo B. Kapadia, M.D.

Associate Professor, Department of Pathology, University of Pittsburgh School of Medicine, Pittsburgh, Pennsylvania

Ivo P. Janecka, M.D.

Professor of Otolaryngology and Neurology, Center for Cranial Base Surgery, Departments of Otolaryngology and Neurological Surgery, University of Pittsburgh, Pittsburgh, Pennsylvania

N asopharyngeal carcinoma (NPCA) is a malignant tumor derived from the surface epithelium of the nasopharyngeal mucosa.[1-9] The definition excludes malignant tumors with evidence of glandular differentiation or mucin production.[2,3] All types of NPCA, however poorly differentiated, have ultrastructural characteristics of a squamous-cell carcinoma (tonofilaments and desmosomes).[2,3] Multiple factors play a role in the etiology of NPCA. They include race, genetically determined susceptibility, and environmental carcinogens of viral and chemical nature. However, the precise role of each of these factors is unknown.[8,9] The incidence of this tumor varies in different countries. People of southern Chinese origin have an unusually high frequency of this tumor (10 to 27 cases per 100,000). A lower incidence is found in Western countries including the United States (USA) (0.2% of all cancers), compared to 18% in Chinese populations.[6-11] Genetic susceptibility has been noted in Chinese patients in the presence of HLA-A2 and less than two antigens at locus B.[9,10] Consumption of nitrosamine-rich salted fish in early childhood and occupational exposure to smoke or dust inhalants may contribute to the high risk in southern Chinese.[9] Second generation Chinese have a lower risk than Asian-born first generation Chinese after emigration to the USA.[3,7,8,11] The ubiquitous Epstein-Barr virus (EBV) has a worldwide association with NPCA, despite geography.[12-14]

High titers of IgA antibodies to EBV-specific antigens, namely, the viral capsid antigen (VCA) and early antigen (EA), are seen in most patients with NPCA and reflect tumor burden.[12-14] A rising titer of anti-EBV antibodies is useful in the diagnosis and monitoring of patients.[8,9,13,14] In addition, EBV-DNA is consistently detectable in biopsy material of NPCA. The keratinizing variety is an exception.[15]

Nasopharyngeal carcinoma occurs in all age groups. The mean age of

---

*Surgical treatment adapted with permission from Janecka IP: in Myers EN (ed): *Operative Otolaryngology-Head and Neck Surgery.* WB Saunders, in preparation. Used by permission.

Advances in Otolaryngology—Head and Neck Surgery®, vol. 9
© 1995, Mosby–Year Book, Inc.

occurrence is about 50 years and males predominate by a ratio of 3:1.[3-8, 16, 17] The most frequent site of origin in the nasopharynx is the lateral wall (80%) in the region of Rosenmüller's fossa.[7, 9, 17] Common initial manifestations are a mass in the neck, middle ear effusion, and nasal obstruction or discharge. The presence of hearing loss, epistaxis, otalgia, headache, and cranial nerve involvement (10% to 12% of cases) are associated with more advanced stages of disease.[6, 8, 17] About 60% to 72% of patients have unilateral or bilateral cervical lymph node metastasis at the time of diagnosis, typically in the apex of the posterior cervical triangle.[8, 17] The primary lesion may be occult. The nasopharynx appears normal in 6% of cases.[17] In one study, the tumor was exophytic in 74.2%, infiltrative in 14.4%, and ulcerative in 7%; in 4.8% the type was not well documented.[7] Computed tomography (CT) provides an accurate assessment of the extent of the tumor, and of skull base erosion by tumor (30.9% of cases). Plain radiography lacks sensitivity and specificity.[18] A distant metastasis is not common at the time of diagnosis (4% to 5%), but is seen in up to 50% of cases during the course of the disease.[7, 17] Common distant metastatic sites include the bone, lung, and liver.

STAGING

In the American Joint Commission on Cancer (AJCC) staging classification for NPCA (Table 1), the primary tumor (T stage) is classified as follows: an invasion of one site of nasopharynx (T1), invasion of more than one site (T2), an invasion of nasal cavity and/or oropharynx (T3), and an invasion of skull and/or cranial nerve(s) (T4).[19] The nodal status (N stage) is classified as follows: a metastasis to a single ipsilateral lymph node, ≤3 cm in maximum dimension (N1); a metastasis in a single ipsilateral lymph node, >3 cm but <6 cm in maximum dimension, or multiple ipsilateral lymph nodes, none >6 cm, or bilateral or contralateral lymph nodes, none >6 cm (N2); and a metastasis in a lymph node >6 cm in maximum dimension (N3).[19]

According to Ho and others, examination of the nasopharynx is difficult in some patients. Therefore, the separation of tumors confined to the nasopharynx into T1 and T2, as recommended by the AJCC, is not practical.[9, 17] The Ho staging system (1978; Table 2) adopts the designation T1 for a primary tumor confined to the nasopharynx; T2 for extension to nasal fossa (T2n), oropharynx (T2o), parapharyngeal region (T2p), or nerves below the skull base; T3 for extension beyond areas of T1 and T2, with involvement of bone below skull base (T3a), of skull base (T3b), cranial nerves (T3c), and orbits, laryngopharynx, or infratemporal fossa (T3d).[9] Nodal status is classified as a nodal metastasis in the upper cervical level (N1), a nodal metastasis between level of the skin crease and the supraclavicular fossa (N2), and a nodal metastasis in the supraclavicular fossa and/or skin involvement (N3).[9] Using Ho's classification, Skinner et al found that at diagnosis, 80% of tumors were T2 or T3. Seventy-five percent of their patients had nodal disease, and 70% had advanced disease (Stage III-V).[17]

A recent modification of the Ho staging classification for NPCA was proposed by Theo et al (1991), with reduction in the number of stages

TABLE 1.

The American Joint Committee on Cancer (AJCC) Classification Nasopharynx—TNM Staging (1992)*

Primary tumor (T)

T1	Tumor limited to one subsite of nasopharynx (superior wall, posterior wall, lateral wall, or anterior wall)
T2	Tumor invades more than one subsite of nasopharynx
T3	Tumor invades nasal cavity and/or oropharynx
T4	Tumor invades skull and/or cranial nerve(s)

Regional lymph nodes (N)

N0	No regional lymph node metastasis
N1	Metastasis in a single ipsilateral lymph node, ≤3 cm in greatest dimension
N2	Metastasis in a single ipsilateral lymph node, >3 cm but <6 cm; or in multiple ipsilateral lymph nodes, none >6 cm; or in bilateral or contralateral lymph nodes, none >6 cm
N3	Metastasis in lymph node >6 cm in greatest dimension

Distant metastasis (M)

M0	No distant metastasis
M1	Distant metastasis

Stage grouping

I	T1	N0	M0
II	T2	N0	M0
III	T3	N0	M0
	T1	N1	M0
	T2	N1	M0
	T3	N1	M0
IV	T4	N0	M0
	T4	N1	M0
	Any T	N2	M0
	Any T	N3	M0
	Any T	Any N	M1

*From Beahrs OH: American Joint Committee on Cancer Manual for Staging of Cancer, 4th ed. Philadelphia, JB Lippincott, 1992, pp 34–35.

without reducing the accuracy in predicting the prognosis.[20] In this modification, the primary tumor (T stage) is classified into early (Ho's T1 + T2n + T2) and advanced (Ho's T2p + T3). Cervical lymph node metastases (N stage) are modified into supraclavicular (Ho's N3) and above supraclavicular (Ho's N1 + N2). According to Theo et al, the Ho staging classification shows a more even distribution of patients among the stages and a greater power in predicting the prognosis than the other classifications.[20] However, there is no single generally accepted classification that would simplify comparison of treatment of NPCA between centers.

Nasopharyngeal carcinoma shows a variability in its histologic differentiation, growth patterns, and tissue reactions.[1-5] The World Health Organization (WHO) histologic classification (first edition, 1978) did

---

TABLE 2.

The Ho Staging System for Nasopharyngeal Carcinoma (1978)*

T Stage
  T1   Confined to nasopharynx
  T2   Tumor extends to nasal fossa (T2n), adjacent muscles of oropharynx
        (T20), parapharyngeal region (T2p) or nerves below skull base
  T3   Extension beyond areas of T1 and T2
  T3a   Bone involvement below skull base
  T3b   Involvement of skull base
  T3c   Cranial nerve involvement
  T3d   Involvement of orbits, laryngopharynx, or infratemporal fossa
N Stage
  N0   No nodes evident
  N1   Nodes entirely within upper cervical level
  N2   Nodes palpable between upper cervical level lower boundary and
        supraclavicular fossa
  N3   Nodes palpable in supraclavicular fossa and/or skin involvement
M Stage
  M0   No evidence of distant metastases
  M1   Definite evidence of distant metastases
Stage grouping
  I   Tumor confined to nasopharynx (T1)
  II   Tumor extends to nasal fossa, oropharynx, or adjacent muscles or nerves
        below the base of skull (T2) and/or N1 involvement
  III   Tumor extends beyond T2 limits or bone involvement (T3) and/or N2
  IV   N3 involvement, irrespective of the primary tumor
  V   Hematogenous metastasis and/or involvement of skin or lymph node(s)
        below the clavicals (M1)

---

*Adapted from Ho JHC: *Int J Radiat Oncol Biol Phys* 4:183–197, 1978.

---

much to standardize the histologic terminology.[1, 2] In this classification, NPCA was divided into three histologic types: (1) a squamous-cell carcinoma, (2) a nonkeratinizing carcinoma, and (3) an undifferentiated carcinoma, depending on the presence or absence of clear evidence of squamous differentiation by light microscopy (Table 3).[1, 2] These types have been referred to in the literature as WHO types 1, 2 and 3, respectively.

In 1991, the second edition of the WHO Histologic Typing of Upper Respiratory Tract Tumors revised the classification of NPCA into two main histologic types, those with or without clear evidence of squamous-cell differentiation, namely, (1) a squamous-cell carcinoma, and (2) a nonkeratinizing carcinoma (Table 4).[21, 22] The latter is further subclassified into two groups, a differentiated nonkeratinizing carcinoma and an undifferentiated carcinoma. The reason for combining the nonkeratinizing-undifferentiated carcinomas into one group is that these subtypes have overlapping histologic features and are not always easily distinguished from each other.[22] Furthermore, they have similar epidemiological and

TABLE 3.

Nasopharyngeal Carcinoma—World Health
Organization Histologic Classification (1978)*

1. Squamous-cell carcinoma
2. Nonkeratinizing carcinoma
3. Undifferentiated carcinoma

*Adapted from Shanmugaratnam K: *International Histological Classification of Tumors*, No. 19. Geneva, World
Health Organization, 1978.

biologic characteristics, especially with respect to their relationship to
EBV.[21, 22]

In the USA, 25% of all NPCA are squamous-cell carcinomas.[3, 8] Histologically, there is evidence of squamous differentiation (intercellular
bridges and/or keratinization) over most of the tumor. The tumor may be
well, moderately, or poorly differentiated.[1, 2, 21, 22] A desmoplastic reaction is often present. This type occurs more commonly in adults and is
rare under the age of 40 years.[1-5] There is absent, or weak, relationship
to EBV.[3] Squamous-cell carcinoma is usually not radiosensitive. The
5-year survival rate of patients with this type of NPCA is only 16% to
22%.[7]

The nonkeratinizing-undifferentiated type of NPCA, with both of its
subtypes, is frequently associated with a cervical lymph node metastasis
and detection of EBV. Tumors in this group display cell differentiation
with a maturation sequence that lacks evidence of squamous differentiation by light microscopy.[1, 2, 21, 22]

The subtype, a differentiated nonkeratinizing carcinoma, is the least
common and constitutes only 12% of all NPCA in the USA.[1-3, 8] Tumor
cells typically have well-defined cell borders and stratified or pavement-like arrangement, reminiscent of a urothelial transitional-cell carcinoma.[1, 2, 21, 22] Tumor cells vary from bland to anaplastic, and have many
nuclear characteristics of the undifferentiated type, such as vesicular
chromatin and a prominent nucleolus.[3, 22] This subtype has a variable re-

TABLE 4.

Nasopharyngeal Carcinoma—World Health Organization
Histologic Classification (1991)*

1. Squamous-cell carcinoma
2. Nonkeratinizing carcinoma
   Differentiated nonkeratinizing carcinoma
   Undifferentiated carcinoma

*Adapted from Shanmugaratnam K: *International Histological Classification of Tumors*, 2nd ed. Heidelberg, Springer-Verlag, 1991.

sponse to radiation therapy with a 5-year survival rate of 30% to 50%.[7]

Undifferentiated carcinoma is the most frequent histologic type in the Chinese population, in young patients under the age of 35, in children, and in blacks but only accounts for 60% of NPCA in the United States.[1-7, 15] The tumor cells have large, round or oval, vesicular nuclei and prominent nucleoli, with indistinct cellular borders, imparting a characteristic syncytial growth pattern (Figs 1 and 2).[1, 2, 21, 22] Spindle-shaped tumor cells may be present. The tumor cells are arranged in irregular, well-demarcated nests (Regaud pattern). They may also be present as isolated cells (a Schmincke pattern) within a non-neoplastic lymphoid stroma, therefore, the historical term "lymphoepithelioma".[1-5, 21, 22] The infiltrating lymphoid element comprises mainly lymphocytes, predominantly T cell in nature.[23, 24] Plasma cells, follicular dendritic cells (S-100+), and eosinophils are also often present. This subtype is highly radiosensitive with a 5-year survival rate of 50% to 60%.[7]

The undifferentiated subtype is easily mistaken histologically for large-cell lymphoma, especially immunoblastic lymphoma.[3-5, 25] Immunohistochemical stains demonstrate reactivity of the carcinoma cells in nearly all cases for cytokeratin, but not for a leukocyte common antigen (LCA). This confirms their epithelial cell origin.[26, 27] In contrast, lymphoma cells would be expected to be positive for LCA and negative for cytokeratin. In a recent study, Sugimoto et al found keratin positivity in

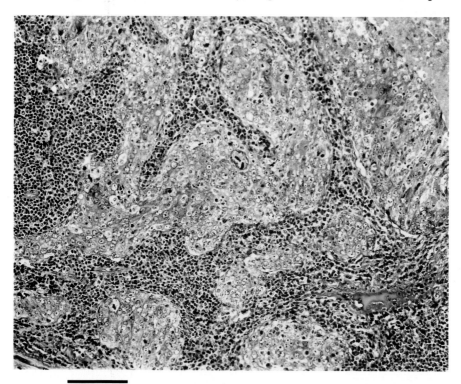

FIGURE 1.

Low-magnification photomicrograph showing a nonkeratinizing undifferentiated NPCA. Note irregular, well-demarcated nests of carcinoma cells in a lymphoid stroma.

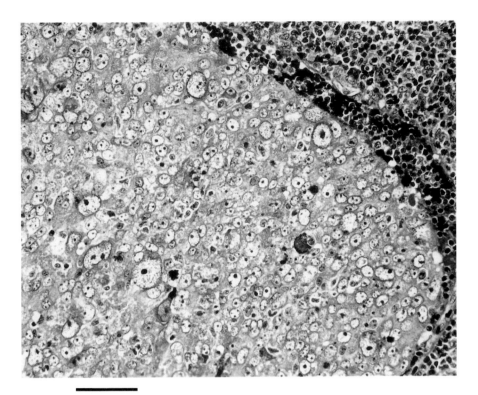

FIGURE 2.
Higher magnification of undifferentiated NPCA. Tumor cells have large round vesicular nuclei of varying sizes with prominent central nucleoli and indistinct cell
borders, imparting a syncytial growth pattern. Note absence of keratinization by
light microscopy.

56 of 58 NPCA (97%), with reactivity for LCA in none (0%). All 16 lymphomas studied were immunoreactive for LCA (100%) and none (0%)
were positive for keratin.[27]

In the presence of an unknown primary, the histologic finding of an
undifferentiated carcinoma in a cervical lymph node biopsy specimen is
highly suggestive of a primary carcinoma of the nasopharynx. This is especially true with upper cervical lymph nodes.[3, 5] Elevated serologic titers of anti-EBV antibodies may also prove useful in the identification of
patients with NPCA with an occult primary.[12-14] However, recent reports
have described the "lymphoepithelioma-like" undifferentiated carcinomas originating in other sites, namely, salivary glands, lung, stomach, and
thymus.[23, 28, 29] Undifferentiated carcinomas from these non-
nasopharyngeal sites have on occasion been associated with EBV but the
consistency of the association is yet to be established.

In most nonkeratinizing-undifferentiated nasopharyngeal carcinomas, EBV-DNA can be detected in formalin-fixed, paraffin-embedded tissue sections, or even in material obtained by fine needle aspiration. This
may be found in the primary tumor or metastasis, using immunohisto-
chemistry or more sensitive molecular techniques (such as in situ hybridization and the polymerase chain reaction).[28-41] The EBV-DNA is absent
in squamous-cell carcinomas.[29, 39] Using in situ hybridization, the pres-

ence of EBV-DNA and expression of the small nuclear EBV-coded RNAs (EBERs) are seen localized to the malignant epithelial cells.[15, 32−41] The non-neoplastic lymphocytes infiltrating the tumor do not contain the EBV genome. Most NPCAs containing EBV-DNA show an unusual pattern of EBV latent gene expression. The nuclear antigen EBNA 1 and, in a lesser proportion of cases (22% to 70%), the latent membrane protein LMP 1 are coexpressed. This is in the absence of EBNA 2, 3, 4, 5, 6, and EBNA-LP.[35, 37, 38, 40] Whether LMP expression correlates with tumor progression has not been learned.

TREATMENT

It is important to tailor the therapeutic modality of NPCA to its histologic type and the anatomic extent. The majority of NPCAs are of the non-keratinizing histologic type which is radiosensitive. These tumors are treated by primary radiation therapy. External beam-supervoltage radiation is the standard therapy.[6, 9, 42−44] The keratinizing type of NPCA and carcinomas of glandular origin, which have limited response to radiation therapy, may be now considered for surgical resection. Advances in cranial base surgery permit resection of nasopharyngeal soft tissue as well as some clival bone. Certain recurrent nonkeratinizing NPCAs may also be amenable to surgical salvage.

SURGICAL TECHNIQUE

Modular craniofacial disassembly is the principal of the facial translocation approach to the nasopharynx. It is based on creation of composite facial units which are designed along key neurovascular anatomic and esthetic lines. The complementary units allow their merger into larger composites without compromising their functionality. It is possible to attach eponyms to the technical variations of facial translocation for ease of communication and comparison. Thus, we can recognize "mini," "standard," "expanded" (vertically, medially, posteriorly), or "bilateral" facial translocation procedures. Complementary craniotomies or craniectomies may be added to these approaches as necessary to assist with three-dimensional tumor resection. Selection of an approach to the nasopharynx is guided by the tumor extent. The surgical technique that has the greatest potential for a three-dimensional tumor resection should be selected. Examples below include those procedures directly applicable to the surgical removal of nasopharyngeal carcinoma.

Standard facial translocation achieves surgical access to the anterolateral skull base. It was originally described in 1989. The ipsilateral facial skin (including the lower eyelid) is displaced laterally and inferiorly with the underlying maxilla (with or without the hard palate). The nasal incision may extend inferiorly to include an upper lip split. Superior incision continues from the nose to the inferior fornix of the lower eyelid, through the lateral canthus horizontally to the preauricular area. In some cases (more anterior tumors) it is possible to conclude this incision about 1.5 cm beyond the lateral canthus after identifying and preserving the most anterior frontal branch of the facial nerve. This then serves as the point of rotation of facial tissues. This is sufficient for access to some para-

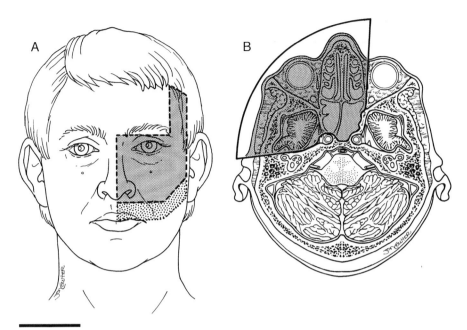

FIGURE 3.
A, schematic outline of standard facial translocation procedure for surgical exposure of nasopharynx. (Stapled area indicates palatal split). **B,** axial delineation of surgical reach.

central tumors. When the entire extent of the horizontal temple incision is needed, the frontal branches of the facial nerve are identified with a nerve stimulator, placed in silicone tubings and transected. During the reconstruction these transected tubings are reconnected and the continuity of the facial nerve branches is reestablished. Osteotomies correlate to

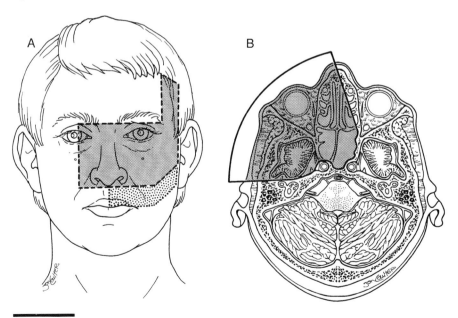

FIGURE 4.
A, facial translocation—medial extension. **B,** surgical reach.

LeFort I-II level or mid-platal when the entire maxilla is being displaced. The inferior orbital nerve is sectioned along the floor of the orbit, tagged, and repaired at the end of the procedure. Rigid fixation is achieved with mini- and microplates. With this technique of facial translocation, good exposure of the anterolateral skull base is achieved especially when the infratemporal fossa is involved as well (Fig 3A, B).

Extended facial translocation—medial incorporates the standard translocation unit plus the nose and the medial one half of the opposite face (up to the infraorbital nerve). This composite facial unit can be rotated at the LeFort I level or include the ipsilateral palate and upper lip split. The skin incisions are similar to the standard technique except the paranasal incision is made on the contralateral side. The surgical exposure includes the ipsilateral infratemporal fossa and central and paracentral skull base bilaterally. The entire clivus is accessible as are the optic

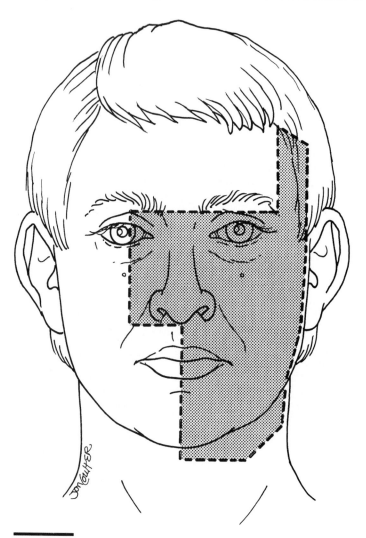

FIGURE 5.
Facial translocation—medial and inferior extension.

nerves, both precavernous internal carotid arteries, and the nasopharynx. The wide communication with the infratemporal fossa allows the placement of the temporalis muscle flap for vascularized reconstruction of the skull base defect. Bony fixation is done with miniplates and a lag screw for the palate. The occlusal plane is reestablished with the help of an orthognathic split. In addition a palatal splint is attached to the maxillary dentition for additional stability and protection of the palatal incision. Temporary silicone intranasal stents are inserted as are bilateral lacrimal stents (Fig 4 A, B).

Extended facial translocation—medial and inferior includes the above procedure with an inferior extension via mandibular split. The lower lip incision is performed in a zigzag fashion to conform to the tension lines of the skin with an extension horizontally into the upper neck. Mandibular osteotomy is performed just medial to the mental foramen. Usually an interdental space is found that is wide enough to permit placement of a reciprocating saw for the osteotomy. This is performed in a step fashion, which then permits more stable reconstructive reapproximation of the bone. Prior to the osteotomy it is wise to select an appropriate miniplate for eventual fixation, contour the mandible, and create drill holes. This assists in the postoperative reestablishment of a normal occlusion. This extended translocation procedure adds a significant inferior as well as upper cervical surgical access (Fig 5).

Bilateral facial translocation combines complete right and left basic translocation units with or without palatal split. The exposure incorporates both infratemporal fossae, the central skull base, and the entire paracentral skull base. Both distal cervical internal carotid arteries (ICAs) are in view as is the full clivus. The palatal split permits a reach to the level of C2–3. If further inferior extension is needed, a mandibular split can be added so a vertical reach to C3–4 is accomplished. A single tempo-

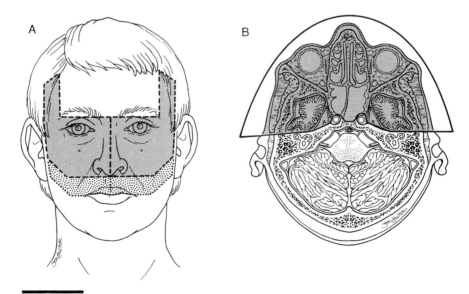

FIGURE 6.
A, facial translocation—bilateral. **B,** surgical reach.

ralis muscle flap is sufficient for the coverage of the surgical defect at the skull base (Fig 6A, B).

STATISTICS

Survival of patients with NPCA is influenced by age, sex, T and N stage at diagnosis, and histologic type.[6–9, 18, 42–47] Patients under the age of 40 have a better prognosis than those aged 40 or older,[9, 42, 45] and women have a significantly better prognosis than men.[43] In a recent analysis of the epidemiology and survival of NPCA in the USA, Burt et al found survival to be independently influenced by age, sex, stage, histology, and grade.[46] According to their analysis, Chinese patients survived longest compared to Filipino, white, and black patients.[46] Of the histologic subtypes, undifferentiated NPCA has the most favorable outcome compared to squamous-cell carcinoma, which has the least favorable prognosis.[1–5, 46]

In a recent study by Bailet et al, which studied patients in the USA, the overall 5- and 10-year survival of 103 patients treated with radiotherapy (1955 to 1990) was 58% and 47%, respectively.[44] In their study, the disease-free survival rate at 3 and 5 years was 45% and 30%, respectively. Local, persistent, or recurrent disease in the nasopharynx was the primary cause of failure (32%), correlating with initial tumor size (T stage).[44] Distant metastases developed in 24% of the patients and correlated with nodal status (N stage) but not T stage. In their study, 79% of patients had local or distal failure by 4 years.[44]

The 5-year actuarial survival rate in a 1978 study by Ho was 83.7% for Stage I, 67.9% for Stage II, 40.3% for Stage III, and 22.3% for Stage IV.[9] A recent study of patients treated during 1976 to 1985 in Hong Kong revealed an overall actuarial 10-year survival rate of 43%.[47] Complete remission lasting more than 6 months was achieved in 83% of patients, but 53% relapsed after a median interval of 1.4 years.[47] The 10-year actuarial local, regional, and distant failure-free rates were 61%, 64%, and 59%, respectively. The incidence of distant failure correlated with N and T stage.[47] Patients treated during 1981 to 1985 had a better overall survival rate, 57% versus 47% at 5 years.[47]

The utility of DNA ploidy in predicting prognosis in this tumor remains controversial.[48, 49] Cheng et al found aneuploidy correlated with diminished survival, 25% versus 55% for diploid tumors at 2 years.[48] In their study, ploidy status emerged as a statistically significant independent variable after correcting for stage, histology, and radiation dose.[48] However, Costello et al were unable to show a significant prognostic influence of cellular DNA content on outcome, with a 5-year survival rate in aneuploid vs diploid NPCA of 42% versus 48%, respectively.[49]

Recent studies have shown a consistent loss of genetic material at two defined loci (RAF-1 and D3S3) on the short arm of chromosome 3 in Chinese patients with NPCA.[50, 51] Choi et al found a consistent presence of the cytogenetic abnormality and EBV genome (especially type A) in the same tumor, suggesting that these findings may represent important genetic events in the multistep genesis of NPCA.[51] The precise role of the virus or cytogenetic abnormality in the pathogenesis of NPCA, however, remains unclear; further studies are necessary to establish the significance of these findings.

REFERENCES

1. Shanmugaratnam K, Sobin LH: Histological typing of upper respiratory tract tumours, in *International Histological Classification of Tumors,* No. 19. Geneva, World Health Organization, 1978.

2. Shanmugaratnam K, Chan SH, de-The, et al: Histopathology of nasopharyngeal carcinoma: Correlations with epidemiology, survival rates, and other biological characteristics. *Cancer* 44:1029–1044, 1979.

3. Weiland LH: Nasopharyngeal carcinoma, in Barnes L (ed): *Surgical Pathology of the Head and Neck.* New York, Marcel Dekker, 1985, pp 453–466.

4. Hyams VJ, Batsakis JG, Michaels L: Squamous cell carcinoma of the nasopharynx mucosa, in Hyams VJ, Batsakis JG, Michaels L (eds): *Tumors of the Upper Respiratory Tract and Ear,* Fascicle 25, second series. Washington, DC, Armed Forces Institute of Pathology, 1986, pp 62–66.

5. Barnes L, Kapadia SB: The biology of selected skull base tumors. *J Neurooncol* 20:213–240, 1994.

6. Neel HB: Nasopharyngeal carcinoma: Diagnosis, staging and management. *Oncology* 6:87–95; 99–102, 1992.

7. Dickson RI: Nasopharyngeal carcinoma: An evaluation of 209 patients. *Laryngoscope* 91:333–354, 1981.

8. Easton JM, Levine PH, Hyams VJ: Nasopharyngeal carcinoma in the United States. A pathologic study of 177 US and 30 foreign cases. *Arch Otolaryngol* 106:88–91, 1980.

9. Ho JHC: An epidemiologic and clinical study of nasopharyngeal carcinoma. *Int J Radiat Oncol Biol Phys* 4:183–197, 1978.

10. Henderson BE, Louie E, Jing JSH, et al: Risk factors associated with nasopharyngeal carcinoma. *N Engl J Med* 295:1101–1106, 1976.

11. Armstrong RW, Armstrong MJ, Yu MC, et al: Salted fish and inhalants as risk factors for nasopharyngeal carcinoma in Malaysian Chinese. *Cancer Res* 43:2967–2970, 1983.

12. Henle W, Henle G: Epstein-Barr virus-specific IgA serum antibodies as an outstanding feature of nasopharyngeal carcinoma. *Int J Cancer* 17:1–7, 1976.

13. Neel HB, Pearson HB, Weiland LH, et al: Anti-EBV serologic tests for nasopharyngeal carcinoma. *Laryngoscope* 90:1981–1990, 1980.

14. Ringborg U, Henle G, et al: Epstein-Barr virus-specific serodiagnostic tests in carcinomas of the head and neck. *Cancer* 52:1237–1243, 1983.

15. Zur Hausen H, Schulte-Hosthausen H, Klein G: EBV DNA in biopsies of Burkitt tumors and anaplastic carcinomas of the nasopharynx. *Nature* 228:1056–1058, 1970.

16. Hawkins EP, Krischer JP, Smith BE, et al: Nasopharyngeal carcinoma in children—a retrospective review and demonstration of Epstein-Barr viral genomes in tumor cell cytoplasm: A report of the Pediatric Oncology Group. *Hum Pathol* 21:805–810, 1990.

17. Skinner DW, Van Hasselt CA, Tsao SY: Nasopharyngeal carcinoma: Modes of presentation. *Ann Otol Rhinol Laryngol* 100:544–551, 1991.

18. Cheung YK, Sham J, Cheung YL, et al: Evaluation of skull base erosiomi nasopharyngeal carcinoma: Comparison of plain radiography and computed tomography. *Oncology* 51:42–46, 1994.

19. Beahrs OH, Henson DE, Hutter RVP, et al (eds): *American Joint Committee on Cancer Manual for Staging of Cancer,* 4th ed. Philadelphia, JB Lippincott, 1992, pp 34–35.

20. Theo PM, Tsao SY, Ho JH, et al: A proposed modification of the Ho stage-classification for nasopharyngeal carcinoma. *Radiother Oncol* 21:11–23, 1991.

21. Shanmugaratnam K, Sobin L: Histological typing of tumors of the upper re-

spiratory tract and ear, in *International Histological Classification of Tumors,* 2nd ed. Heidelberg, Springer-Verlag, 1991.

22. Shanmugaratnam K, Sobin LH: The World Health Organization histologic classification of tumors of the upper respiratory tract and ear. A commentary on the Second Edition. *Cancer* 71:2689–2697, 1993.

23. Weiss LM, Gaffey MJ, Shibata D: Lymphoepithelioma-like carcinoma and its relationship to Epstein-Barr virus. *Am J Clin Pathol* 96:156–158, 1991.

24. Jondal M, Klein G: Classification of lymphocytes in nasopharyngeal carcinoma (NPC) biopsies. *Biomedicine* 23:163–165, 1975.

25. Carbone A, Micheau C: Pitfalls in microscopic diagnosis of undifferentiated carcinoma of the nasopharyngeal type (lymphoepithelioma). *Cancer* 50:1344–1351, 1982.

26. Madri JA, Barwick KW: An immunohistochemical study of nasopharyngeal neoplasms using keratin antibodies: Epithelial versus nonepithelial neoplasms. *Am J Surg Pathol* 6:143–149, 1982.

27. Sugimoto T, Hashimoto H, Enjoji M: Nasopharyngeal carcinoma and malignant lymphomas: An immunohistochemical analysis of 74 cases. *Laryngoscope* 100:742–748, 1990.

28. Weiss LM, Movahed LA, Butler AE, et al: Analysis of lymphoepithelioma and lymphoepithelioma-like carcinomas by in situ hybridization. *Am J Surg Pathol* 13:625–631, 1989.

29. Niedobitek G, Hansman ML, Herbst H, et al: Epstein-Barr virus and carcinomas: Undifferentiated carcinoma but not squamous cell carcinomas of the nasopharynx are regularly associated with the virus. *J Pathol* 165:17–24, 1991.

30. Feinmesser R, Miyazaki I, Cheung R, et al: Diagnosis of nasopharyngeal carcinoma by DNA amplification of tissue obtained by fine-needle aspiration. *N Engl J Med* 326:17–21, 1992.

31. Chan MKM, Huang DP, Ho YH, et al: Detection of Epstein-Barr virus-associated antigen in fine needle aspiration smears from cervical lymph nodes in the diagnosis of nasopharyngeal carcinoma. *Acta Cytol* 33:351–354, 1989.

32. Klein G, Giovanella BC, Lindahl T, et al: Direct evidence for the presence of Epstein-Barr virus DNA and nuclear antigen in malignant epithelial cells from patients with poorly differentiated carcinoma of the nasopharynx. *Proc Natl Acad Sci U S A* 71:4737–4741, 1974.

33. Akoa I, Sato Y, Mukai K, et al: Detection of Epstein-Barr virus DNA in formalin-fixed, paraffin-embedded tissue of nasopharyngeal carcinoma using polymerase chain reaction and in situ hybridization. *Laryngoscope* 101:279–283, 1991.

34. Brousset P, Butet V, Chittal S, et al: Comparison of in situ hybridization using different nonisotopic probes for detection of Epstein-Barr virus in nasopharyngeal carcinoma and immunohistochemical correlation with anti-latent membrane protein antibody. *Lab Invest* 67:457–464, 1992.

35. Fahraeeus R, Fu HL, Ernberg I, et al: Expression of Epstein-Barr virus-encoded proteins in nasopharyngeal carcinoma. *Int J Cancer* 42:329–338, 1988.

36. Feinmesser R, Feinmesser M, Freeman JL, et al: Detection of occult nasopharyngeal primary tumours by means of in situ hybridization. *J Laryngol Otol* 106:345–348, 1992.

37. Niedobitek G, Young LS, Sam CK, et al: Expression of Epstein-Barr virus genes and of lymphocyte activation molecules in undifferentiated nasopharyngeal carcinomas. *Am J Pathol* 140:879–887, 1992.

38. Stewart JP, Arrand JR: Expression of the Epstein-Barr virus latent membrane protein in nasopharyngeal carcinoma biopsy specimens. *Hum Pathol* 24:239–242, 1993.

39. Torre GD, Pilotti S, Donghi R, et al: Epstein-Barr virus genome in undifferen-

tiated and squamous cell nasopharyngeal carcinomas in Italian patients. *Diagn Mol Pathol* 3:32–37, 1994.

40. Young LS, Dawson CW, Clark D, et al: Epstein-Barr virus gene expression in nasopharyngeal carcinoma. *J Gen Virol* 69:1051–1065, 1988.

41. Wu T-C, Mann RB, Epstein JI, et al: Abundant expression of EBER 1 small nuclear RNA in nasopharyngeal carcinoma. A morphologically distinctive target for detection of Epstein-Barr virus in formalin-fixed paraffin-embedded carcinoma specimens. *Am J Pathol* 138:1461–1469, 1991.

42. Qin D, Hu Y, Yan J, et al: Analysis of 1379 patients with nasopharyngeal carcinoma treated by radiation. *Cancer* 61:1117–1124, 1988.

43. Wang CC: Accelerated hyperfraction radiation therapy for carcinoma of the nasopharynx. Techniques and results. *Cancer* 63:2461–2467, 1989.

44. Bailet JW, Mark RJ, Abemayor E, et al: Nasopharyngeal carcinoma: Treatment results with primary radiation therapy. *Laryngoscope* 102:965–972, 1992.

45. Sham JST, Choy D: Prognostic factors of nasopharyngeal carcinoma: A review of 759 patients. *Br J Radiol* 63:51–58, 1990.

46. Burt RD, Vaughan T, McKnight B: Descriptive epidemiology and survival analysis of nasopharyngeal carcinoma in the United States. *Int J Cancer* 52:549–556, 1992.

47. Lee AW, Poon YF, Foo W, et al: Retrospective analysis of 5037 patients with nasopharyngeal carcinoma treated during 1976–1985: Overall survival and patterns of failure. *Int J Radiat Oncol Biol Phys* 23:261–270, 1992.

48. Cheng DS, Campbell BH, Clowry LJ, et al: DNA content in nasopharyngeal carcinoma. *Am J Otolaryngol* 11:393–397, 1990.

49. Costello F, Mason BR, Collins RJ, et al: A clinical and flow cytometric analysis of patients with nasopharyngeal carcinoma. *Cancer* 66:1789–1795, 1990.

50. Huang DP, Lo KW, Choi PHK, et al: Loss of heterozygosity on the short arm of chromosome 3 in nasopharyngeal carcinoma. *Cancer Genet Cytogenet* 54:91–99, 1991.

51. Choi PHK, Suen MWM, Huang DP, et al: Nasopharyngeal carcinoma: Genetic changes, Epstein-Barr virus infection, or both. A clinical and molecular study of 36 patients. *Cancer* 72:2873–2878, 1993.

Gastroesophageal Reflux Disease in the Pediatric Population

Andrew J. Hotaling, M.D.
Associate Professor Otolaryngology, Head and Neck Surgery and Pediatrics, Loyola University Medical Center, Maywood, Illinois

Andrew B. Silva, M.D.
Resident, Department of Otolaryngology, Head and Neck Surgery, Loyola University Medical Center, Maywood, Illinois

G astroesophageal reflux (GER) is a common disorder in the pediatric population with symptoms ranging from benign postprandial vomiting in the first year of life to failure to thrive (FTT), esophagitis, and airway obstruction. The purpose of this chapter is to review GER, focusing attention on airway manifestations.

Every child must be evaluated thoroughly. Reflux alone can cause disease, but in certain patient populations, it has a much higher morbidity and mortality. These populations include those with tracheoesophageal fistula (TEF), esophageal atresia, colonic interposition, bronchopulmonary dysplasia, recurrent pneumonia, subglottic stenosis, neurologic impairment, and, possibly, cystic fibrosis.

During the last several decades, we have learned that GER affects children differently than adults due to the anatomy and physiology of a developing child in contrast to the adult. Consequently, the pathophysiology, pathogenesis, and manifestations of GER are different in children. Koufman reported that the pediatric otolaryngologic manifestations of pathologic GER differ from the adult population because children have a higher incidence of life-threatening airway complications.[1]

DEFINITION

GER is defined as the retrograde passage of gastric contents into the esophagus. The pH can be acidic, basic, or neutral. Gastroesophageal reflux is either physiological (normal) or pathologic (disease). Physiological GER, defined as GER, is usually asymptomatic, rarely occurs during sleep, and is frequent in the upright position postprandially.[2] Pathologic reflux is symptomatic, can be recognized and quantified diagnostically, can cause pathologic changes in the upper aerodigestive tract (UADT) and is defined as gastroesophageal reflux disease (GERD).

The newborn population is subdivided into different gestational age

Advances in Otolaryngology—Head and Neck Surgery®, vol. 9
© 1995, Mosby–Year Book, Inc.

groups at birth: premature newborn (<38 weeks old), term infant (38 to 42 weeks old), and a post-term infant (>42 weeks old). The neonatal period is 0 to 28 days old, infancy is 28 days to 12 months old, and a toddler is 12 to 36 months old.

In children, 24-hour pH-probe studies have been used to obtain normative values for different pediatric age groups.[3] The total percentage of the study time with pH <4 and the number of reflux episodes >5 minutes have proved to be the best discriminating parameters between reflux patients and controls.[4] A threshold pH of <4 has been used to define acidic GER.[5-7] Because the total average percentage of time that a normal pediatric esophagus remains <4 is 3% to 11%, a value of 7% has been used as a threshold for this parameter.[3] However, there is a subgroup of 3 to 9-month-old normal infants with pH <4 for 9% to 10% of the test time; therefore, some centers use a threshold value of 10%.[8]

Gastroesophageal reflux affects each child differently. The amount of reflux required to be pathologic in one patient may not be pathologic in another. Kennedy was one of the first authors to document the presence of GERD with concomitant respiratory disease in adults who did not manifest the typical symptoms of GER, termed silent GERD.[9] The greatest diagnostic challenge exists in the asymptomatic patient with silent GERD.

EPIDEMIOLOGY

Gastroesophageal reflux is common in infants during the first year of life. Physiological reflux occurs in 1:500 births and has a male to female ratio of 1.27:1.[10, 11] Carre reported on the natural history of GERD in 53 untreated patients with a "partial thoracic stomach" in his 1959 landmark paper.[11] Sixty percent of infants improve after they are weaned from a liquid diet to a solid diet, 30% improve by the age of 4, 5% develop esophageal strictures, and 5% die from marasmus or pneumonia. Kibel reported on the natural history of vomiting in 93 infants with GER, reported 46 vomiting at 2 months, 6 at 4 months, 4 at 6 months, and 1 at 12 months.[12]

Esophageal acid clearance improves during the first year of life. The number of episodes lasting >5 minutes decreases while the total number of episodes remains unchanged.[3] Boix-Ochoa et al studied 680 infants manometrically and found that lower esophageal sphincter (LES) pressure normalized by 6 to 7 weeks of age, regardless of gestational age or weight.[13] Vandenplas et al screened 509 healthy infants for sudden infant death syndrome (SIDS) and reported that the reflux index, defined as the percentage of time that the pH is <4, was 13% at birth, 8% at 12 months, and averaged 10% during the first year of life.[8] The pH-probe data normalizes after one year, with the incidence of GER in infants (8%) approaching that in adults (7%).[8]

As a general rule, physiological reflux should improve after a solid diet is achieved and certainly by the end of the first year of life when the majority of infants outgrow GER.[14] Patients with persistent GER after the age of 3 usually require medical or surgical treatment in order to control GER and have a less favorable prognosis with a higher rate of GERD-related complications.[15]

ANATOMY AND PHYSIOLOGY

The dual functions of the UADT in the child are to maintain adequate gas exchange with the environment and provide enough nutritional intake to support growth. The average infant grows 10 inches and triples birth weight in one year. During the second year, a child will grow 5 inches and quadruple birth weight.

THE NORMAL SWALLOW

The process of deglutition requires complex neuromuscular coordination between the oral cavity, pharynx, larynx, and esophagus. The swallow is divided into four stages: oral preparatory, oral, pharyngeal, and esophageal. Initially, the infant's deglutition is based on a suck and swallow mechanism. The oral preparatory stage does not exist in the unweaned infant, with the transition naturally occurring in the first year of life. These topics are reviewed in more detail elsewhere.[16, 17]

SALIVARY FUNCTION

Saliva is produced by the major and minor salivary glands to lubricate the oral cavity, moisten the bolus to facilitate swallowing, provide a source of secretory IgA for immune protection, and initiate enzymatic digestion. Saliva, with a high concentration of bicarbonate ions, is basic and helps to maintain the pH balance in the oral cavity and esophagus and neutralizes acidic reflux in the distal esophagus.

GASTRIC PHYSIOLOGY

Gastroesophageal reflux can be acidic, basic, or neutral in pH. While each of these types of reflux can be pathologic, acidic reflux is by far the most common. To prevent reflux, the LES must first passively relax, allowing the bolus to pass into the stomach, and then actively contract to prevent reflux. The stomach is then responsible for receiving, mixing, digesting, and delivering the bolus to the duodenum, efficiently emptying its contents and preventing a rise in intragastric pressures.

Acid production is modulated through the neural and hormonal systems. The gastric mucosa is populated by different cell types, which secrete local and systemic substances affecting gastric physiology, and contains a rich submucosal vagal parasympathetic innervation responsible for motility and acid secretion.

The gastric mucosa contains mast, parietal, chief, mucous, and surface epithelial cells. Hydrochloric acid (HCl) and intrinsic factor are secreted by the parietal cell located in the gastric body. The chief cell secretes the pre-enzyme pepsinogen, which is activated by a pH <3 into pepsin, a powerful proteolytic enzyme. The antral G cell secretes the peptide hormone gastrin.

Acid secretion is stimulated when histamine, gastrin, and acetylcholine bind the corresponding parietal cell membrane receptors. Acid production is greater when the H2-receptor is activated simultaneously with either the gastrin or acetylcholine receptor. Receptor binding triggers calcium entry into the cell and production of cyclic adenosine monophosphate, thus activating the hydrogen-potassium pump at the apical cell border. The pump exchanges a potassium ion for a hydrogen ion, resulting in the secretion of HCl. This mechanism is the final common pathway for acid secretion and explains why proton pump inhibitors (omeprazole) are so effective in decreasing basal acid output.

Gastric acid production during eating is divided into three phases: cephalic, gastric, and intestinal. The cephalic phase is mediated by vagal stimulation by the sight, smell, or thought of food, which trigger acid production. The cephalic phase through vagal stimulation directly affects the parietal cell and releases gastrin, together totalling 20% to 30% of acid production in response to a meal. The gastric phase of acid secretion is provoked by vagal excitation, antral distention, and protein contacting the antral mucosa. These factors release gastrin from the antral G cells, constituting 60% to 70% of acid output. The intestinal phase of acid secretion is not well understood; however, the presence of chyme in the proximal small intestine can stimulate 5% to 10% of acid output from a meal.

Three feedback mechanisms inhibit gastric acid secretion. First, vagal stimulation decreases postprandially. Second, an antral pH <2.5 inhibits the release of gastrin. Third, chyme entering the duodenum inhibits acid production by stimulating the release of secretin and cholecystokinin, hormones that stimulate bicarbonate production and act to competitively inhibit gastrin at the parietal cell level, respectively.

The stomach has a well-developed mucosal barrier resistant to autodigestion. Its mucosa contains mucous cells secreting a viscous gel, rich in bicarbonate ions. Below the mucosa is a well-developed capillary plexus able to increase nutrient blood flow in response to injury.

The stomach's defensive barriers are far more developed than those of the esophagus. The esophageal mucosa is lined by a stratified squamous epithelium, relatively devoid of mucous-secreting glands compared with the mucosa of the stomach. The esophagus is also unable to secrete a protective viscous bicarbonate-rich gel. These factors render the esophagus more susceptible to the damaging effects of gastric acid.

In summary, acid suppression will decrease mucosal damage, produce an alkaline environment, and prevent the enzymatic activation of pepsin, a potent esophageal mucosal irritant. Gastric alkalization stimulates gastrin secretion which increases the lower esophageal sphincter pressure (LESP).

NONACIDIC REFLUX

Nonacidic esophageal reflux can be either alkaline or mixed and is diagnosed using a pH-probe. Alkaline reflux has a pH >7 to 7.5 and is attributed to gastroduodenal reflux into the esophagus.[18, 19] Mixed reflux occurs when both acidic and alkaline reflux episodes are recorded during a pH-probe study.[18] False-positive results have been attributed to oral or esophageal bacterial overgrowth, which causes an alkaline environment in the esophagus.[18]

Trypsin, a pancreatic enzyme, pepsin, a parietal cell enzyme, and bile salts, secreted by the gallbladder, can all produce mucosal damage at various pH levels, dictated by enzyme kinetics. Trypsin and deconjugated bile salts produce the greatest injury in an alkaline environment while pepsin and conjugated bile salts produce the greatest injury in an acidic environment.[18]

Higher gastric concentrations of bile acids in patients with gastric ulcers or patients' postgastrectomy have been reported.[20] Bile causes cellular damage by increasing hydrogen ion permeability and acting as a detergent, dissolving intraluminal membranes.

In order to determine the true incidence of alkaline reflux, Malthaner et al, using a pH-probe, studied 111 consecutive children referred for symptoms of GERD and reported 10 (9%) had no reflux, 56 (50%) had acid reflux, 27 (24%) had mixed reflux, and 18 (16%) had alkaline reflux.[18] Endoscopic biopsy specimens from 8 of the 16 patients with pure alkaline reflux demonstrated 4 (50%) with esophagitis. Vandenplas et al reported nine children with alkaline or mixed reflux with histologic evidence of esophagitis.[19]

In contrast, in a editorial comment by Jolley on Malthaner and coworkers' results, he stated that he has performed over 1,500 pH recordings and was unable to document alkaline reflux in any child who did not have an gastroduodenal obstruction, a partial gastrectomy, or a gastric drainage procedure.[18] These patients may represent a high risk group in whom a high index of suspicion is needed to diagnose alkaline GERD.

THE REFLUX BARRIER

The reflux barrier is composed of anatomic and physiological barriers. The easiest way to conceptualize the barrier is to follow the path of refluxate from the stomach to the pharynx.

ANATOMIC BARRIERS

The anatomic barrier is composed of five discrete anatomic structures which prevent GER from entering the distal esophagus: the diaphragmatic crura, phrenoesophageal ligament, gastroesophageal angle with its mucosal flap valve, and the intra-abdominal esophagus.

Animal studies involving partial excision of the diaphragm suggest that it is responsible for 25% of LES competence.[21] The phrenoesophageal ligament, a fibroelastic membrane fixing the esophagus in the diaphragmatic hiatus, may assist in holding or pulling the esophagus inferiorly, thus helping to establish an intra-abdominal esophageal segment.[22] The gastroesophageal (GE) angle is created as the esophagus enters the cardia, creating a 180 degree circumferential mucosal fold that aids in preventing reflux in the presence of a low LESP in adults.[23] The length of the intra-abdominal esophagus is paramount in preventing GER because, according to the physical laws that govern the behavior of soft tubes, the greater the length of the tube, the lower the external pressure required to collapse the tube, preventing reflux.[24]

PHYSIOLOGIC BARRIERS

Lower Esophageal Sphincter

The LES, the distal 3 cm to 4 cm of the esophagus, is one of the most important deterrents to GER. While the proximal one-third of the esophagus is voluntary striated muscle, the distal two-thirds is involuntary smooth muscle. Histologically, the LES is identical to its proximal smooth muscle counterpart but can be localized radiographically and manometrically.

During the first few weeks of life, the abdominal esophagus is short, and the GE angle is wide, predisposing the infant to reflux. Physiologically, maturation occurs by the 6th to 7th week of life, regardless of birth weight or gestational age. The normal LESP for children younger than 7 years of age is 11.8 ± 3.6 mm Hg.[25]

The LESP is controlled by neural impulses and circulating peptides and exhibits a greater responsiveness to cholinergic stimulation than the rest of the esophagus. Nonadrenergic inhibitory fibers may play a role in neural control.[26] Dopamine receptors have been described in the LES,[27] the blockade of which may explain the increased LESP with antidopaminergic agents (metoclopramide). Other factors that affect the LESP are listed in Table 1.

Esophageal Acid Clearance

Inappropriate transient lower esophageal sphincter relaxations (TLESRs) form the basis for physiological reflux across a normal LES.[3] Esophageal peristalsis and salivary flow are responsible for esophageal acid clearance and neutralization. Increased salivary flow has been recorded as a physiological response to esophageal acidification.[28]

TABLE 1.
Factors that can Affect Lower Esophageal Pressure*

PULMONARY MEDICATIONS THAT DECREASE LESP	MEDICATIONS THAT INCREASE LES
Theophylline	Norepinephrine
Isopsoteresol	Phenylephrine
Beta-adrenergic agonists	Cholinergic agonists
OTHER MEDICATIONS THAT DECREASE LESP	Alpha-adrenergic agonists
Alcohol	Histamine
Anticholinergic agonists	Protein meal
Alpha antagonists	Gastric altealinization
Dopamine	Gastrin
Calcium channel blockers	Metoclopramide
Narcotics	Indomethacin
Drazapan	MEDICATIONS THAT HAVE NO EFFECT ON LESP
Atropine	Propranolol
Secretin	
Glucagon	
Cholecystokinin	
Carminatives	
Chocolate	
Dietary fats	

LESP = lower esophageal pressure; LES = lower esophageal sphincter.
*Adapted from Blount BW: *Am Fam Physician* 37:201–216, 1988.

Physiological reflux was experimentally simulated in 27 adults by installing a 15 mL bolus of 0.1 normal HCl acid into the distal esophagus.[29] These patients were able to clear the bolus with a single peristaltic wave; however, it took an average of nine swallows until the pH returned to 4, the level defined as the acid clearance time (ACT). Salivary stimulation by an oral peppermint lozenge reduced the ACT by 50% while oral aspiration of saliva markedly prolonged the ACT.

The degree of GER is affected by the child's state of alertness, being more common while awake; however, the duration of the longest reflux episode occurs during sleep.[30] Vandenplas et al reported that the incidence of GER in infants >4 months of age correlated directly with an increased state of alertness and activity.[3]

The majority of postprandial GER episodes occur secondary to TLESRs in children,[3] and are triggered by gastric distention, possibly by vagal and/or parasympathetic pathways.[31, 32] Transient lower esophageal sphincter relaxations occurred at a rate of 0.6 per hour, accounting for 10% of fasting and 45% of postprandial reflux episodes.[33] Refluxate is efficiently cleared from the esophagus by secondary peristaltic waves with swallowed saliva neutralizing the juxtamucosal acidic environment.

Nocturnal pediatric esophageal motility studies demonstrated that the stage of sleep affects esophageal acid clearance, with primary esophageal contractions decreasing as the stage of sleep increases. Secondary contractions also decrease as the stage of sleep increases but normalize in REM sleep, resulting in a decreased volume of saliva reaching the distal esophagus.

Epithelial Resistance

The esophageal epithelium has layered protection, with a superficial mucous layer that prevents cellular contact of large molecules, including pepsin. A layer of unstirred water, with a high concentration of bicarbonate derived from swallowed saliva, lies below the mucus, preventing penetration of hydrochloric acid. If cellular damage does occur, the subepithelial capillary system is capable of removing waste products, providing nutrients for repair, and helping to restore the acid-base balance.

Upper Esophageal Sphincter

Anatomically, the upper esophageal spincter (UES) and the cricopharyngeus muscle are synonymous, receiving motor, sensory, parasympathetic, and sympathetic innervation from the pharyngeal plexus, cranial nerves IX and X, and the sympathetic cervical ganglion. The UES is tonically contracted, increasing basal tone in response to esophageal acidification, and relaxing with vagal input.[34]

Physiological manometric studies of the UES are difficult to perform due to asymmetrical contraction. The side-to-side pressure is lower than the anteroposterior pressure. The UES has a diurnal pressure cycle, being lowest with sleep.[35]

PATHOPHYSIOLOGY

The pathogenesis of GERD is multifactorial in origin and includes decreased LESP, TLESRs, delayed acid clearance, impaired mucosal barrier, delayed gastric emptying, UES dysfunction, and neuromuscular immaturity. It is appreciated that reflux of any pH level is capable of causing GERD.

LOWER ESOPHAGEAL SPHINCTER PRESSURE

The normal resting pressure of the LES is 11.8 ± 3.6 mm Hg in children <7 years of age.[25] In healthy children, the myogenic tone of the LES is able to overcome the intraesophageal–intragastric pressure gradient to prevent reflux. This pressure gradient between the stomach (+6 mm Hg to 10 mm Hg) and the esophagus (−6 mm Hg to 10 mm Hg) reflects positive intra-abdominal and negative intrapleural pressures.

There are three mechanisms that help maintain the normal pressure gradient: the myogenic tone of the LES, normally in an intra-abdominal location; increases in intra-abdominal pressure accentuating the GE angle; and, most importantly, increases in intra-abdominal pressure collapsing the distal abdominal esophagus/LES. If these mechanisms are altered, the child is more prone to reflux.

Sleeping infants with GERD have an increased number and greater duration of reflux episodes compared with asymptomatic sleeping infants.[30] The majority of these episodes occur during inappropriate TLESRs, unassociated with swallowing. Werlin et al reported that 34% of reflux episodes were associated with TLESRs in 27 children between the ages of 5 days and 2 years.[36] The etiology of these TLESRs is still unknown, but they occur in response to an afferent vagal pulmonary pathway triggered by inspiration.[37] Both the presence of esophagitis and the postprandial state increase the frequencies of TLESRs.[38]

INADEQUATE MUCOSAL BARRIER

A defective mucosal barrier exposes the mucosa to refluxate. However, exposure is not the only factor responsible for esophagitis. Decreased tissue resistance and bilious and/or pancreatic secretions in the refluxate are also involved in the pathogenesis of esophagitis.[4]

DELAYED ESOPHAGEAL ACID CLEARANCE

Delayed esophageal acid clearance can result from decreased rates of nocturnal swallowing and/or an inadequate arousal stimulus from sleep. Swallowing increases esophageal acid clearance by initiating peristalsis and delivering saliva. The normal infant swallows less during sleep than awake, and the infant with pathologic GER swallows even less than the infant with physiological reflux while asleep.[38] The normal infant increases swallowing frequency from 0.46 to 3.5 per minute during sleep reflux episodes while the pathologic child is unable to do so, only increasing swallowing from 0.45 to 0.49.[38] Defective esophageal motility also results in delayed acid clearance. Infants with severe reflux esophagitis have been reported to have a decreased peristaltic amplitude and abnormal contractility patterns.[38, 39]

UPPER ESOPHAGEAL SPHINCTER PRESSURE

The final barrier is the UES. Traditional thinking has blamed reflux on an abnormally low upper esophageal sphincter pressure (UESP).[40] However, both Sondheimer[34] and Striano et al[41] have been unable to demonstrate a difference in the resting UESP of children with and without reflux. Recently, Willing et al studied 53 symptomatic children with dual sleeve manometry without sedation, locating one probe in the UES and the other in the distal esophagus.[42] Esophageal distention with reflux caused an increase in the resting UESP; however, abrupt relaxations of the UES occurred during 54% of the reflux episodes, accounting for pharyngoesophageal reflux and possible laryngeal acid exposure.

DELAYED GASTRIC EMPTYING

Delayed gastric emptying may play a role in the pathogenesis of GERD by raising intragastric pressures and triggering TLESRs. Feeding, age, presence of severe pathology, and alterations of gastroduodenal motility can all influence gastric emptying. There is disagreement in the literature concerning the role of gastric emptying in patients with GERD, and reports of normal, delayed, and accelerated gastric emptying times can be found.[39, 43-47]

COMPLICATIONS OF GASTROESOPHAGEAL REFLUX

Both esophageal and extraesophageal complications can result from GERD (Table 2). Early recognition and treatment is critical in order to reduce the patient's morbidity and mortality. The reader is referred to several excellent reviews of esophageal complications.[48-51]

TABLE 2.
Direct and Indirect Sequelae of GERD*

Esophageal	Laryngeal	Miscellaneous
Ulceration	Laryngospasm	Atypical chest pain
Stricture	Cough	Hiccups
Bleeding	Reflux laryngitis	Torticollis
Barrett's mucosa	Apnea	Sleep disturbance
Adenocarcinoma	ALTE	Otitis media
Dysphagia	SIDS	Otalgia
	Subglottic stenosis	
	Bradycardia	
	Croup	
Oropharyngeal	Pulmonary	Nutritional
Dental erosions	Aspiration pneumonitis	Failure to thrive
Burning mouth syndrome	Pulmonary abscess	Feeding difficulty
Pharyngitis	Bronchiectasis	Protein-losing
Globus sensation	Bronchopulmonary dysplasia	enteropathy
	Chronic bronchitis	Anemia
	Asthma	
	Recurrent pneumonia	

*Adapted from Koufman JA: *Laryngoscope* 101(suppl 53):1–78, 1991.

RESPIRATORY COMPLICATIONS OF GASTROESOPHAGEAL REFLUX

There is longstanding concern over the role that reflux plays in causing respiratory disease. William Osler observed in 1884 that "asthmatics learnt not to eat a large meal before bed if they were going to avoid their nighttime asthma".[52] In 1960 a review of 1,300 surgical cases of esophageal disease found a high incidence of chronic respiratory disease.[53] In 1962, Kennedy introduced the term "silent GERD," describing a group of patients with documented but silent GER and respiratory disease.[9]

Gastroesophageal reflux disease has been implicated in the pathogenesis of asthma,[54, 55] stridor,[56, 57] apnea,[58] chronic pulmonary diseases,[54] reflux laryngitis,[59] apparent life-threatening events (ALTEs),[60] and SIDS.[61] The pathophysiology of GER-related airway disease may include three mechanisms:

1. Macroaspiration with chemical pneumonitis
2. Microaspiration with chemical pneumonitis or stimulation of laryngeal protective reflexes, possibly involved in the pathogenesis of apnea or ALTE
3. Stimulation of esophageal receptors causing bronchial hyperactivity

A relation between GERD and respiratory disease was established by Halpern et al who demonstrated that the mean duration of reflux episodes during sleep (ZMD) corresponded directly with the presence of respiratory symptoms in children with GERD.[62] Others report children whose difficult-to-control pulmonary disease improves or resolves with control of GERD.[63–65]

Stridor

Reflux has been identified as a causative agent in the pathogenesis of pediatric stridor.[56, 66] Repeated micro- or macroaspirations can cause an indolent inflammatory process in the laryngotracheal tree, decreasing intraluminal diameter. Repeated acidic insults to the laryngotracheal tree can cause erosions, exposed cartilage, granulation tissue, subglottic stenosis, and posterior glottic scarring.

Orenstein et al described a 9-day-old infant with episodic reflux documented by pH-probe and concurrent stridor, each episode of which resolved after esophageal acid clearance.[66] The infant was subsequently treated with a prokinetic agent, and the stridor resolved. To our knowledge, this report is the first that describes a cause and effect relationship between GER and stridor.

Contencin et al. used a two-channel pH-probe to study normal children and children with recurrent stridor.[56] The most significant parameter was the total time that the pH was <6 in the pharynx, described as the "pharyngeal acidity index" (PAI). Defining GERD as a PAI >1%, the specificity was 83%, and the sensitivity was 100%.

Nielson et al reported seven infants with GERD and continuous stridor undergoing simultaneous pH-probe and cardiorespiratory testing.[57] GER preceded stridor and hypercarbia. Five patients responded to medical management; three required fundoplication.

Asthma

The association between asthma and GER has been known for over 50 years, since Bray first proposed a vagally-mediated reflex mechanism in its pathogenesis.[67] Subsequently, various studies have demonstrated that GER has a higher prevalence in asthmatics.[54, 68, 69] A temporal relationship between GER episodes and wheezing has also been reported.[70]

Asthma can predispose a patient to GER. High negative intrapleural pressures generated during inspiration will amplify the existing pressure gradient between the esophagus and the stomach, increasing the reflux gradient. Chronic hyperinflation will flatten and stretch the diaphragmatic crura, shortening the intra-abdominal esophagus, thus facilitating LES incompetence. Many asthma medications decrease LESP (see Table 1). Finally, there may be a reflex relaxation of the LES mediated through bronchial receptors triggered by inspiration.[37]

Gastroesophageal reflux can exacerbate asthma by two mechanisms. First, micro- or macroaspiration of gastric contents can cause an indolent upper respiratory tract inflammatory reaction. Radionucleotide scintiscanning has documented pulmonary aspiration of gastric contents on the day following administration of a labeled meal in adult patients with GER and chronic pulmonary disease.[71]

The second mechanism is by reflex bronchoconstriction, triggered by distal esophageal acidification. Bronchoconstriction was induced in young asthmatic animals after acid instillation into the tracheobronchial tree.[72] Perfusion of diluted HCl into the distal esophagus reproduced wheezing in some asthmatics,[73] and, in asymptomatic asthmatics, caused increased bronchial hypersensitivity as measured by methacholine challenge.[74, 75] These studies have been criticized because microaspiration of acid may be a cause for symptoms. However, in animal models, vagal nerve section obliterates this bronchoconstrictive response to acidification, supporting a vagally-mediated reflex mechanism. Topical anesthesia or antacid neutralization of the esophagus also eliminates this response.[76]

APNEA

A direct cause and effect relationship between GER, apnea, ALTEs, and SIDS has not been established. Gastroesophageal reflux disease can cause obstructive apnea from aspirated material, stimulation of the laryngeal chemoreceptor reflexes, altered pulmonary gas exchange, and bronchial anaphylaxis to aspirated milk antigens.[55]

The laryngeal chemoreceptor reflex is of special interest to the otolaryngologist. Stimulation of the superior laryngeal nerve (SLN) at the laryngeal inlet can cause the following: apnea, bradycardia, hypotension, peripheral vasoconstriction, blood flow redistribution, and swallowing.[77] Arousal typically terminates this sequence, but, in the presence of hypoxemia, an apneic event can become pathologic.[78] Thus, if a reflux event occurs in the presence of hypoxemia, an exaggerated laryngeal chemoreceptive reflex leading to airway obstruction can ensue.

Gastroesophageal reflux disease has been implicated in the pathogenesis of cardiac and respiratory events such as bradycardia and apnea. Eight normal near-term infants underwent distal esophageal acid perfusion to simulate a reflux episode. Compared to saline infusion, there was significant prolongation of the RR interval on the electrocardiogram, an increase in respiratory cycles followed by a missed breath, and a significant increase in the number and duration of EEG arousals.[58]

Apparent Life-Threatening Event

An apparent life-threatening event ALTE is defined as an apneic event during the first year of life with a combination of apnea, color change, altered muscle tone, choking, or gagging.[79] Various pediatric series demonstrate a high incidence of asymptomatic reflux (46% to 87%),[79] a high incidence of symptomatic reflux (42% to 95%),[79-81] and a significant correlation between the duration of esophageal acidification and length of the apneic event.[81] One series identified GERD as the etiology of 26% of ALTEs.[82] Vagal hyperactivity has been implicated in the pathogenesis of ALTEs. Bethmann et al report that 67% of patients having an ALTE event had vagal overactivity and 62% had GERD; only 45% and 42% of controls had these factors, respectively.[60] The association of reflux and vagal activity was observed in 42% of the ALTE group versus 18% of controls. Vagal overactivity is treatable with atropine-like drugs.

Sudden Infant Death Syndrome

Gastroesophageal reflux disease has been implicated in the pathogenesis of SIDS,[83, 84] defined as the sudden death of an infant <1 year of age, unexplained by autopsy. In 10% of the children with ALTEs, GER was implicated.[38]

Sudden infant death syndrome is the leading cause of postnatal death between 1 and 12 months of life, with an incidence of 1 to 2:1000 live births.[85] One hypotheses for these deaths is reflux-induced bradycardia.[83]

Recently, Wetmore has proposed that acid-induced laryngospasm may be responsible for SIDS, demonstrating that instillation of acid into the larynx provoked laryngospasm, mimicking apnea in an animal model.[84] Spitzer et al reported a subgroup of infants experiencing awake apnea correlating to reflux episodes documented by pH-probe.[86] Veereman-Wauters et al. reported that 49 of 130 patients had an ALTE soon after feeding; 34 of 49 had pathologic reflux.[82] Possible pathophysiologic mechanisms include laryngospasm mediated through the SLN afferents and recurrent laryngeal nerve efferents.[84] Central apnea can be mediated by SLN afferents and phrenic nerve efferents.[84] Stimulation of the SLN could result in apnea and, possibly, SIDS, as seen in an animal model.[84]

Twenty-four–hour pH monitoring has been used to identify patients with GERD, considered to be at higher risk for SIDS. Jolley et al studied 499 patients with reflux for one year, reporting a 9.1% incidence of reflux-related or SIDS deaths in infants with a type 1 reflux pattern (this pattern consists of a continuously high frequency of reflux episodes and is often seen in the setting of a low LESP or a large hiatal hernia) and a prolonged ZMD score treated medically compared to no deaths in the group undergoing anti-reflux surgery.[61, 87] They concluded that surgery may be indicated in this high risk group.

Reflux Laryngitis

Reflux laryngitis is a well-recognized phenomena in adults[88] and children.[59] Acidic refluxate can cause laryngeal inflammation, edema, ulceration, and/or granulation, interfering with laryngeal function and causing hoarseness, cough, and a globus sensation. Putnam et al reported a child with hoarseness with GER whose symptomatology resolved after medical treatment.[59] Any child with unexplained hoarseness should be evaluated for GER.

Cystic Fibrosis

Cystic fibrosis (CF) is a autosomal recessive disorder of pancreatic insufficiency, malabsorption, and chronic pulmonary disease. The role that GERD plays in CF is controversial although reflux is common in this population.[89] Reflux may occur because of chronic coughing, a flattened diaphragm, or esophageal dysfunction.[89, 90] Recently, TLESRs have been blamed for the majority of GER[91] and have been linked to a pulmonary afferent/vagal efferent reflex pathway initiated by lung inflation.[37]

Gastroesophageal reflux disease can complicate respiratory and nutritional problems in the CF patient. However, as GER has been shown to improve with age while CF worsens, the role of GER in the CF population remains controversial.[92]

EVALUATION OF GASTROESOPHAGEAL REFLUX

HISTORY AND PHYSICAL EXAMINATION

The diagnosis of GERD can be difficult. A complete history is obtained, including birth, past medical, feeding, airway, and reflux history. Establishing a cause and effect relationship between GER episodes and the airway symptoms remains difficult. Reflux may be asymptomatic or "silent," and the clinician must maintain a high index of suspicion. The manifestations of GERD are listed in Table 2.

Recently, Orenstein et al developed a 161 item questionnaire covering demographics, symptoms, and possible causative etiologic factors for GER, requiring 20 minutes for the parent to complete.[93]

Twenty-five percent to 35% of patients will receive an incorrect diagnosis and undergo inappropriate medical or surgical treatment if the symptom-based diagnosis alone is used.[94] Diagnostic testing is usually necessary to make the diagnosis of GERD.

A physical exam including growth curve is performed. While these findings are usually nonspecific, a complete head and neck examination is included. The upper and lower airway should be auscultated.[69]

DIAGNOSTIC TESTING

The specificity and sensitivity of the more common tests used to confirm the diagnosis of GER are listed in Table 3. The diagnostic error can be reduced by confirming GER on two different tests.

BLOOD WORK

Routine blood counts and chemistries are useful to evaluate the nutritional state and to screen for anemia.

RADIOLOGICAL TESTS

Barium Studies

The barium esophagram with a small bowel follow through remains useful to demonstrate the anatomy and function of the upper gastrointesti-

TABLE 3.
Reliability of Diagnostic Tests for Gastroesophageal Reflux*

Test	Author 1: Jaimieson GG, Duranceau A		Author 2: Riechter JE, Castell DO		
	Sensitivity + (Abnormality in Disease)	Specificity + (Normalcy in Health)	Sensitivity % (Abnormality in Disease)	Specificity % (Normalcy in Health)	Studies Reviewed
Barium esophagram	+	++	40%	85%	3
Esophagoscopy	++	+++	95%	41%	2
Esophageal biopsy	+++	+++	77%	91%	5
Lipid-laden macrophage	+++	unknown	—	—	—
Scintiscan	++	+++	61%	95%	3
pH monitoring	++++	++++	88%	98%	3

*Adapted from Jaimieson GG, Duranceau A: *Gastroesophageal reflux.* Philadelphia, WB Saunders Co, 1988, p 281, and from Riechter JE, Castell DO: *Ann Intern Med* 97:93, 1982.
++++ = excellent; +++ = good; ++ = fair; + = poor.

nal tract. It detects anatomic abnormalities that cause or exacerbate GER such as a tracheoesophageal fistula (TEF), vascular anomalies, or gastric outlet obstruction. While it can demonstrate esophageal pathology such as strictures and mucosal erosions, the shortcoming of the barium esophagram with a small bowel follow through is that it represents only a snapshot in time with consequent low sensitivity and specificity for GERD.[96]

Sonography

Gastric sonography has been advocated for as an initial diagnostic test for GERD with a specificity of 87.5% and a sensitivity of 100% compared to pH monitoring in children.[97] While convenient, noninvasive, and without risk of radiation, sonography can detect only reflux, not esophagitis.

Radionuclide Scintiscan (Milk Scan)

The gastroesophageal scintiscan typically requires the patient to swallow a liquid (milk) tagged with a gamma-emitting radionucleotide. The passage of the bolus in the postprandial period is monitored with a gamma camera and quantified with a computer. The presence of GER of any pH can be identified and quantified, and the rate of gastric emptying determined. One study reports that 1-hour tests are as reliable as 2 hour tests.[98] The scan can be repeated later to detect the presence of aspiration over the lung fields. The sensitivity of the gastroesophageal scintiscan is 90%, providing accurate, rapid, and noninvasive diagnosis and quantitating GER in a physiological manner.[99] It can also be used to assess improvement of GERD with therapy.

MOTILITY STUDIES

Manometry can be used to locate the LES, identify motility disorders, correctly position the pH-probe, and record the pressures within the upper gastrointestinal tract. However, a normal LESP does not exclude the diagnosis of GERD.[25] Recently, the technology to perform manometry on an outpatient basis has been developed.[100, 101] Ambulatory pH-probe studies will reflect a more physiological test than laboratory conditions and will have better diagnostic capabilities for reflux.[100]

pH STUDIES

The gold standard for diagnosis of GER is a 24-hour pH-probe using a single or double electrode system. A symptom observational log during the study aids in the temporal relationship between reflux and symptomatology.

Varty et al suggested that the pH study be used to identify patients requiring surgery.[102] Their study group consisted of 57 children with GERD, who had failed medical management and underwent a pH-probe study. They were able to predict which children would require surgical control of their GERD if they used a cutoff point of >18% of study time that the patient had a pH <4, with different specificities and sensitivities depending upon the subpopulation that was studied. For the subpopulation of patients who had GERD without any concomitant illnesses, the values were 92% and 70%, respectively, and for the subpopulation of children who had GERD secondary to esophageal atresia, TEF, or neurologic conditions, the values were 80% and 86%, respectively.

The weakness of a pH study is its inability to diagnose neutral or basic reflux. A normal pH study does not rule out GER. Cucchiara et al reported that in children with GERD, 20% had normal acid exposure times and 30% had a normal number of reflux episodes >5 minutes.[4] A false-negative test can occur in the following situations: neutral reflux, basic reflux, refluxed gastric contents buffered by the infant's milk, or increased salivary flow from nasogastric tube stimulation.[103]

INVASIVE TESTS

Esophageal endoscopy is an excellent diagnostic modality that allows visualization of the esophageal mucosa to detect edema, erythema, erosions, stricture, and Barrett's mucosa. Endoscopic biopsy is also performed as there is a 40% incidence of histological esophagitis with normal-appearing mucosa on endoscopy.[99, 104]

The upper airway is inspected with microlaryngoscopy and bronchoscopy. Interarytenoid edema, vocal cord changes, and mucosal abnormalities or edema can be detected and biopsy specimens obtained if suspicious. The subglottis can be evaluated for stenosis, and the arytenoids palpated to determine mobility. Aspiration of tracheobronchial secretions may detect lipid-laden macrophages (LLMs). While LLMs can be attributed to a variety of irritative phenomena, the sensitivity of LLMs for GER is 85%.[105] However, their absence does not rule out GER.

TREATMENT

The treatment protocol for GERD involves three phases. Phase I involves alterations in lifestyle and diet, phase II involves pharmacologic treatment, and phase III involves surgical treatment. Not every patient will undergo an orderly stepwise escalation of treatment to control GERD. Life-threatening complications may require direct surgical evaluation and control. Typically, however, the patient with GERD responds well to less aggressive therapy.

PHASE I: LIFESTYLE MODIFICIATION

Lifestyle modification should be the initial form of treatment in children without life-threatening complications of GERD. In the young child, treatment may include smaller, more frequent meals and head elevation when recumbent. In the infant, both dietary modification and positioning may be very helpful. Dietary modifications promoting gastric emptying include formulas with medium-chain triglycerides, whey-hydrolysate or soy,[106] and/or lower osmolality.[107]

Body positioning is an integral component in the treatment of GERD. By having the head of the bed elevated, gravitational forces will aid in preventing reflux. Originally, the seated position was recommended for the infant until the 1980s when data showed that this position actually worsened GER.[108, 109] Traditionally, the 30 degree prone position is preferred to the horizontal prone position.[108, 110] However, a recent study demonstrated that the horizontal prone position is as effective as the 30 degree prone position in reducing GER and is easier to use as a harness is not required to keep the child from sliding down the incline.[111]

PHASE II: PHARMACOLOGIC TREATMENT

The goal of the pharmacologic treatment is to relieve symptoms, promote esophageal healing, and prevent progression of disease. If the symptomatology persists through phase I, pharmacologic management is indicated. Goals are acid reduction, cytoprotection, improved motility, and improvement of LES tone. It should be noted that there are no drugs with FDA approval for use in young children with GERD.

Cytoprotective Agents

Antacids are commonly used in the treatment of GER to neutralize acid, reduce acidic mucosal injury, and prevent the activation of pepsin. There are few side effects. Preparations with alginic acid are especially helpful, forming a thick viscous foam over the gastric contents and acting as an additional reflux barrier. Sucralfate is also cytoprotective, as it coats areas of denuded esophageal and gastric mucosa with a nearly acid-impermeable layer. A liquid preparation is now available for use in esophagitis.

H2 Receptor Antagonists

Cimetadine and ranitidine are the most commonly used H2 receptor antagonists in the treatment of GERD in children. Because the parietal cell contains histamine, gastrin, and acetylcholine receptors, which are all capable of stimulating acid secretions, H2 receptor antagonists are not 100% effective. These agents reduce acid secretion by competitively blocking the H2 receptor. There is no effect on LESP or gastrointestinal motility. Esophageal mucosal healing rates are inversely proportional to the severity of esophagitis. Fifty percent to 70% of symptomatic adult patients have partial or total relief, but symptom relief does not correlate with esophageal healing.[112] Esophageal healing is proportional to the length of treatment up to 12 weeks.[112]

Proton Pump Inhibitor

Omeprazole is a new agent which inhibits the last step in acid production, the parietal cell potassium/hydrogen ATPase enzyme. In adults, it blocks 90% of the daily acid production in comparison to 70% with the H2 receptor antagonists.[113] A recent British study reported omeprazole's efficacy in the treatment of severe esophagitis in 15 infants and children, including 8 neurologically impaired children, refractory to H2 blockers and prokinetic agents.[114] Treatment doses ranging from 0.7 mg/kg to 3.3 mg/kg were sufficient to control the symptoms and allow esophageal healing.

Prokinetic Agents

Metaclopramide is a dopamine antagonist which increases gastric emptying, improves esophageal peristalsis, and raises LESP.[115] Its exact mechanism of action is unknown, but its extrapyramidal and sedative side effects are related to its central dopaminergic antagonism.

Cisapride is a new selective cholinergic agent lacking the antidopinergic activity of metaclopramide and, thus, its side effects. Cisapride has been successful in controlling reflux in both term[92] and preterm[116] infants. It facilitates the release of acetylcholine from the myenteric plexus, controls severe regurgitation in infants, and has an excellent safety profile and low toxicity.[117] It effectively decreases the total percentage of reflux time, gastric emptying time, and gastric distention.[43] It is also effective in the treatment of chronic respiratory disease in children with GERD.[118]

PHASE III: SURGICAL TREATMENT

The surgical treatment of GERD is reserved for patients that fail maximal medical management.[119] Its goals are to restore the natural integrity of the LES, to improve the gastroesophageal valve function, and to maintain normal deglutition. The Nissen fundoplication is the most common surgical procedure for medically refractory GERD.

The anatomical basis of this repair rests on its ability to accomplish three goals: restore the competence of the cardia by increasing the length and pressure of the LES, decrease the esophageal diameter, and resist gastric distention with a 360-degree wrap, requiring a higher opening pressure for reflux to occur.[120] The Nissen fundoplication has a 85% to 90% symptom control rate with a 1% mortality rate.[119, 121]

THE NEUROLOGICALLY IMPAIRED CHILD

There is a high incidence of GERD in neurologically impaired children (NIC).[122] Halpern et al reported a 69% incidence of GER in NIC versus a 47% incidence in normal children.[123] These children are difficult to manage, and surgical treatment is often necessary because of the high failure rate with medical management. Symptoms may recur postoperatively, with 71% of NIC having recurrent GER symptoms within 1 year of fundoplication.[124]

TREATMENT PROTOCOL

The majority of patients seen for otolaryngologic consultation will have airway manifestations of GERD. There have been several treatment paradigms presented in the literature.[125] A suggested treatment paradigm follows. Each patient should undergo a thorough history and physical examination, including flexible fiberoptic nasopharyngoscopy. In addition, a screening battery of tests is suggested: airway films, chest radiograph, and barium esophagram with a small bowel follow through.

From this initial evaluation, the clinician will have a high or low suspicion of GERD or conclude that the child has life-threatening airway complication. The typical history of a life-threatened patient includes cyanosis or apnea, often with feeding, stridor, ALTE, or a sibling with SIDS. A child for whom the clinician has a high level of suspicion typically has frequent regurgitation, difficulty with feeding, FTT, anemia, evidence of laryngeal inflammation, or a positive radiologic study. Suggested treatment paradigms are shown in Figures 1 to 3.

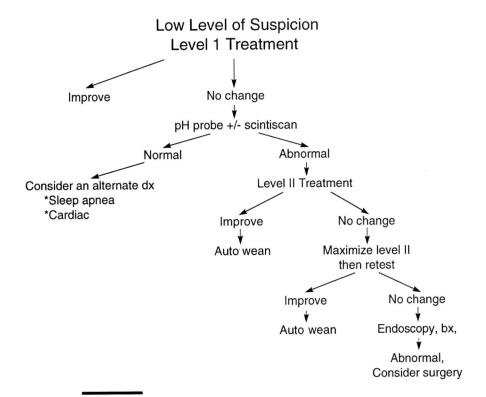

FIGURE 1.

Suggested treatment paradigm for airway symptomatic children with low suspicion for GERD. dx, diagnosis; bx, biopsy.

As with any protocol, there are shortcomings. Not every patient will fit neatly into a treatment arm. Each child should be treated individually, modifying the protocol as needed. In addition, a pH-probe and nuclear scintiscan are complementary, not interchangeable tests. If one test is negative, the other should be performed before an alternate diagnosis (i.e., obstructive sleep apnea or cardiac disease) is considered. If a child improves at any point during treatment, that level of treatment can be maintained, weaning the treatment as the child gains weight and outgrows the tendency to reflux.

For a low level of suspicion, phase I treatment should be instituted. If a child fails to improve, pH-probe and/or nuclear scintiscan should be obtained. Patients with positive studies should start phase II treatment. If there is still no improvement, the treatment doses should be maximized, and a repeat study considered to see if there has been improvement on maximal medical therapy. A resistant child may undergo panendoscopy and consideration for an antireflux procedure if there is no improvement.

With a high level of suspicion, the child should begin with a pH-probe or nuclear scintiscan. If positive, patients start phase I and II treatments simultaneously. If the child fails to improve, phase II treatment is maximized and a repeat study performed to assess progress. If the child remains refractory to treatment, panendoscopy should be performed, and consideration of a antireflux procedure should be discussed with the parents.

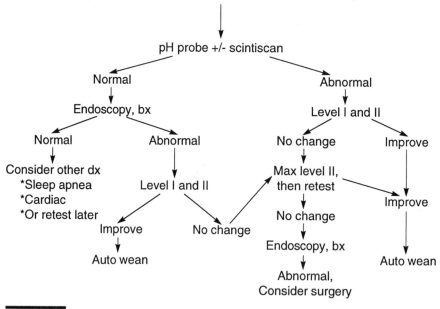

FIGURE 2.

Suggested treatment paradigm for airway symptomatic children with a high suspicion for GERD including special population children (tracheoesophageal fistula, bronchopulmonary dysplasia, esophageal atresia, colonic interposition, recurrent pneumonia, subglottic stenosis, neurologic impairment, and cystic fibrosis). *dx* = diagnosis; *bx* = biopsy.

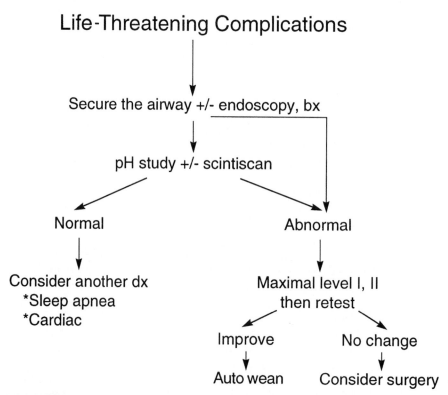

FIGURE 3.

Suggested treatment paradigm for children with life-threatening airway complications of GERD (cyanosis or apnea, often with feeding, stridor, ALTE, or a sibling with SIDS). *dx*, diagnosis; *bx*, biopsy.

With life-threatening airway complications, the number one priority is to evaluate the airway. The patient is admitted to an intensive care unit and may require urgent endoscopic evaluation. After the airway has been evaluated and/or secured, a pH-probe or nuclear scintiscan can be performed. Children with positive study should be treated with both phase I and maximized phase II treatment plans. Treatment failures are candidates for an antireflux procedure.

REFERENCES

1. Koufman JA: The otolaryngologic manifestations of gastroesophageal reflux disease (GERD), in Myers EN, Bluestone CD, Brackmann DE, Krause CJ (eds): *Advances in Otolaryngology-Head and Neck Surgery,* vol 7. St. Louis, Mosby, 1993, pp 115–147.
2. Demeester TR, Johnson LF, Joseph GJ, et al: Patterns of gastroesophageal reflux in health and disease. *Ann Surg* 184:459–470, 1976.
3. Vandenplas Y, Sacre-Smits L: Continuous 24-hr esophageal pH monitoring in 285 asymptomatic infants 0–15 months old. *J Pediatr Gastroenterol Nutr* 6:220–224, 1987.
4. Cucchiara S, Stiano A, Casali LG, et al: Value of 24-hr intraesophageal pH monitoring in children. *Gut* 31:129–133, 1990.
5. Schindlbeck NE, Ippisch H, Klauser AG, et al: What pH threshold is best in esophageal pH monitoring? *Am J Gastroenterol* 86:1138–1141, 1991.
6. Zhu H, Pace F, Sangaletti O, et al: pH Fluctuations versus reflux episodes in patients with gastroesophageal reflux disease: Their optimal thresholds and significance in diagnosis. *Digestion* 51:152–160, 1992.
7. DeMeester TR, Wang CI, Winans CS: Comparison of clinical tests for the detections of gastroesophageal reflux (abstract). *Eur Surg Res* 11(suppl 2):13, 1979.
8. Vandenplas Y, Goyvaerts H, Helven R, et al: Gastroesophageal reflux as measured by 24-hr pH monitoring in 509 healthy infants screened for risk of sudden infant death syndrome. *Pediatrics* 88:834–840, 1991.
9. Kennedy JH: "Silent" gastroesophageal reflux: An important but little known cause of pulmonary complications. *Dis Chest* 42:42–45, 1962.
10. Peeters S, Vandenplas Y: Sex ratio of gastroesophageal reflux in infancy. *J Pediatr Gastroenterol Nutr* 13:314, 1991.
11. Carré IJ: The natural history of the partial thoracic stomach (hiatous hernia) in children. *Arch Dis Child* 34:344–353, 1959.
12. Kibel MA: Gastroesophageal reflux and failure to thrive in infancy, in Gells SS (ed.): *Gastroesophageal Reflux 76th Ross Conference on Pediatric Research.* Columbus, OH, Ross Laboratories, 1979, pp 39–42.
13. Boix-Ochoa J, Canals J: Maturations of the lower esophagus. *J Pediatr Surg* 11:749–756, 1976.
14. Balistreri WF, Farrell MK: Gastroesophageal reflux in infants. *N Engl J Med* 309:790–792, 1983.
15. Treem WR, Davis PM, Hyams JS: Gastroesophgeal reflux in the older child: Presentation, response to treatment and long-term follow-up. *Clinical Pediatrics* 30:435–440, 1991.
16. Weiss MH: Dysphagia in infants and children. *Otolaryngol Clin North Am* 21:727–735, 1988.
17. Logemann JA: *Evaluation and Treatment of Swallowing Disorders.* San Diego, College-Hill Press, 1983.
18. Malthaner R, Newman KD, Parry R, et al: Alkaline gastroesophageal reflux in infants and children. *J Pediatr Surg* 26:986–991, 1991.

19. Vandenplas Y, Loeb H: Alkaline gastroesophageal reflux in infancy. *J Pediatr Gastroenterol Nutr* 12:448–452, 1991.
20. Goldstein JL, Schlesinger PK, Mozwecz HL, et al: Esophageal mucosal resistance. *Gastroenterol Clin North Am* 19:565–587, 1990.
21. Rodmark T, Petterson GB: The contribution of the diaphragm and an intrinsic sphincter to the gastroesophageal anti-reflux barrier. An experimental study in the dog. *Scand J Gastroenterol* 24:85–94, 1989.
22. Watanabe Y, Lister J: Development of the human fetal-esophageal membrane and its role in the anti-reflux mechanism. *Surg Today Jpn J Surg* 23:722–727, 1993.
23. Hill LD, Kraemer SJ: Does modern technology belong in GI surgery: A step from subjective perception to objective information. *World J Surg* 16:341–342, 1992.
24. Bonavina L, Evander A, DeMeester TR, et al: Length of a distal esophageal sphincter and competency of the cardia. *Am J Surg* 151:25–34, 1986.
25. Boix-Ochoa J: Diagnosis and management of gastroesophageal reflux in children. *Surg Annu* 13:123–137, 1981.
26. Castell DV: Physiology and pathophysiology of the lower esophageal sphincter. *Ann Otol Rhinol Laryngol* 84:569–575, 1975.
27. Willems J, Buylaert W, LaFebure R, et al: Neuronal dynamic receptors on autonomic ganglia and sympathetic nerves and dynamic receptors in the gastrointestinal system. *Pharmacol Rev* 37:165–216, 1985.
28. Helm JF, Dodds WJ, Hogan WJ: Salivary response to esophageal acid in normal subjects and patients with reflux esophagitis. *Gastroenterology* 92:1393–1397, 1987.
29. Helm JF, Dodds WJ, Riedel DR, et al: Determinants of esophageal acid clearance in normal subjects. *Gastroenterology* 85:607–612, 1983.
30. Vandenplas Y, Wolf DD, Deneger M, et al: Incidence of gastroesophageal reflux in sleep, awake, fasted, and portable periods in asymptomatic and symptomatic infants. *J Pediatr Gastroenterol Nutr* 7:177–180, 1988.
31. Holloway RH, Hongo M, Berger K, et al: Gastric distention: A mechanism for postprandial gastroesophageal reflux. *Gastroenterology* 89:779–784, 1985.
32. Martin CJ, Patrikios J, Dent J: Abolition of gas reflux and transient lower esophageal sphincter relaxation by vagal blockade in the dog. *Gastroenterology* 92:890–896, 1986.
33. Mittal RK, McCallum RW. Characteristics and frequency of transient relaxations of the lower esophageal sphincter in patients with reflux esophagitis. *Gastroenterology* 95:593–599, 1988.
34. Sondheimer JM: Upper esophageal sphincter and pharyngoesophageal motor function in infants with and without gastroesophageal reflux. *Gastroenterology* 85:301–305, 1983.
35. Shapiro GG, Christie DL, Pierson WE, et al: Gastroesophageal reflux in asthmatic children. *J Allergy Clin Immunol* 61:137, 1978.
36. Werlin SL, Dodds WJ, Hogan WJ, et al: Mechanisms of gastroesophageal reflux in children. *J Pediatr* 97:244–249, 1980.
37. Boyle JT, Altschuler SM, Patterson BL, et al: Reflex inhibition of the lower esophageal sphincter (LES) following stimulation of pulmonary vagal afferent receptors. *Gastroenterology* 90:1353, 1986.
38. Sondheimer JM: Clearance of spontaneous gastroesophageal reflux in awake and sleeping infants. *Gastroenterology* 97:821–826, 1989.
39. Hillemeier AC, Grill BB, McCallum R, et al: Esophageal and gastric motor abnormalities in gastroesophageal reflux during infancy. *Gastroenterology* 84:741–746, 1983.

40. Gerhardt DC, Castell DO, Winship DH, et al: Esophageal dysfunction in esophageal regurgitation. *Gastroenterology* 78:893–897, 1980.
41. Striano A, Cucciara S, De Visia B, et al: Disorders of upper esophageal sphincter motility in children. *J Pediatr Gastroenterol Nutr* 6:892–898, 1987.
42. Willing J, Davidson GP, Dent J, et al: Effect of gastroresophageal reflux on upper oesophageal sphincter mobility in children. *Gut* 34:904–910, 1993.
43. Carroccio A, Iacono G, Voti GL, et al.: Gastric emptying in infants with gastroesophageal reflux: Ultrasound evaluation before and after cisapride administration. *Scand J Gastroenterol* 27:799–804, 1992.
44. Andres J, Hansely LS, Mathias JR: Measurement of gastric emptying in infants with technetium-99m labeled solid-phase meal. *Pediatr Res* 14:495, 1980.
45. Papaila JG, Wiolmot D, Grosfeld J, et al: Increased incidence of delayed gastric emptying in children with gastroesophageal reflux. *Arch Surg* 124:933–936, 1989.
46. Jolley SG, Leonard JC, Tunell WP: Gastric emptying in children with gastroesophageal reflux: An estimate of effective gastric emptying. *J Pediatr Surg* 22:923–926, 1987.
47. Euler AR, Byrne WJ: Gastric emptying times of water in infants and children: Comparisons of those with and without gastroesophageal reflux. *J Pediatr Gastroenterol Nutr* 2:595–598, 1983.
48. O'Neill JA, Betts J, Ziegler MM, et al: Surgical management of reflux strictures of the esophagus in childhood. *Ann Surg* 196:453–460, 1982.
49. Catto-Smith AG, Machida H, Butzner JD, et al: The role of gastroesophageal reflux in pediatric dysphagia. *J Pediatr Gastroenterol Nutr* 12:159–165, 1991.
50. Rode H, Millar AW, Brown RA, et al: Reflux strictures of the esophagus in children. *J Pediatr Surg* 27:462–465, 1992.
51. Cheu HW, Grosfeld JL, Heifetz SA, et al: Persistence of Barrett's esophagus in children after antireflux surgery: Influence on follow-up care. *J Pediatr Surg* 27:260–266, 1992.
52. Osler WB: *The Principle of Medicine.* New York, Appleton, 1982.
53. Belsey R: The pulmonary complication of esophageal disease. *Br J Dis Chest* 54:342–348, 1960.
54. Berquist W, Rachelefsky GS, Kadden M, et al: Gastroesophageal reflux-associated recurrent pneumonia and chronic asthma in children. *Pediatrics* 68:29–35, 1981.
55. Mansfield LE: Gastroesophageal reflux and asthma. *Postgrad Med* 86:265–269, 1989.
56. Contencin P, Narcy P: Gastropharyngeal reflux in infants and children—A pharyngeal pH monitoring study. *Arch Otolaryngol Head Neck Surg* 118:1028–1030, 1992.
57. Nielson DW, Heldt GP, Tooley WH: Stridor and gastroesophageal reflux in infants. *Pediatrics* 85:1034–1039, 1990.
58. Ramet J, Egreteau L, Cruzi-Dascalova L, et al: Cardiac, respiratory, and arousal responses to an esophageal acid infusion test in near-term infants during active sleep. *J Pediatr Gastroenterol Nutr* 15:135–140, 1992.
59. Putnam PE, Orenstein SR: Hoarseness in a child with gastroesophageal reflux. *Acta Paediatr* 81:635–686, 1992.
60. Bethmann O, Couchard M, Ajuriaguerra M, et al: Role of gastroesophageal reflux and vagal overactivity in apparent life-threatening events: 160 cases. *Acta Paediatr* 389(suppl 82):102–104, 1993.
61. Jolley SG, Halpern LM, Tunell WP: The risk of sudden infant death from gastroesophageal reflux. *J Pediatr Surg* 26:691–696, 1991.

62. Halpern LM, Jolley SG, Tunell WP, et al: The mean duration of gastroesophageal reflux during sleep as an indicator of respiratory symptoms from gastroesophageal reflux in children. *J Pediatr Surg* 26:688–690, 1991.

63. Hoyoux CL, Forget P, Lanrechts L, et al: Chronic bronchopulmonary disease and gastroesophageal reflux in children. *Pediatr Pulmonol* 1:149–153, 1985.

64. Andze GO, Brandt ML, Vil DL, et al: Diagnosis and treatment of gastroesophageal reflux in 500 children with respiratory symptoms: The value of pH monitoring. *J Pediatr Surg* 26:295–300, 1991.

65. Chen PH, Chang MH, Hsu SC: Gastroesophageal reflux in children with chronic recurrent bronchopulmonary infection. *J Pediatr Gastroenterol Nutr* 13:16–22, 1991.

66. Orenstein SR, Orenstein DM, Whitington PF: Gastroesophageal reflux causing stridor. *Chest* 84:301–302, 1983.

67. Bray GW: Recent advances in the treatment of asthma and hay fever. *Practitioner* 133:368–379, 1934.

68. Gustafsson PM, Kjellman NIM, Tibbling L: Oesophageal function and symptoms in moderate and severe asthma. *Acta Paediatr Scand* 75:729–736, 1986.

69. Euler AR, Byrne WJ, Ament ME, et al: Recurrent pulmonary disease in children: A complication of gastroesophageal reflux. *Pediatrics* 63:47–51, 1979.

70. Martin ME, Grunstein MM, Larsen GL: The relationship of gastroesophageal reflux to nocturnal wheezing in children with asthma. *Ann Allergy* 49:318–322, 1982.

71. Crausaz FM, Faver G: Aspiration of solid food particles into lungs of patients with esophageal reflux and chronic bronchial disease. *Chest* 93:376–378, 1988.

72. Bancewicz J, Bernstein A, Pierry A, et al: Surgery for gastroesophageal reflux in asthmatic patients. *Br J Dis Chest* 75:320, 1981.

73. Davis RS, Larsen GL, Grunstein MM: Respiratory response to intraesophageal acid infusion in asthmatic children during sleep. *J Allergy Clin Immunol* 72:393–398, 1983.

74. Moote DW, Lloyd DA, McCourtie DR, et al: Increase in gastroesophageal reflux during methacholine-induced bronchospasm. *J Allergy Clin Immunol* 78:619–623, 1986.

75. Herve P, Denjean A, Jian R, et al: Intraesophageal perfusion of acid increases the bronchomotor response to methacholine and to isocapnic hyperventilation in asthma subject. *Am Rev Respir Dis* 134:986–989, 1986.

76. Mansfield, LE, Stein MR: Gastroesophageal reflux and asthma: A possible reflux mechanism. *Ann Allergy* 41:224–226, 1978.

77. Wennergren G, Bjure J, Hertzberg T, et al: Layngeal reflex. *Acta Paediatr* 389(suppl 82):53–56, 1993.

78. Lanier B, Richardson MA, Cummings C: Effect of hypoxia on laryngeal reflux apnea-implications on sudden infant death. *Otolaryngol Head Neck Surg* 91:597–604, 1983.

79. Newman LJ, Russe J, Glassman MS, et al: Patterns of gastroesophageal reflux (GER) in patients with apparent life-threatening events. *J Pediatr Gastroenterol Nutr* 8:157–160, 1989.

80. Sacré L, Vandenplas Y: Gastroesophageal reflux associated with respiratory abnormalities during sleep. *J Pediatr Gastroenterol Nutr* 9:2833, 1989.

81. See CC, Newman LJ, Berezine S, et al: Gastroesophageal reflux-induced hypoxia in infants with apparent life-threatening events. *Am J Dis Child* 143:951–954, 1989.

82. Veereman-Wauters G, Bochner A, Caillie-Bertrand MV: Gastroesophageal re-

flux in infants with a history of near-miss sudden infant death. *J Pediatr Gastroenterol Nutr* 12:319–323, 1991.

83. Kenigsberg K, Griswold PG, Buckley BJ, et al: Cardiac effects of esophageal stimulation: Possible relationship between gastroesophageal (GER) and sudden infant death syndrome (SIDS). *J Pediatr Surg* 18:542–545, 1983.

84. Wetmore RF: Effects of acid on the larynx of the maturing rabbit and their possible significance to the sudden infant death syndrome. *Laryngoscope* 103:1242–1254, 1993.

85. Ariagno RL, Glotzbach SF: Sudden infant death syndrome, in Rudolph AM (ed): *Pediatrics*, 19th ed. Norwalk, CT, Appleton and Lange, 1991, pp 850–858.

86. Spitzer AR, Boyle JT, Tuchman DN, et al: Awake apnea associated with gastroesophageal reflux: A specific clinical syndrome. *J Pediatr* 104:200–205, 1984.

87. Jolley SG, Herbst JJ, Johnson DG: Patterns of postcibal gastroesophageal reflux in symptomatic infants. *Am J Surg* 138:946–950, 1979.

88. Jacob P, Kahrilas PJ, Iterzon G: Proximal esophageal pH-metry in patients with "reflux laryngitis". *Gastroenterology* 100:305–310, 1991.

89. Scott RB, O'Loughlin EV, Gall DG: Gastroesophageal reflux in patients with cystic fibrosis. *J Pediatr* 106:223–227, 1985.

90. Bendig DW, Seilheimer DK, Wagner ML: Complications of gastroesophageal reflux in patients with cystic fibrosis. *J Pediatr* 100:536–540, 1982.

91. Cucchiara S, Santamaria F, Andreotti MR, et al: Mechanisms of gastroesophageal reflux in cystic fibrosis. *Arch Dis Child* 66:617–622, 1991.

92. Malfoot A, Dab I: New insights on gastroesophageal reflux in cystic fibrosis by longitudinal follow up. *Arch Dis Child* 66:1339–1345, 1991.

93. Orenstein SR, Cohn JF, Shalaby TM, et al: Reliability and validity of an infant gastroesophageal reflux questionnaire. *Clin Pediatr* 32:472–484, 1993.

94. Costantini M, Crookes PF, Bremner RM, et al: Value of physiologic assessment of frequent symptoms in a surgical practice. *Surgery* 114:780–786, 1993.

95. Tolia V, Calhoun JA, Kuhns LR, et al: Lack of correlation between extended pH monitoring and scintigraphy in the evaluation of infants with gastroesophageal reflux. *J Lab Clin Med* 115:559–563, 1990.

96. Leonidas JC: Gastroesophageal reflux in infants: Role of the upper gastrointestinal series. *American Journal of Roentgenology* 143:1350–1351, 1984.

97. Riccabona M, Maurer U, Lackner H, et al: The role of sonography in the evaluation of gastroesophageal reflux-correlation to pH-metry. *Eur J Pediatr* 151:655–657, 1992.

98. Tolia V, Kuhns L, Kauffman R: Correlation of gastric emptying at one and two hours following formula feeding. *Pediatrics* 45:341–342, 1970.

99. Fisher RS, Mamud LS, Roberts GS, et al: Gastroesophageal (GE) scintiscanning to detect and quantitate GE reflux. *Gastroenterology* 70:301–308, 1976.

100. Barham CP, Gotley DC, Miller R, et al: Ambulatory measurement of oesophageal function: Clinical use of a new pH and motility recording system. *Br J Surg* 79:1056–1060, 1992.

101. Bumm R, Feussner H, Holscher AH, et al: Interaction of gastroesophageal reflux and esophageal motility: Evaluation by ambulatory 24-hr manometry and pH-metry. *Dig Dis Sci* 37:1192–1199, 1992.

102. Varty K, Evans D, Kapila L: Paediatric gastro-esophageal reflux: Prognostic indicators from pH monitoring. *Gut* 34:1478–1481, 1993.

103. Tovar JA, Angulo JA, Gorostiaga L, et al: Surgery for gastroesophageal reflux in children with normal pH studies. *J Pediatr Surg* 26:541–545, 1991.

104. Ismail-Beigi F, Horton PF, Pope CF: Histological consequences of gastro-esophageal reflux in man. *Gastroenterology* 58:163–174, 1970.

105. Nussbaum E, Maggi JC, Mathis R, et al: Association of lipid-laden macrophages and lactose assay as markers of aspiration in neonates with lung disease. *J Pediatr* 110:190–194, 1987.

106. Tolia V, Lin CHM, Kuhns LR: Gastric emptying using three different formulas in infants with gastroesophageal reflux. *J Pediatr Gastroenterol Nutr* 15:297–302, 1992.

107. Duke JC, Sekar KC, Torres R: Does increased osmolarity increase the exposure of an infant's esophagus to reflux? *Clin Res* 38:(50), 1990.

108. Meyers WF, Herbst JJ: Effectiveness of positioning therapy for gastroesophageal reflux. *Pediatrics* 69:768–772, 1983.

109. Orenstein SR, Whitington PF, Orenstein DM: The infant seat as treatment for gastroesophageal reflux. *N Engl J Med* 309:760–763, 1983.

110. Vandenplas Y, Sacre-Smits L: Seventeen-hour continuous esophageal pH monitoring in the newborn: Evaluation of the influence of position in asymptomatic and symptomatic babies. *J Pediatr Gastroenterol Nutr* 4:356–361, 1985.

111. Orenstein SR: Prone positioning in infant gastroesophageal reflux: Is elevation of the head worth the trouble? *J Pediatr* 114:184–187, 1990.

112. Sontag SJ: The medical management of reflux esophagitis: Role of antacids and acid inhibition. *Gastroenterol Clin North Am* 19:683–713, 1990.

113. Sharma BK, Walt RP, Pounder RE, et al: Optimal dose of oral omeprazole for maximal 24 hour decrease of intragastric acidity. *Gut* 5:957–964, 1984.

114. Gunasekaran TS, Hassal EE: Efficacy and safety of omeprazole for severe gastroesophageal reflux in children. *J Pediatr* 123:148–154, 1993.

115. Vasundhara T, Calhoun J, Kuhns L, et al: Randomized, prospective double-blind trial of metaclopramide and placebo for gastroesophageal reflux in infants. *J Pediatr* 115:141–145, 1989.

116. Justo RN, Gray PH: Fundoplication in preterm infants with gastroesophageal reflux. *J Paediatr Child Health* 27:250–254, 1991.

117. Van Eyben M, Ravensteyn H: Effect of cisapride on excessive regurgitation in infants. *Clin Ther* 11:669–677, 1989.

118. Malfroot A, Vandenplas Y, Verlinden M, et al: Gastroesophageal reflux and unexplained respiratory disease in infants and children. *Pediatr Pulmonol* 3:208–213, 1987.

119. Fung KP, Seagram G, Pasieka J, et al: Investigation and outcome of 121 infants and children requiring Nissen fundoplication for management of gastroesophageal reflux. *Invest Med* 13:237–246, 1990.

120. Little AG: Mechanisms of action of antireflux surgery: Theory and fact. *World J Surg* 16:320–325, 1992.

121. Little AG, Ferguson MK, Skinner DB: Reoperation for failed antireflux operations. *J Thorac Cardiovasc Surg* 91:511–517, 1986.

122. Wheatley MJ, Wesley JR, Tkach DM, et al: Long-term followup of brain-damaged children requiring feeding gastrostomy: Should antireflux procedure always be done? *J Pediatr Surg* 26:301–305, 1991.

123. Halpern LM, Jolley SG, Johnson DG: Gastroesophageal reflux: A significant association with central nervous system disease in children. *J Pediatr Surg* 26:171–173, 1991.

124. Martinez LDA, Ginn-Pease ME, Caniano DA: Sequelae of antireflux surgery in profoundly disabled children. *J Pediatr Surg* 27:267–273, 1992.

125. Burton DM, Pransky SM, Kat RM, et al: Pediatric airway manifestations of gastroesophageal reflux. *Ann Otol Rhinol Laryngol* 101:742–749, 1992.

New Concepts in Nonsurgical Facial Nerve Rehabilitation

H. Jacqueline Diels, O.T.R.

Facial Rehabilitation Specialist, Neuromuscular Retraining Clinic, Department of Rehabilitation Medicine, University of Wisconsin Hospital and Clinics, Madison, Wisconsin

"The face is the image of the soul."
—Cicero[1]

Facial paralysis has been primarily considered a cosmetic inconvenience with associated functional problems. In reality, facial paralysis is a disability of communication. As human beings, our primary form of nonverbal communication relies upon minute changes in facial expression that reveal our innermost feelings. Just as an aphasic person cannot communicate verbally after a stroke, the patient with facial paralysis cannot convey the normal social signals of interpersonal communication. Although therapeutic treatment for aphasia is commonplace, nonsurgical rehabilitation for facial paralysis has been neglected, by and large, and patients have been "left to their own devices."[2] Those who work with patients with facial paralysis are acutely aware of the need for rehabilitating both the physiological and psychosocial aspects of this disability. Restoring function and expression to the highest level possible results in improved health, self-esteem, self-acceptance, acceptance by others, and quality of life.

Neuromuscular retraining (NMR) is gaining recognition as an effective element for optimal recovery from facial nerve paresis. Retraining techniques have been developed for treating sequelae that range from flaccidity to mass action and synkinesis, improving facial motor control, and enhancing patient satisfaction and outcomes.

Neuromuscular retraining for facial paralysis is a growing field of practice in the United States and Canada.[3] Physical, occupational, and speech therapists trained specifically in facial NMR provide important elements in the continuity of care for the patient with facial paralysis.

Treatment begins with a thorough clinical evaluation. Realistic goals are established and a comprehensive, individualized home program is developed. This is accomplished through specific NMR techniques and augmented sensory feedback (including surface electromyography [EMG]) within an educational model.

This chapter will introduce the concept and practice of NMR for facial paralysis. Qualities that differentiate NMR from other nonsurgical

Advances in Otolaryngology—Head and Neck Surgery®, vol. 9
© 1995, Mosby–Year Book, Inc.

therapies will be discussed. Appropriate candidates for treatment will be identified and optimal timelines for referral presented. Specific techniques for treating flaccid paralysis as well as synkinesis will be outlined.

PHYSIOLOGICAL AND PSYCHOSOCIAL CONSEQUENCES OF FACIAL PARALYSIS

The psychological effects associated with facial paralysis are related to the physical manifestations, including impaired eye closure and lacrimation, difficulty with oromotor functions of speech and mastication, hypotonus resulting in flaccidity, hypertonus resulting in synkinesis or mass action, and disfigurement with decreased emotional expression.

Loss of ability to move the face can be devastating. In a survey conducted by the Acoustic Neuroma Association, facial paralysis was reported to be the most significant problem experienced after acoustic neuroma resection.[4] Psychological adjustment to facial paralysis varies with each individual[5] and does not necessarily correlate with degree of dysfunction. Depression, guilt, anger, hostility, anxiety, rejection, and paranoia have been noted after facial paralysis.[6] Patients may be considered mentally deficient[7] and experience difficulties with interpersonal relationships, employability, making friends, and coping with looks of disgust or horror in others' faces.[8]

A variety of surgical procedures have been developed for rehabilitation of the face after paralysis, including techniques designed to reduce synkinesis.[2, 9-14] No method has been found that can restore normal expression.[9] Though the integrity of the facial nerve may be intact postoperatively, its continuity is not necessarily an indicator of functional outcome,[15] and what may be thought of as a good result by the surgeon, may not be noted as such by the patient.[16] The addition of NMR for further improving physical and psychological function in the patient with incomplete recovery is a natural complement to surgical treatment for refining facial movement.

HISTORY OF NONSURGICAL TREATMENT FOR FACIAL PARALYSIS

Physical and occupational therapists have been treating facial paralysis for decades. As early as 1927, physical therapy for treatment of Bell's palsy was advocated[17] using treatment methods that have become "standard" in the decades since. Treatment modalities, originally developed for and successfully used on the extremities, were applied to the face. Gross facial exercises,[18, 19] massage, electrical stimulation, and prosthetic devices or taping to lift a drooping, flaccid face were the treatments of choice.[20-22] These nonspecific procedures continue to be recommended and practiced today.

TRADITIONAL THERAPY TECHNIQUES

Electrical Stimulation

Electrical stimulation continues to be widely used in the treatment of facial paralysis[20, 23] although there is mounting evidence that it may be contraindicated. It has been suggested that electrical stimulation may interfere with neural regeneration following peripheral nerve injury[24, 25] and studies proving its efficacy with facial muscles are lacking in the literature. A 1984 report by the National Center for Health Services Research concluded that "Electrotherapy treatment for Bell's palsy . . . has no demonstrable beneficial effect in enhancing the functional or cosmetic outcomes in patients with Bell's palsy".[26]

Additionally, patients who undergo acute electrical stimulation may demonstrate more synkinesis and mass action than those who do not.[27] It is difficult to produce an isolated contraction of the facial muscles using electrical stimulation because of their small size and proximity to each other. The contraction produced causes mass action which reinforces abnormal motor patterns and can be painful.[20]

Gross Exercises

Gross facial exercises are another staple in the therapy repertoire. However, because of their nonspecificity, gross exercises typically given to patients reinforce abnormal movement patterns.[28] Instructions such as "close your eyes as hard as you can," "smile broadly," or "pucker your lips" do not produce the desired facial symmetry and control required for normalized facial function. The use of maximum effort exercises recruits excessive motor units, producing patterns that differ from typical facial expressions which are gentle and fluid.

WHY NONSPECIFIC THERAPY IS INEFFECTIVE

The ineffectiveness of traditional therapy methods for facial paralysis stems from their nonspecificity and lack of adaptation to the unique characteristics of facial muscle.

FACIAL MUSCLES DIFFER FROM SKELETAL MUSCLES

Facial muscles differ from most other skeletal muscles in several significant ways. Facial muscles

- Lack muscle spindles.[29-32]
- Have small motor units.[30, 33]
- Are relatively slow to degenerate.[10, 34]
- Receive emotional as well as volitional neural inputs.[35]

Muscle Spindles

The muscle spindle is the physiological mechanism by which a muscle contraction is produced in response to a shortening of its fiber during a percutaneous stretch.[36] Therapeutic facilitory techniques such as quick stretch, vibration, and tapping rely upon the muscle spindle to stimulate muscle contraction.[37] Because facial muscles lack spindles, the use of these techniques to elicit a contraction is ineffective.

Small Motor Units

A motor unit is defined as one motoneuron and all of the muscle fibers it innervates.[38] The ratio of muscle fibers to motoneurons determines the refinement of a movement. In the facial muscles the ratio is approximately

25 muscle fibers to one motoneuron allowing great complexity of movement compared with limb muscles, which have a much higher ratio (e.g., 2,000 muscle fibers to one motoneuron in the gastrocnemius).[33] The intricacy of movement that can be achieved by the facial muscles should preclude the use of maximum effort exercises, where motor units other than those targeted are recruited because of overflow.[39]

Resistance to Degeneration

Facial muscle appears to resist degeneration postdenervation for longer periods of time than other skeletal muscle, and may remain viable for 3 or more years.[10, 34] Because of this unique characteristic, the use of electrical stimulation to maintain viability of facial muscle during regeneration is unfounded.

Cortical Connections for Emotional Expression

There is a well-established distinction between volitional and emotional facial movements.[35] Volitional movements of the face use different upper motor neuron pathways (pyramidal tract) than those used for emotional movements (extrapyramidal motor system). The use of emotional inputs during NMR may be helpful to reestablish more natural motor control after paralysis.

Lack of Specific Clinical Training

Most therapists receive no specialized training in facial muscle anatomy, physiology, or specific facial therapy techniques. The patient with peripheral facial nerve paralysis has been treated ineffectively in the past; therapy has been initiated too early and terminated too soon, before neural recovery has taken place. The naturally occurring spontaneous recovery of patients with Bell's palsy reinforced the seeming "appropriateness" of whatever treatment modality was used. After 6 to 12 months, patients who did not regain function were classified as "chronic" with no further therapy attempted. No techniques were described for treating the aberrant, unsynchronous facial movements that characterize synkinesis. Given the nonspecific nature of the therapy provided, it is not surprising that many clinicians found the treatment of facial paralysis to be frustrating and ineffective.[40]

HISTORY OF FACIAL NEUROMUSCULAR RETRAINING

Specific NMR techniques for facial paralysis appeared in the literature 30 years ago.[41–45] Patients demonstrated improved facial function using EMG feedback to modify the manner in which they contracted their muscles. A comprehensive review of case studies using similar techniques is presented by Balliet.[46] More recent studies have included both acute (less than 1 year post) and postacute patients, and the effect of spontaneous recovery of function could not be ruled out.[47, 48]

In 1982, Balliet and associates described a comprehensive clinical program that combined EMG feedback, mirror exercises, and detailed, individualized home exercise programs and demonstrated improved function with patients more than 2 years postfacial nerve injury.[46] The authors hypothesized that brain plasticity, the capacity of the central nervous system to modify its organization to bring about lasting functional change, explained the acquisition of new motor behaviors in the post-acute patient.

In 1991, Ross and co-workers[49] compared two treatment groups with a third control group that received no treatment. All patients were more than 18 months postinjury in order to control for spontaneous recovery effect. After comprehensive evaluation, one group was trained with EMG and mirror feedback, while the second group used mirror feedback alone. Patients were reevaluated after 1 year of treatment. A significant difference was found between the treatment groups and the control group. Patients in both treatment groups demonstrated improvements in facial motor control, excursion of movement, and decreased synkinesis. The control group showed no change, or decreased function. A follow-up study 1 year later concluded that gains acquired during treatment had been maintained without continued therapy.[50]

It is clear from research thus far, that the application of NMR techniques *specifically designed for the treatment of facial paralysis* can effectively reduce sequelae after facial nerve injury.

NEUROMUSCULAR RETRAINING FOR FACIAL PARALYSIS

"Rehabilitation can not be administered to the patient, in contrast to the treatment for many other disorders. The psychosocial and educational aspects of the rehabilitation process are thus of very great importance. In spite of the existence of biological bases for recovery, it does not occur without the appropriate environment, the attitude, and the involvement of the patient."[51]

Neuromuscular retraining for facial paralysis is a marriage of neurophysiology, psychology, therapeutic science, learning theory, and art. Neuromuscular retraining is a problem solving approach to treatment using selective motor training to facilitate symmetrical movement and control undesired gross motor activity (synkinesis). Tools such as surface EMG (sEMG) feedback and specific mirror exercises provide augmented sensory information to enhance neural adaptation and learning.[38] The application of learning theory maximizes motivation through individualized instruction and active patient participation. Because each patient presents a different functional profile, there are no generic lists of exercises. Treatment is based on individual function, and as a result, each treatment program is different.

Patient education is the most basic aspect of the therapeutic process and lays the necessary foundation for learning the selective movement patterns that will improve motor function. The facial therapist provides training in basic facial anatomy, physiology, and kinesiology pertinent to each patient's specific situation. To familiarize them with muscle terminology and actions, patients receive the following graphic (Fig 1) depicting the major facial muscle groups, branches of the facial nerve, and the angles of muscular pull.

As each muscle group is evaluated the patient observes the action of that group in the mirror, bilaterally. Most people are not conscious of the specific movements involved in normal facial expression. To identify the

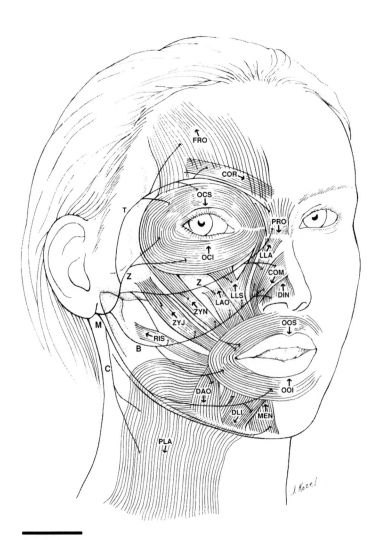

FIGURE 1.

Diagrammatic representation of the muscles of facial expression and branches of the facial nerve. *FRO = musculus frontalis, COR = m. corrugator, PRO = m. procerus, OCS = m. orbicularis oculi superioris, OCI = m. orbicularis oculi inferioris, DIN = m. dilator naris, COM = m. compressor naris, LLA = m. levator labii alaeque nasi, LLS = m. levator labii superioris, LAO = m. levator anguli oris, ZYJ = m. zygomaticus major, ZYN = m. zygomaticus minor, RIS = m. risorius, OOS = m. orbicularis oris superioris, OOI = m. orbicularis oris inferioris, DAO = m. depressor anguli oris, DLI = m. depressor labii inferioris, MEN = m. mentalis,* and *PLA = platysma.* Facial nerve branches: *T = temporal, Z = zygomaticus, B = buccal, M = mandibular,* and *C = cervical.* (Modified from Balliet R: Facial Paralysis and Other Neuromuscular Dysfunctions of the Peripheral Nervous System, in Payton OD (ed): *Manual of Physical Therapy,* Churchill Livingstone, New York, 1989. Used by permission.)

correct response, patients are instructed to perform small, specific movements on the contralateral side. The exploration of facial movement is a time of discovery for the patient as she or he identifies the specific areas of function and dysfunction and begins to formulate strategies to improve facial movement.

GENERAL TREATMENT PRINCIPLES

Treatment is based on functional profile rather than etiology. Techniques to facilitate movement and inhibit abnormal patterns refine motor control, coordination, and complexity of movement. Although each patient's program differs, there are common aspects in the treatment of all patients.

Slow Execution

Initiating movements slowly and gradually allows the patient to observe and modify the angle, strength, and speed of the excursion as it occurs.[52] As a result, new motor control strategies are systematically developed and learned.[39] Movements performed rapidly will revert to the previous, abnormal motor pattern.

Small Movements

Small movements preserve isolated responses of the facial muscles by limiting motor unit recruitment to those muscles targeted.[39] Large movements recruit successively greater numbers of motor units as well as neighboring muscles (overflow), diminishing accuracy.[39] Improved coordination develops as small movements are practiced accurately.

Symmetry

Patients are instructed in symmetrical excursion of movements to reinforce the normal physiological response. Attempts to produce symmetrical movements initially include limiting excursion on the contralateral side. If the contralateral side is allowed to dominate, activity on the involved side could be diminished.[46]

ACTION-ORIENTED AND COST-EFFECTIVE THERAPY

Just as no surgical technique provides the patient with normal, synchronous facial movement, NMR cannot restore normal function. However, these action-oriented techniques enable patients to "become their own best therapist,"[53] and assume control of their recovery, which results in improved physical function, increased self-esteem, and satisfaction.[54]

Treatment schedules are based on individual patient needs that vary widely. Factors such as motivation, compliance, need for sEMG feedback, and geographic location affect scheduling. Treatment sessions may range from 2 hours per month (for local patients) to an intensive treatment session of 9 to 12 hours spaced over 3 to 4 days, every 6 months (for patients traveling a great distance). This differs significantly from a typical therapy schedule in which patients are treated on a weekly basis. A limited schedule can be maintained in a NMR program because the therapist provides educational rather than "hands on" treatment and the patient directly controls the practice of his or her own therapy program at home.

A patient may be involved in NMR for 3 years or longer. It has been estimated that the average ratio of home practice to supervised clinical instruction is about 20:1.[38] Structuring therapy in this manner results in a cost-effective service delivery system that reduces the number of billed clinic hours while increasing the overall number of treatment hours. Patients return to the clinic periodically to refine movement patterns, learn new exercises, document progress and establish new treatment goals.

INDICATIONS FOR TREATMENT

Patients who have facial paralysis, paresis or synkinesis as the result of the conditions listed in Table 1 may be appropriate candidates for facial NMR.

OPTIMAL TIME FOR REFERRAL

Recognition of the many benefits of NMR is growing, although currently there are only a few centers in the United States and Canada which specialize in NMR for facial paralysis.[3]

Patients should be referred to therapists trained in specific facial NMR techniques when visible signs of functional return become apparent (e.g., increasing facial tone, minimal motion), or as soon as synkinesis is noted.

Postsurgery or Trauma

The optimal time to refer patients for facial NMR occurs as soon as there are subtle signs of recovery, such as increased tone or slight movements. If there has been significant damage to the facial nerve, Wallerian degeneration occurs. After formation of the growth cone, regeneration occurs at the rate of 1 mm per day.[33, 36] The reinnervation process varies with each individual, and can occur from 3 to 18 months postsurgery or postinjury,[55] although most patients referred for NMR begin to demonstrate movement in 5 to 12 months.[56] Facial NMR initiated before evidence of

---

TABLE 1.
Etiologies Treated

Postsurgical tumor resection
   Acoustic neuroma (vestibular schwannoma)
   Meningioma
   Facial nerve neuroma
   Glomus tumors
   Cholesteatoma and others
Bell's palsy
Herpes zoster oticus (Ramsay Hunt syndrome)
Traumatic injury
Guillain-Barré syndrome
Congenital
   Asymmetrical crying facies
   Moebius syndrome with incomplete paralysis
   Microsomia and other paresis
Carcinoma
Postoperative repair
   Primary graft
   Neural anastomosis (XII-VII, XI-VII)
   Cross facial nerve graft
   Muscle transposition (*musculus temporalis* or *m. masseter*)
   Free muscle graft (*m. gracilis, m. pectoralis minor*)

reinnervation may be detrimental,[49] resulting in frustration for the patient and therapist.

If no visible movement is noted by 12 months after beginning NMR, the patient should still be referred for evaluation. Often, recovery has begun slowly and has gone undetected. A trial course of NMR should be undertaken to facilitate movement. If no movement is noted by 18 months after onset of paralysis, other surgical rehabilitation options should be explored.

Bell's Palsy, Ramsay Hunt Syndrome
Approximately 70% of patients with Bell's Palsy recover complete function spontaneously with another 15% demonstrating "satisfactory" recovery.[2, 57] Facial NMR is deferred until 3 months postonset because of the high probability that spontaneous recovery will occur before that time. If paralysis persists after 3 months, recovery may be incomplete with the development of synkinesis,[2, 57] and patients should be referred for NMR. Electrical stimulation is not indicated at any time.[26]

Congenital
Children with congenital facial paralysis can be referred for evaluation at any time, however, treatment should not begin until the child is cognitively aware of the problem and can actively participate in treatment (usually by 7 or 8 years of age). Neuromuscular retraining is an especially effective treatment for asymmetric crying facies (see case study number 3). In other cases of congenital paralysis (moebius syndrome, birth trauma, microsomia), variable success has been obtained with children who demonstrate some degree of motion on evaluation. Those who demonstrate complete paralysis are not appropriate candidates for NMR until surgical rehabilitation has been completed.

Synkinesis
Synkinesis has been defined as "an abnormal synchronization of movement occurring with voluntary and reflex activity of muscles that normally do not contract together".[58] Several hypotheses attempt to explain this phenomenon.[59, 60] Synkinesis can vary in severity from subtle to severe and in its worst form, mass action, can result in gross deformity with any attempted facial movement.

Patients should be referred for NMR as soon as synkinesis appears, although *there is no time limit when facial retraining can begin for the treatment of synkinesis.* With proper instruction, improvements can be made at any time, even years after onset. People 40 or more years postonset have demonstrated significant reduction in synkinesis through NMR.[61] Table 2 summarizes ideal guidelines for referral to facial NMR.

PATIENT SELECTION CRITERIA
The following criteria determine which patients are good candidates for facial NMR.

Neural Supply
There must be direct (intact nerve) or indirect (graft, anastomosis, muscle transfer, etc.) neural supply to the facial muscles. If the facial nerve has

TABLE 2.
Optimal Time for Referral

Etiology	Referral Timeline

Acoustic neuroma
Meningioma
Facial nerve neuroma
Traumatic injury
Glomus tumor
Guillain-Barré syndrome
Postoperative nerve graft,
  anastomosis or muscle transfer
Carcinoma (parotid gland tumors)
	As minimal facial movement becomes
	  apparent
	or
	As synkinesis begins to develop
	or
	By 12 months postonset if no movement

Bell's palsy
Herpes zoster oticus (Ramsay Hunt
  syndrome)
	At 3 months postonset if paralysis or
	  paresis persists
	or
	If there is evidence of synkinesis

Congenital	May refer at any time for evaluation; however, NMR is deferred until patient develops cognitive abilities to participate in the program
Synkinesis	As soon as synkinesis is noted (there is no outside time limit)

been sacrificed with no subsequent repair, NMR is not indicated until surgical rehabilitation has been completed.

Motivation

The patient must be persistent, disciplined, and compliant to achieve benefits with facial NMR. Practice sessions require intense concentration for a minimum of 30 to 60 minutes per day.[49] Consistency of practice is paramount to the learning process. As is the case for the serious student committed to learning the new skills required to play a musical instrument, there must be sufficient motivation to practice daily. Motivation is renewed as specific functional goals are achieved.

Cognition

Adequate cognitive function is necessary for the precise and accurate practice of the program, allowing the patient to observe and modify movement patterns based on self-analysis of responses.[46] Cognitive and attention deficits such as those often associated with brain injury or cerebrovascular accident (CVA) may limit successful participation in a NMR program. Only with accurate observation and problem solving skills are patients able to learn more appropriate motor control strategies.[39]

GOALS OF TREATMENT

The goals of facial NMR are consistent with the goals of surgical rehabilitation,[9, 62] that is, improved eye closure to decrease corneal exposure, improved oromotor function for speech and mastication, improved facial tone, symmetry, and volitional and spontaneous movement.

Specific, individual goals are identified during the initial evaluation, and most often include increased eye closure, improved smile, and lip function. They may also include decreased facial tightness, twitching, or abnormal eye closure during speech (synkinesis). Realistic and attainable goals are established by the patient and therapist before proceeding with treatment and are revised as progress is achieved.

EVALUATION METHODS

CLINICAL INSTRUMENTS

Evaluation of facial function has been the topic of much discussion.[63-65] The definitive evaluation tool must be objective, sensitive to subtle dynamic changes, and easy to administer, however, this instrument has not yet been developed.

The adoption of the International Grading scale in 1984 established a universal measuring system, developed for the needs of physicians and surgeons.[66] However, for the practitioner of facial NMR, the International scale does not detect the subtle changes that occur during the course of treatment.[47] Other methods, such as measuring facial landmarks,[67] and the more complicated facial grading systems,[68] are cumbersome and difficult to apply consistently. The Facial Grading System is a new tool currently undergoing multicenter trials. It is easy to administer and sensitive to small functional changes that occur during the course of treatment.[69]

Whatever tools are used, each muscle group must be evaluated to determine available volitional movement (excursion), spontaneous movement, and presence of synkinesis/mass action.

VIDEOTAPE

There is no substitute for videotape evaluation as an objective measure of facial motion. Videotape captures sequential facial movements as they occur, allowing the therapist and patient to review movements in detail and compare progress over time. Patients are asked to perform specific facial movements using an established protocol (Table 3).[68]

PHOTOGRAPHS

Photographic evaluation allows the patient to easily compare one treatment session to the next. Because functional change occurs slowly, having photos in hand enables the patient to see small changes over time that otherwise may not be readily visible. Patients should view photographs reflected in a mirror to preserve the relative position of the paralyzed side.

SELF-ASSESSMENT

Patient self-assessment is an important aspect of the evaluation process because it provides insight into the patient's self-esteem. Ultimately, it is the patient's self-perception that determines the success of treatment.

TABLE 3.
Videotape Protocol*

Muscles	Volitional Movement
FRO	Raise your eyebrows
COR, PRO	Bring eyebrows down and together
OCS, OCI,	Gently close eyes
OCS, OCI	Squint your lower eyelids up
OCS, OCI	Close your eyes tightly
DIN	Flare nostrils
RIS, ZYJ, ZYN, LAO, LLS	Smile evenly with your lips together
RIS, ZYJ, ZYN, LAO, LLS	A big wide smile with your lips apart
LLS, LAO	Raise your upper lip while wrinkling your nose
LLS, LAO	Raise your left or right upper lip while wrinkling your nose (start with noninvolved side)
RIS	Move the corner of your mouth back toward your ear (start with noninvolved side)
OOS, OOI	Pucker your lips
OOS, OOI	Press your lips together
OOS, OOI	Pull your lips back and in over your teeth
OOS, OOI	Push your lips out as far as they will go
OOI, DAO, DLI	Roll your lower lip out and down
DAO, DLI	Turn the corners of your mouth downward
DAO, DLI	Pull your lower lip down to expose lower teeth
MEN	Tighten your chin
PLA	Tighten your neck

*Modified from Balliet R: Facial paralysis and other neuromuscular dysfunctions of the peripheral nervous system, in Payton OD (ed): *Manual of Physical Therapy*. New York, Churchill Livingstone, 1989. Used by permission.

ESSENTIAL ELEMENTS FOR EFFECTIVE NEUROMUSCULAR RETRAINING

PROPER TREATMENT ENVIRONMENT

A quiet, individual room where therapy is conducted without distractions, establishes the proper learning environment.[39, 68] Anyone who has worked with patients with facial paralysis is aware of the social stigma associated with this disability. Privacy is essential to create a "safe" environment for the patient who is embarrassed by his or her appearance. In this setting, psychosocial issues can also be discussed.

SENSORY FEEDBACK

Optimal learning depends on making maximal use of sensory information. Accurate, proportional, and immediate sensory feedback provides the information required for modification and learning of new motor patterns.[38, 70] Visual (mirror) feedback is the most commonly used type of feedback in the clinic and at home. Inexpensive and portable, mirrors provide the patient with immediate feedback regarding performance. Proprioception provides internal facial position sense and is essential for accurate exercise practice and generalization of movements outside of the clinical setting.

SURFACE EMG FEEDBACK

Just as intraoperative EMG facial nerve monitoring has led to modifications in surgical techniques by providing the surgeon with specific feedback,[71] sEMG monitoring of facial muscles during NMR can lead to modification of facial movement patterns by providing the patient with feedback regarding motor performance. It is an important tool in NMR of facial paralysis.[48, 49, 68, 70]

Also referred to as EMG biofeedback or EMG rehabilitation, its purpose is "to bring the normally unconscious control of specific muscles under conscious control."[72] Surface EMG feedback provides the patient with immediate information regarding the rate and strength of the muscle contraction in real time. As part of a NMR program, sEMG feedback is used as an evaluative, as well as therapeutic tool to:

- Increase activity in weak muscles.
- Decrease activity in hyperactive muscles.
- Improve coordination of muscle groups.

Surface electrodes placed on the skin over the muscle(s) being monitored detect electrical activity produced by the muscle contraction. The amplified signals are displayed on a video monitor. Patients observe this feedback and vary the manner in which they produce a specific movement until the desired pattern is achieved. By correlating information from sEMG feedback with mirror and proprioceptive feedback, the patient learns to reproduce the new movement patterns outside of the clinical setting and within the context of the home exercise program.

Specific protocols for the use of sEMG feedback have been outlined elsewhere.[68, 70, 73] All stress the importance of achieving normalized resting tone (in cases of hypertonicity or synkinesis), symmetry, and isolated responses (Fig 2).

HOME PROGRAM

Clinic treatment sessions are designed to identify, develop, and refine the movement patterns that will be of greatest benefit to each patient. Patients practice these movement patterns repeatedly in the clinic to assure accuracy. Through the home program, patients *consistently* practice the strategies learned in the clinic. The home program usually requires 30 to 60 minutes of concentrated practice per day. No specific number of repetitions are given. Several "good trials" of an exercise practiced with complete focus and concentration are better than many trials done without adequate attention, or by rote.[68] Each trial is analyzed and modified based on self-observation.

Patients record detailed instructions and observations in a notebook or on audiotape as the home program is developed. A videotape record-

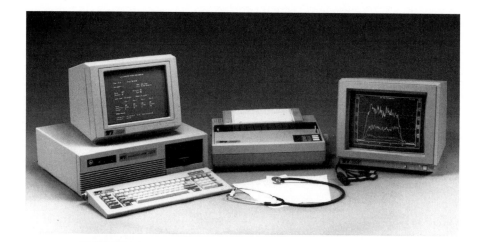

FIGURE 2.

The neuroEducator II, produced by Therapeutic Alliances Inc. (Fairborn, Ohio), has been developed specifically for neuromuscular retraining and provides information from 4 channels simultaneously. Especially helpful in the treatment of synkinesis, homologous muscles are monitored bilaterally with the primary movement represented by a trace of one color and the synkinetic movement represented by another. Immediate comparison can be made enabling the patient to modify motor strategy on the next trial.

ing demonstrating the patient performing his own exercises is made for home reference, especially if return visits to the clinic are infrequent. The video aids in correct practice and serves as a baseline to measure functional progress between treatment sessions.

SPECIFIC TECHNIQUES FOR TREATING FLACCID PARALYSIS AND SYNKINESIS

Clinically, facial paralysis falls into two categories:

- Flaccid paralysis (complete facial paralysis) or paresis.
- Synkinesis or mass action (varying degrees of motor weakness accompanied by abnormal, unsynchronous facial movements).

The two types of paralysis require different treatment strategies.

FLACCID PARALYSIS/PARESIS

The therapist determines the presence of activity using clinical evaluation methods and sEMG. Slight movement that is undetectable by the patient or physician is made visible by sEMG feedback which reinforces the proper movement pattern and illustrates the presence of muscle activity to the patient. Retraining strategies begin with slow, small, symmetrical movements that are continued during home program practice. The patient should be followed monthly to record changes, modify the home program, and monitor for the development of synkinesis. Detailed protocols for the treatment of flaccid paralysis, including sEMG training, have been outlined elsewhere.[68, 70]

Decreased facial sensation, often associated with facial paralysis, limits awareness of the affected side and may hinder the ability to learn new motor behaviors.[74] Sensory reeducation techniques can be applied to enhance awareness.[68, 74]

SYNKINESIS/MASS ACTION

The primary feature of the treatment of synkinesis is inhibition of the unwanted, aberrant movements that occur with volitional and spontaneous movements. Abnormal, synkinetic movement may have the effect of working antagonistically, like a tug-of-war, against the normal, primary movement. For example, a patient who demonstrates zygomatic activity trying to smile, but also has synkinesis of the platysma, has limited zygomatic excursion. Instead of the characteristic upward curl at the angle of the mouth (a smile), she or he has a drawing down at the angle of the mouth (a grimace). By inhibiting the synkinesis of the platysma, the zygomaticus gains a more normal range of motion without the antagonistic effect of the platysma. The result is a more natural smile.

Any of the facial muscle groups can be involved in synkinesis to varying degrees. The challenge is to identify the sites of synkinesis and teach the patient effective inhibition techniques. As inhibition of synkinesis takes place, the range of the primary movement gradually extends, increasing excursion, strength, and isolated motor control simultaneously.

Reduce Resting Tone

Increased facial tone, tightness, or rigidity may be noted in any area of the affected face and is most likely caused by increased background muscle activity.[59] Signs may include increased nasolabial fold (*musculi levators, m. zygomaticus*), decreased palpebral fissure (*m. orbicularis oculi*), retraction of the corner of the mouth (*m. zygomaticus, m. risorius*), dimpling of the chin (*m. mentalis* and/or depressors), drawing down of the corner of the mouth (depressors and platysma), and banding of the neck (platysma). Abnormal tone of the lips may present as thinning or "puffiness."

Because normal movement can not be superimposed on abnormal tone,[39, 75] the first stage of NMR for the patient with synkinesis is to decrease hypertonus. Therapists begin by making patients aware that facial stiffness or tightness is caused by increased muscle activity at rest. General relaxation training and sEMG feedback[47, 68] are effective tone reduction techniques.

Massage mobilizes the tissues of the affected side where thickening and immobility are observed.[76, 77] Using the opposite thumb on the inside of the cheek and the second and third digit on the facial skin, patients are taught to draw the tissues toward the mouth. Patients will often encounter a trigger point, an area of discrete pain caused by focal contraction of that motor unit, which will resolve with maintained deep pressure.[78] Patients report increased comfort and mobility after several weeks of practice.

Inhibition of Synkinesis

With attention focused on the precise movement pattern, the patient initiates the primary movement slowly, monitoring the area of synkinesis from the start. As synkinesis becomes visible, the primary movement is maintained while the synkinetic response is reduced. This difficult process requires complete concentration in order to "release" the synkinetic area. Once this is achieved, the patient then relaxes the primary movement. The exact timing of this sequence is essential for dissociation of synkinesis from primary movement (Fig 3).

As the patient becomes proficient in performing the exercise, inhibition of synkinesis requires less concentration, and excursion of the primary movement increases as control is learned. Initially, this movement pattern can only be accomplished volitionally, however, in time, these patterns are demonstrated spontaneously.[47, 68]

BOTULINUM TOXIN INJECTION FOR REDUCING SYNKINESIS.—Botulinum toxin (Botox) injections have been found to reduce aberrant contractions of the facial muscles by blocking the acetylcholine receptor sites at the synapse.[48, 79, 80] Botox temporarily paralyzes targeted areas of synkinesis, (usually m. orbicularis oculi inferioris, platysma and m. mentalis) with effects lasting from 4 to 6 months.[79] When combined with NMR, Botox provides a "window of opportunity" during which the patient can practice more normal movement patterns without synkinetic interference. In some cases, patients experience decreased synkinesis after the injection effects have worn off.[81]

XII-VII ANASTOMOSIS

Neuromuscular retraining for the patient with a hypoglossal (XII) anastomosis is similar to treatment of synkinesis. However, the motor nucleus of the XIIth cranial nerve must learn to control the facial musculature.

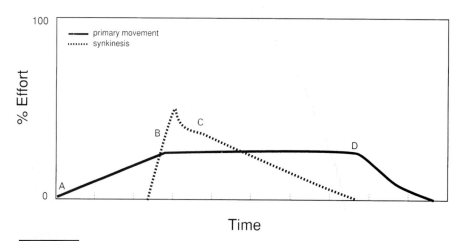

FIGURE 3.

Recommended strategy for inhibition of synkinesis. The patient initiates the primary movement **(A)** while monitoring area of synkinesis. As synkinesis becomes apparent **(B)**, the patient maintains activity of the primary mover while releasing the synkinesis **(C)**. After the synkinesis is inhibited, the patient relaxes the primary movement **(D)**. The duration of this process is typically 10 to 20 seconds.

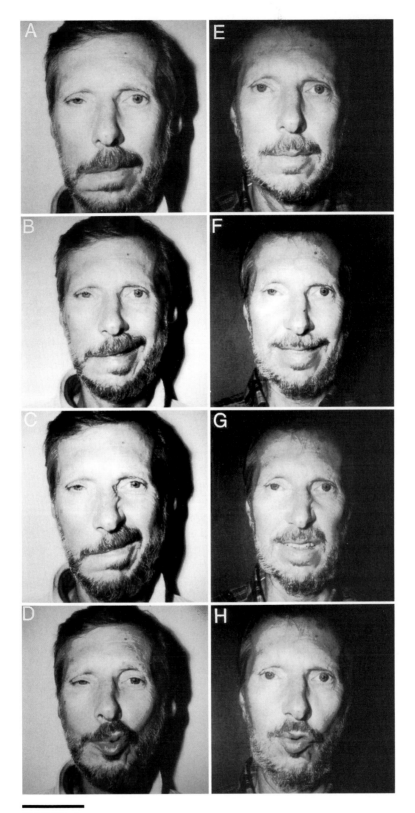

FIGURE 4.

Case study #1. Photographic evaluation, 15 months post–right-acoustic neuroma resection. Pretreatment: Resting tone **(A)**, smile **(B)**, snarl **(C)**, pucker **(D)**. Reevaluation of same movements after 3 years of participation in facial NMR **(E-H).**

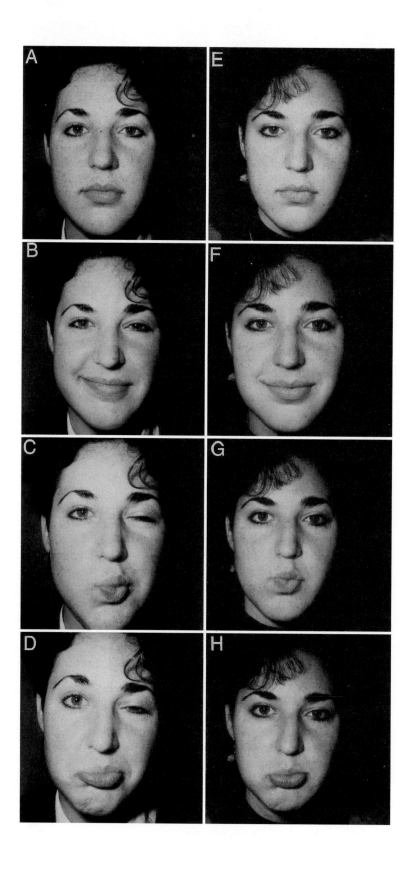

Two additional steps to those described for synkinesis are required to improve motor control:

1. The patient allows movement of the tongue to initiate facial movement, but only until she or he begins to make minimal movements of the face without activating the tongue.
2. The patient learns to inhibit facial movement while the tongue moves. This step reduces the aberrant facial movement seen during speech and mastication.

These difficult procedures require intense concentration. As the patient becomes adept at performing these movement patterns, she or he can begin to dissociate tongue from facial movements. These techniques are also effective with spinal accessory-facial nerve (XI-VII) anastomosis, substituting shoulder movement for tongue movement.

DURATION AND PROGRESSION OF TREATMENT AND FOLLOW-UP

The entire course of NMR typically lasts from 12 months to 3 years. Exercises progress as successive short-term goals are attained during this relatively slow process. Long-term goals may take years to achieve, therefore it is unrealistic to expect this process to occur quickly.[38]

Videotape and photographic reevaluations are completed approximately every 6 months or as significant functional change is noted. Patients actively participate in comparing the initial to subsequent evaluations, identifying new problem areas and establishing new goals.

REFERRAL TO OTHER MEDICAL SPECIALISTS

During the course of NMR, it may be necessary to refer patients to other health care providers. Prolonged lack of eye closure and lacrimation may lead to ophthalmologic referral for gold weight, spring placement, or other procedure. Plastic surgeons may be consulted for nerve grafting, muscle transposition, or related procedures. In cases of severe depression, psychology or psychiatry referrals may be indicated. Rehabilitation specialists may be able to assist patients with vestibular problems. Audiologists can provide hearing assistive devices. Timely referrals to appropriate health care providers are essential in providing optimal care for the patient with facial paralysis.

FIGURE 5.
Case study #2. Photographic evaluation, 12 months post—left-facial paralysis resulting from Lyme disease. Pretreatment: Resting tone **(A)** smile **(B)**, pucker **(C)**, pout **(D)**. Note normal resting tone, decreased excursion of left smile with mild synkinesis of left OCS/OCI and severe synkinesis of left OCS/OCI during lip movements. Reevaluation of same movements 6 months after beginning facial NMR **(E-H)**. Note improved excursion of smile and decreased synkinesis around eye with improved symmetry.

CASE STUDIES

CASE #1

R.R. is a 53-year-old chief executive officer of an advertising agency who underwent resection of a right, 3.5 cm acoustic neuroma in March, 1986. The facial nerve was reported to be intact postoperatively. The patient experienced complete right facial paralysis which persisted until 15 months postoperatively, at which time facial NMR was initiated. Initial evaluation revealed a flaccid paralysis with decreased resting tone, eye closure (medial and lateral tarsorrhaphies had been performed), and volitional and spontaneous facial movements. Trace movement was observed in the right cheek musculature (Fig 4, A–D).

The initial clinic visit was 4 days (total 12 hours) during which time evaluation was completed and the home program was developed. Surface EMG feedback was utilized to evaluate and train minimal, symmetrical facial movements. Clinic treatment sessions (3 to 4 hours in duration) were conducted approximately every 8 weeks during the first year, quarterly during the second year, and only twice during the third year of treatment.

During the course of treatment, gradual increases occurred in excursion of movement. The patient developed minimal synkinesis during year two. During year three, spontaneous occurrence of new motor patterns was noted. Eye closure had improved sufficiently to partially reverse the tarsorrhaphies. On average, voluntary movements increased from 10% to 80% (Fig 4,E–H).

In a follow-up meeting two years after completing treatment, the patient and his wife felt that function continued to improve although he no longer practiced the exercises. The patient was extremely motivated and compliant with the daily home program throughout the entire 3-year course of NMR, and was extremely pleased with the overall result.

CASE #2

C.B. is a 19-year-old female university student with left facial paralysis resulting from Lyme disease. The patient experienced complete left facial paralysis postonset with gradual recovery beginning two months postonset. She was referred for facial NMR one year postonset. Initial evaluation revealed slightly increased resting tone, complete eye closure, and slightly decreased smile with mild synkinesis noted. Attempted lip movements were accompanied by severe synkinesis of m. orbicularis oculi which resulted in almost complete eye closure (Fig 5,A–D).

The home program consisted of small selective movements practiced with inhibition of synkinesis. She attended clinic sessions once a month for the first 6 months and demonstrated a significant reduction in synkinesis during that time (Fig 5,E–H). Clinic visits decreased to once every 3 months with continued good compliance. The entire course of neuromuscular retraining lasted 2 years with improvements noted in volitional and spontaneous excursion of movement. The patient continued to demonstrate mild synkinesis of m. orbicularis oculi during broad, spontaneous laughter. She was extremely motivated and compliant with the home program, and was pleased with the treatment outcome.

CASE #3

L.C. is a bright and motivated 8-year-old girl with history of congenital asymmetric crying facies. She was referred by a plastic surgeon for NMR before considering an invasive procedure. Her parents reported concern that the patient was being teased by classmates about her "crooked smile." During the initial 2-day treatment session, evaluation and patient education were completed.

A

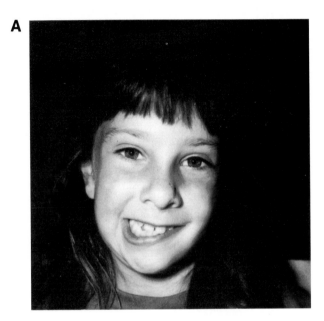

B

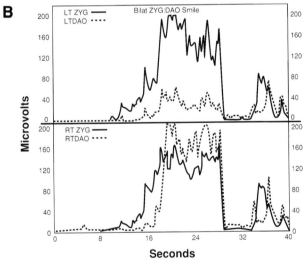

FIGURE 6.

Case study #3. Eight-year-old girl with congenital left asymmetric crying facies. Pretreatment evaluation of smile **(A)**. Initial trial of movement with sEMG monitoring of zygomatic *(ZYG)* and lip depressors *(DAO)* revealed relative hyperactivity of contralateral (right) depressors **(B)**.   *(Continued.)*

Initial evaluation revealed all facial muscle groups were functioning within normal limits, with the exception of the left lip depressors in which no activity was noted. The patient demonstrated an asymmetrical smile with relative hyperactivity of the contralateral depressors (Fig 6,A). The goal of treatment was to achieve a symmetrical smile. Because the patient lacked depressors on the ipsilateral side, treatment was designed to inhibit the relative overactivity of the contralateral depressors in order to achieve symmetry. Surface EMG feedback was used to compare the ratio of zygomatic to depressor activity bilaterally during smile.

Initial sEMG readings demonstrated relative hyperactivity of the contralateral (right) depressors (Fig 6,B). The patient was instructed to at-

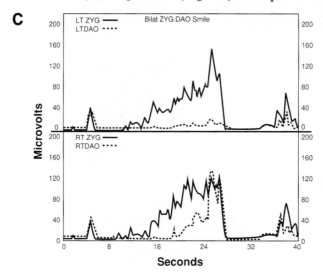

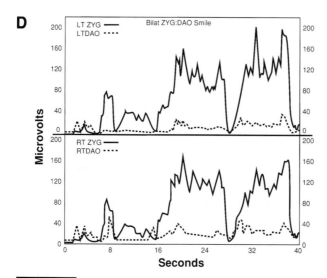

FIGURE 6 (cont.).

Note within normal limits (WNL) zygomatic activity bilaterally. Second trial of smile with attempted inhibition of right depressors **(C)**. Surface EMG graph after 30 minutes of practice **(D)**.

E

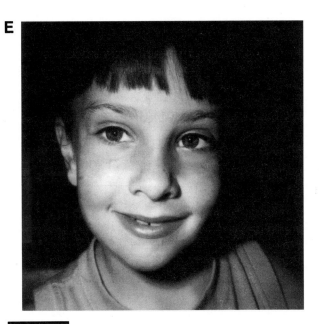

FIGURE 6 (cont.).
Note symmetrical values bilaterally, which correlate with post-treatment photograph demonstrating inhibition of right depressors with symmetrical smile **(E)**. *LT* = left; *RT* = right.

tempt to reduce the depressor activity in the next trial (Fig 6C). During the following 30 minutes, the patient used sEMG feedback to improve her facial responses. She succeeded in inhibiting the contralateral depressor activity to a level at which it was symmetrical with the affected side (Fig 6,D). This level of sEMG activity correlated with a visible, symmetrical smile (Figure 6,E). The patient learned to produce the desired response using mirror feedback, and then using only proprioceptive feedback. Her home program consisted of producing slow, symmetrical movements with and without the mirror, with her parents providing additional feedback initially. In a follow-up telephone conversation 18 months later, the parents reported generalization of the new movement pattern to outside activities about 90% of the time. The only time they noticed the "old" pattern was when the patient cried. The patient did not return for additional treatment and surgery was not performed.

ACKNOWLEDGMENTS

Grateful appreciation for support and assistance is extended to Robert Anderson, Joan Parent, Linda Petersen, and John Diels.

REFERENCES

1. Cicero, in Stevenson B (ed): *Macmillan Book of Proverbs, Maxims and Famous Phrases.* New York, Macmillan, 1948, p 738.
2. Anderson RG: Facial nerve disorders. *Select Read Plast Surg* 6:1–34, 1991.
3. Proceedings of Facial Neuromuscular Retraining Symposium, Toronto, June 1993, unpublished.

4. Schaitkin B: Facial weaknesses #1 problem for most acoustic neuroma patients. *Acoustic Neuroma Association NOTES* 38:1–5, 1991.

5. Macgregor FC: Facial disfigurement: Problems and management of social interaction and implications for mental health. *Aesthetic Plast Surg* 14:249–257, 1990.

6. Twerski A, Twerski B: The emotional impact of facial paralysis, in May M (ed): *The Facial Nerve.* New York, Thieme, 1986, pp 788–794.

7. Hoos L, Devriese PP: The management of psychological problems of patients with facial paralysis, in Portmann M (ed): *Facial Nerve.* New York, Masson Publishing, 1985, pp 337–340.

8. Elks MA: Another look at facial disfigurement. *J Rehab* (Jn Fb Mr):36–40, 1990.

9. Hoffman WY: Reanimation of the paralyzed face. *Otolaryngol Clin North Am* 25:649–667, 1992.

10. Gagnon NB, Molina-Negro P: Facial reinnervation after facial paralysis: Is it ever too late? *Arch Otorhinolaryngol* 246:303–307, 1989.

11. Rubin LR: Reanimation of total unilateral facial paralysis by the contiguous facial muscle technique, in Rubin LR (ed): *The Paralyzed Face.* St. Louis, Mosby, 1991, pp 156–177.

12. Harii K: Microneurovascular free muscle transplantation, in Rubin LR (ed): *The Paralyzed Face.* St. Louis, Mosby, 1991, pp 178–200.

13. May M: Surgical rehabilitation of facial palsy: Total approach, in May M (ed): *The Facial Nerve.* New York, Thieme, 1986, pp 695–777.

14. Fisch U: Extracranial surgery for facial hyperkinesis, in May M (ed): *The Facial Nerve.* New York, Thieme, 1986, pp 509–523.

15. Jackler RK, Pitts LH: Acoustic neuroma. *Neurosurg Clin North Am* 1:199–223, 1990.

16. Moffat DA, Croxson GR, Baguley DM, et al: Facial nerve recovery after acoustic neuroma removal. *J Laryngol Otol* 103:169–172, 1989.

17. Elsom JC: The treatment of nerve palsies. *Arch Phys Ther x-ray Rad* 8:293–295, 1927.

18. Craig M: *Miss Craig's Face Saving Exercises.* New York, Random House, 1970.

19. Kendall FP, McCreary EK: *Muscles Testing and Function,* ed 3. Baltimore, Williams & Wilkins, 1983, pp 235–267.

20. Cole J, Zimmerman S, Gerson S: Nonsurgical neuromuscular rehabilitation of facial muscle paresis, in Rubin LR (ed): *The Paralyzed Face.* St. Louis, Mosby, 1991, pp 107–112.

21. Melvin JL: *Rheumatic Disease: Occupational Therapy and Rehabilitation.* Philadelphia, FA Davis, 1977, pp 40–42.

22. Chusid JG: *Correlative Neuroanatomy and Functional Neurology.* Los Altos, Calif, Lange Medical, 1982, pp 99–101.

23. Farragher DJ: Electrical stimulation: A method of treatment for facial paralysis, in Rose FC, Jones R, Vrbova G (eds): *Neuromuscular Stimulation: Basic Concepts and Clinical Implications,* vol 3. New York, Demos, 1989, pp 303–306.

24. Cohan CS, Kater SB: Suppression of neurite elongation and growth cone motility by electrical activity. *Science* 232:1638–1640, 1986.

25. Brown MC, Holland RL: A central role for denervated tissues in causing nerve sprouting. *Nature* 282:724, 1979.

26. Waxman B: Electrotherapy for Treatment of Facial Nerve Paralysis (Bell's Palsy). *Health Techn Assess Rep* 3:27, 1984.

27. Ross B, Freedman C, Bednarek K: Personal communication, 1993.

28. Balliet R, Lewis L: Hypothesis: Craig's "face saving exercises" exercises may cause facial dysfunction. Edmonton, Alberta, Canadian Acoustic Neuroma Association, April 1985.

29. Shahani BT, Young RR: Blink reflexes in orbicularis oculi, in Desmedt JE (ed): *New Developments in Electromyography and Clinical Neurophysiology*, vol 3. Basel, Karger, 1973, pp 641–659.

30. Brodal A: *Neurological Anatomy: In Relation to Clinical Medicine*, ed 3. New York, Oxford University Press, 1981, pp 495–508.

31. Dubner R, Sessle BJ, Storey AT: *The Neural Basis of Oral and Facial Function*. New York, Plenum Press, 1978, pp 222–229.

32. Basmajian JV, DeLuca CJ: *Muscles Alive: Their Functions Revealed by Electromyography*, ed 5. Baltimore, Williams & Wilkins, 1985, pp 458–465.

33. May M: Microanatomy and pathophysiology of the facial nerve, in May M (ed): *The Facial Nerve*. New York, Thieme, 1986, pp 63–74.

34. Belal A: Structure of human muscle in facial paralysis: Role of muscle biopsy, in May M (ed): *The Facial Nerve*. New York, Thieme, 1986, pp 99–106.

35. Rinn WE: The neuropsychology of facial expression: A review of the neurological nad psychological mechanisms for producing facial expression. *Psychol Bull* 95:52–77, 1984.

36. Werner JK: *Neuroscience, a Clinical Perspective*. Philadelphia, WB Saunders, 1980.

37. Trombly CA: Motor control therapy, in Trombly CA (ed): *Occupational Therapy for Physical Dysfunction*, ed 2. Baltimore Williams & Wilkins, 1983, pp 59–72.

38. Bach-y-Rita P, Lazarus JV, Boyeson MG, et al: Neural aspects of motor function as a basis of early and post-acute rehabilitation, in DeLisa (ed): *Principles and Practice of Rehabilitation Medicine*. Philadelphia, JB Lippincott, 1988, pp 175–195.

39. Kottke FJ: Therapeutic exercise to develop neuromuscular coordination, in Kottke FJ, Lehmann JF (eds): *Krusen's Handbook of Physical Medicine and Rehabilitation*, ed 4. Philadelphia, WB Saunders, 1990, pp 452–479.

40. Anderson D: Personal communication, 1990.

41. Marinacci AA, Horande M: Electromyogram in neuromuscular re-education. *Bull Los Angeles Neurol Soc* 25:57–71, 1960.

42. Brown DM, Nahai F, Wolf S, et al: Electromyographic biofeedback in the re-education of facial palsy. *Am J Phys Med Rehabil* 57:183–190, 1978.

43. Daniel B, Guitar B: EMG feedback and recovery of facial and speech gestures following neural anastomosis. *J Speech Hear Disord* 43:9–20, 1978.

44. Jankel WR: Bell's Palsy: Muscle re-education by electromyograph feedback. *Arch Phys Med Rehabil* 59:240, 1978.

45. Booker HE, Rubow RT, Coleman PJ: Simplified feedback in neuromuscular retraining: An automated approach using electromyographic signals. *Arch Phys Med Rehabil* 50:621–625, 1969.

46. Balliet R, Shinn JB, Bach-y-Rita P: Facial paralysis rehabilitation: Retraining selective muscle control. *Int Rehab Med* 4:67–74, 1982.

47. Brudny J, Hammerschlag PE, Cohen NL, et al: Electromyographic rehabilitation of facial function and introduction of a facial paralysis grading scale for hypoglossal-facial nerve anastomosis. *Laryngoscope* 98:405–410, 1988.

48. May M, Croxson GR, Klein SR: Bell's palsy: Management of sequelae using EMG rehabilitation, botulinum toxin, and surgery. *Am J Otol* 10:220–229, 1989.

49. Ross B, Nedzelski JM, McLean JA: Efficacy of feedback training in long-standing facial nerve paresis. *Laryngoscope* 101:744–750, 1991.

50. Ross B, Nedzelski JM: Feedback training for facial nerve paresis: Are improvements sustained? *Laryngoscope*, in press.

51. Bach-y-Rita P, Bach-y-Rita EW: Biological and psychosocial factors in recovery from brain damage in humans. *Can J Psychol* 44:160, 1990.

52. Desmedt JE: Size principle of motoneuron recruitment and the calibration of muscle force and speed in man, in Desmedt JE (ed): *Motor Control Mechanisms in Health and Disease*. New York, Raven Press, 1983, pp 227–251.

53. Balliet R: Facial paralysis and other neuromuscular dysfunctions of the peripheral nervous system, in Payton OD, DiFabio RP, Paris SV, et al (eds): *Manual of Physical Therapy*, New York, Churchill Livingstone, 1989, p 198.

54. Diels HJ, Balliet R, Bednarek K: Facial paralysis questionaire. 1992, unpublished.

55. Sataloff RT, Myers DL, Kremer FB: Management of cranial nerve injury following surgery of the skull base. *Otolaryngol Clin North Am* 17:577–589, 1984.

56. Diels HJ: Unpublished data.

57. May M, Podvinec M, Ulrich J, et al: Idiopathic (Bell's) palsy, herpes zoster cephalicus and other facial nerve disorders of viral origin, in May M (ed): *The Facial Nerve*. New York, Thieme, 1986, pp 365–399.

58. May M: Microanatomy and pathophysiology of the facial nerve, in May M (ed): *The Facial Nerve*. New York, Thieme, 1986, p 72.

59. Valls-Sole J, Tolosa ES, Pujol M: Myokymic discharges and enhanced facial nerve reflex responses after recovery from idiopathic facial palsy. *Muscle Nerve* 15:37–42, 1992.

60. Montserrat L, Benito M: Facial synkinesis and aberrant regeneration of facial nerve, in Jankovic J, Tolosa E (eds): *Advances in Neurology*, vol 49. New York, Raven Press, 1988, pp 211–224.

61. Diels HJ: Unpublished data

62. Papel ID: Rehabilitation of the paralyzed face. *Otolaryngol Clin North Am* 24:727–738, 1991.

63. House JW: Facial nerve grading systems. *Laryngoscope* 93:1056–1069, 1983.

64. Ohyama M, Obata E, Furuta S, et al: Face EMG topographic analysis of mimetic movements in patients with Bell's palsy. *Acta Otolaryngol (Stockh)* 446(suppl):47–56, 1988.

65. Johnson PC, Brown H, Kuzon WM Jr, et al: Simultaneous quantitation of facial movements: The maximal static response assay of facial nerve function. *Ann Plast Surg* 32:171–179, 1994.

66. House JW, Brackmann DE: Facial nerve grading system. *Otolaryngol Head Neck Surg* 93:146–147, 1985.

67. Burres SA: Facial biomechanics: The standards of normal. *Laryngoscope* 95:708–714, 1985.

68. Balliet R: Facial paralysis and other neuromuscular dysfunctions of the peripheral nervous system, in Payton OD, DiFabio RP, Paris SV, et al (eds): *Manual of Physical Therapy*. New York, Churchill Livingstone, 1989, pp 175–213.

69. Ross BG, Fradet G, Nedzelski JM: Development of a sensitive clinical facial grading system. *Eur Arch Otorhinolaryngol Suppl* S180–S181, 1994.

70. Brudny J: Biofeedback in facial paralysis: Electromyographic rehabilitation, in Rubin LR (ed): *The Paralyzed Face*. St. Louis, Mosby, 1991, pp 247–264.

71. Leonetti JP, Brackmann DE, Prass RL: Improved preservation of facial nerve function in the infratemporal approach to the skull base. *Otolaryngol Head Neck Surg* 101:74–78, 1989.

72. Winstein CJ: Motor learning considerations in stroke rehabilitation, in Duncan PW, Badke MB (eds): *Stroke Rehabilitation: The Recovery of Motor Control*. St. Louis, Mosby, 1987, p 124.

73. Balliet R: Motor control strategies in the retraining of facial paralysis, in Portmann M (ed): *Facial Nerve*. New York, Masson Publishing, 1985, pp 465–469.

74. Novak CB, Ross B, Mackinnon SE, et al: Facial sensibility in patients with unilateral facial nerve paresis. *Otolaryngol Head Neck Surg* 109:506–513, 1993.

75. Bobath B: *Adult Hemiplegia: Evaluation and Treatment*, ed 2. London, William Heinemann Medical Books, 1978.

76. Schram G, Burres S: Non surgical rehabilitation after facial paralysis, in Portmann M (ed): *Facial Nerve*. New York, Masson Publishing, 1985, pp 461–464.

77. Barat M: Principles of rehabilitation in facial paralysis, in Portmann M (ed): *Facial Nerve*. New York, Masson Publishing, 1985, pp 66–67.

78. Manheim CJ, Lavett DK: *The Myofascial Release Manual*. Thorofare, NJ, Slack, 1989, pp 75–80.

79. Mountain RE, Murray JAM, Quaba A: Management of facial synkinesis with clostridium botulinum toxin injection. *Clin Otolaryngol* 17:223–224, 1992.

80. Borodic GE, Pearce LB, Cheney M, et al: Botulinum A toxin for treatment of aberrant facial nerve regeneration. *Plast Reconstr Surg* 91:1042–1045, 1993.

81. Diels HJ: Unpublished data.

Infections of the Fascial Spaces of the Head and Neck in the Pediatric Population

Robert F. Yellon, M.D.

Assistant Professor of Otolaryngology, Department of Pediatric Otolaryngology, Children's Hospital of Pittsburgh; Department of Otolaryngology, University of Pittsburgh School of Medicine, Pittsburgh, Pennsylvania

B ecause life-threatening complications can still occur even in the antibiotic era, familiarity with the important anatomic, etiologic, bacteriologic and clinical factors, as well as selection of the best diagnostic and therapeutic modalities required for care of infections of the fascial spaces of the head and neck in children is essential. The increasing prevalence of patients with immunodeficiency or prior antibiotic treatment may result in unusual clinical presentations and pathogens, making the correct diagnosis and treatment even more important, yet more elusive.

ETIOLOGY OF HEAD AND NECK SPACE INFECTIONS

Infection of the retropharyngeal space frequently originates from infection in the nose, paranasal sinuses, or nasopharynx that spreads to the retropharyngeal lymph nodes. Pharyngeal trauma can also lead to infection of the retropharyngeal and lateral pharyngeal spaces. Infection or trauma of the tonsils, laryngotracheal complex, hypopharynx, and esophagus can result in visceral and pretracheal space infection. Tuberculous infection of the vertebral bodies (Pott's abscess), as well as nontuberculous infection, can cause prevertebral (retropharyngeal) space infections.

Adenotonsillitis is a source of lateral pharyngeal space infection. Infection of the petrous apex may extend into the lateral pharyngeal space. Bezold's abscess (Fig 1) occurs when infection in the mastoid tip erodes through the cortex and lies between the mastoid tip and mandible, and may extend into the lateral pharyngeal space (Fig 2). Of course, tonsillitis precedes peritonsillar space infection, which may extend into the lateral pharyngeal space. Iatrogenic causes of lateral pharyngeal space infections include local anesthesia for tonsillectomy and superior alveolar nerve block.

Infections of mandibular teeth and gingiva may be the cause of infections of the mandibular, submandibular, masticator, parotid, and lateral pharyngeal spaces. Infections of maxillary or mandibular teeth are the usual cause of infection in the buccal space, which may also occur sec-

Advances in Otolaryngology—Head and Neck Surgery®, vol. 9
© 1995, Mosby–Year Book, Inc.

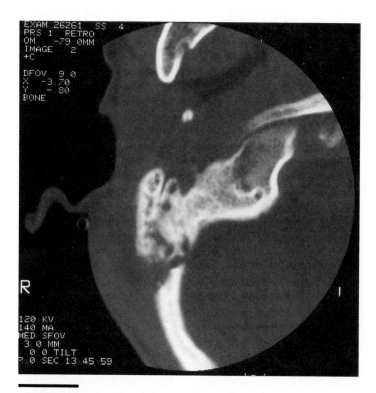

FIGURE 1.

Axial computed tomographic scan of the right temporal bone of a child with Bezold's abscess showing erosion of mastoid cortex.

ondary to infection of the parotid gland or overlying skin, or from adenitis of nodes overlying the adjacent masseter muscle. In young children, buccal space infection may arise secondary to blood-borne *Haemophilus influenzae.* Canine space infection results from canine tooth root abscess that erodes through the anterior cortex of the maxilla. Infections of the parotid space and space of the submandibular gland may follow sialoadenitis or suppuration of lymph nodes in these spaces, or from calculi or tumors encroaching on the ductal system.

Infection of cystic hygromas, and branchial apparatus remnants can spread into adjacent deep neck spaces. Carotid sheath infection may occur by extension from infected adjacent deep neck spaces, suppurative adenitis, intravenous drug abuse, central venous catheter placement, and hypercoagulable states. Deep neck space infections may also arise secondary to their anatomic connections with abscesses in the mediastinum.

BACTERIOLOGY OF INFECTIONS OF HEAD AND NECK SPACES

Of 117 children (N = 78 cultures) with head and neck space infections seen at Children's Hospital of Pittsburgh from 1986 to 1992 (Table 1), the gram-positive aerobic pathogens beta-hemolytic Streptococci (18%) and *Staphylococcus aureus* (18%) were most prevalent. The anaerobic pathogens *Bacteroides melaninogenicus* (16.7%) and *Veillonella* species (14%) predominated.[1] *Haemophilus parainfluenzae,* a gram-negative pathogen, was found in 14% of cultures. If all gram-negative pathogens are included,

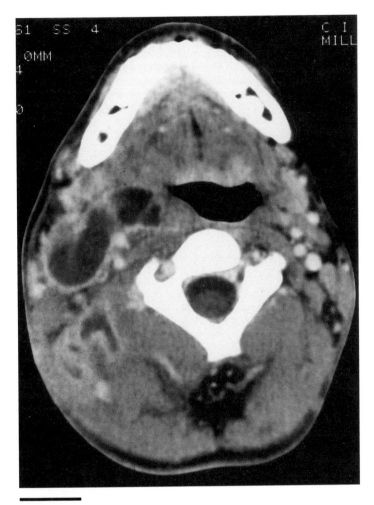

FIGURE 2.

Axial computed tomographic scan of the neck showing right lateral pharyngeal space abscess associated with Bezold's abscess seen in Figure 1.

these organisms were present in 17.9% of cultures. Beta-lactamase production by aerobic pathogens was found in 22% of cultures. Many abscesses are polymicrobial, and many of the anaerobes also produce beta-lactamase.[2, 3]

Mycobacterium tuberculosis, atypical mycobacteria[4] and cat scratch disease can also cause infection of cervical nodes with significant adenopathy and occasional abscesses. Infections caused by atypical mycobacteria and the cat scratch bacillus, *Rochalimaea henselae*,[5] tend to differ from the infections caused by the usual pathogens in that fever and pain are usually absent. The fever and massive adenopathy associated with Kawasaki's disease may simulate bacterial neck space infection, but may be differentiated by associated findings of conjunctivitis, strawberry tongue, rash, desquamation of hands and feet, and coronary artery vasculitis. Other causes of adenopathy in children include viruses, fungi, brucellosis, plague, tularemia, lymphogranuloma venereum, post-transplant lymphoproliferative disease, sarcoidosis, drug reaction (phenytoin), and malignancy.[6]

TABLE 1.

Bacteriology of Head and Neck Space Infections in 78 Infants and Children at Children's Hospital of Pittsburgh: January 1986 through June 1992

	Number of Cases (%)
Beta hemolytic *Streptococcus*	14 (18)
Staphylococcus aureus	14 (18)
Bacteroides melaninogenicus	13 (16.7)
Veillonella species	11 (14)
Haemophilus parainfluenzae	11 (14)
Bacteroides intermedius	6 (7.7)
Micrococcus species	6 (7.7)
Peptostreptococcus species	4 (5)
Fusobacterium species	4 (5)
Candida albicans	4 (5)
Staphylococcus coagulase negative	2 (2.6)
Beta *Streptococcus* group C	2 (2.6)
Haemophilus haemolyticus	2 (2.6)
Haemophilus influenzae (non-typable)	2 (2.6)
Bacteroides bivius	2 (2.6)
Eikenella corrodens	2 (2.6)
Escherichia coli	1 (1.3)
Alpha hemolytic *Streptococcus**	34 (44)
Neisseria species*	17 (22)
Diphtheroid species*	9 (11.5)
Other†	16 (20.5)
No growth	7 (9)

*Normal oropharyngeal flora
†Other organisms consisted of 16 species considered to be normal oropharyngeal flora (one isolate of each species)

ANTIMICROBIAL THERAPY FOR HEAD AND NECK SPACE INFECTIONS

When the diagnosis of infection of the head and neck spaces is made, intravenous antibiotics are indicated, after appropriate cultures are obtained. In selected patients such as adolescents with peritonsillar abscesses that have been drained with relief of trismus and good oral intake, oral antibiotics may be adequate. Because β-lactamase producing bacteria are common, agents that inhibit β-lactamase or are β-lactamase stable are more desirable than penicillin. Clindamycin is an appropriate choice for gram-positive organisms and anaerobes. It is not recommended if gram-negative organisms are suspected, in which case clindamycin plus cefuroxime is preferred. In our series (see Table 1),[1] gram-negative aerobic pathogens were found in 17.9% of cultures from 78 children with head and neck space infections. Ampicillin-sulbactam is also recommended as it has excellent in vitro activity against these pathogens.[7-9] The optimum duration for antimicrobial therapy has not been studied, but 10 days to 14 days is recommended. When the patient has improved sufficiently, for oral therapy, amoxicillin-clavulanate, cefuroxime-axetil or cefprozil are good choices. For children with drug allergy, the combination of erythromycin and sulfisoxazole, or clindamycin are appropriate.

DIAGNOSTIC STUDIES

Complete blood count with differential, prothrombin time, partial thromboplastin time, electrolytes, and possibly urine specific gravity, are appropriate for most patients suspected to have head and neck space infections. Throat, blood, and sputum cultures may be needed.

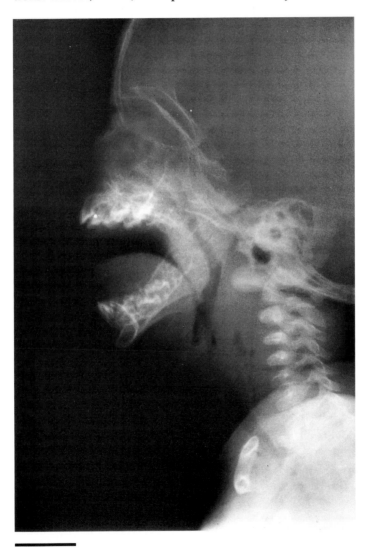

FIGURE 3.
Lateral neck film of a child with retropharyngeal space abscess showing significant thickening of prevertebral soft tissues and gas in the retropharyngeal space.

Anteroposterior and lateral soft tissue radiographs of the neck and pharynx may be indicated, and should be taken with the child's neck in extension and in inspiration, or there may be spurious thickening of the retropharyngeal and retrotracheal spaces, especially in young children When the film is taken properly, if the retropharyngeal space measures more than 7 mm and the retrotracheal space more than 13 mm, an infection in this space is probable.[10] When a retropharyngeal abscess is present, there is usually loss of the normal curvature with straightening of the cervical spine. The presence of gas in the soft tissues confirms the presence of an abscess (Fig 3). Panorex films may identify mandibular bone erosion or dental infection. A chest radiograph will rule out pneumonia or mediastinal involvement.

If questions still exist concerning the presence of a possible abscess versus cellulitis/adenopathy, further imaging techniques may be indicated. In patients with selected head and neck space infections such as the cooperative adolescent with a possible peritonsillar abscess, needle aspiration (NA) will be diagnostic if frank pus is aspirated, thus obviating the need for imaging studies. When imaging studies are required, axial and coronal computed tomography (CT) should be performed with 4 mm to 5 mm sections from the cranial base to the upper mediastinum,[11] which delineates both osseous and soft tissue structures. Intravenous contrast may identify an abscess as a "rim enhancing lesion," with a low density center. A gas-fluid level or bubbles also indicate abscess. Intravenous contrast also helps to delineate vascular structures and lymph node anatomy.

In our study of 117 head and neck space infections treated at the Children's Hospital of Pittsburgh,[1] a series of 16 CT scans were available from children who had also undergone either open surgical exploration or NA. The sensitivity of CT in our study for detection of head and neck space abscesses when reviewed by a neuroradiologist in a blinded fashion, was 91%, with a specificity of 60%. Positive predictive value of CT for abscess was 83% (Table 2). The two false-negative cases underwent NA only, and thus it is possible that abscesses that may have been present were not detected.

Some authors have recommended the use of magnetic resonance imaging (MRI) to distinguish head and neck abscesses from cellulitis/ade-

TABLE 2.

Sensitivity and Specificity of CT Scans in Distinguishing Cellulitis vs. Abscesses in Head and Neck Space Infections in 16 Infants and Children at Children's Hospital of Pittsburgh; January 1986 through June 1992*

	Abscess Found at Surgery	
CT Scan	**Yes**	**No**
Positive	10	2
Negative	1	3

*Sensitivity = 10/11 (91%); Specificity = 3/5 (60%); Positive Predictive Value = 10/11 (83%); Negative Predictive Value = 3/4 (75%)

nopathy. Magnetic resonance imaging has the advantage of examination in multiple planes including axial, coronal and sagittal. Five millimeter sections using T1-weighted sequences delineates major anatomic structures, whereas the inflammatory tissue has low to intermediate signal intensity. T2-weighted images can characterize inflammatory tissue and abscess cavities, as these tissues have high intensity signals. Gadolinium-DTPA contrast may identify abscess cavities with "rim enhancement" of the abscess wall. There appears to be no advantage of CT versus MRI with the exception that sagittal sections using MRI may be particularly valuable for evaluation of retropharyngeal and lateral pharyngeal spaces.[11]

Ultrasonography (US) has also been recommended to differentiate between cellulitis/adenopathy versus abscess during head and neck space infections (Fig 4). One study in children[12] compared US versus CT in the diagnosis of retropharyngeal adenopathy/cellulitis versus abscess. All ten

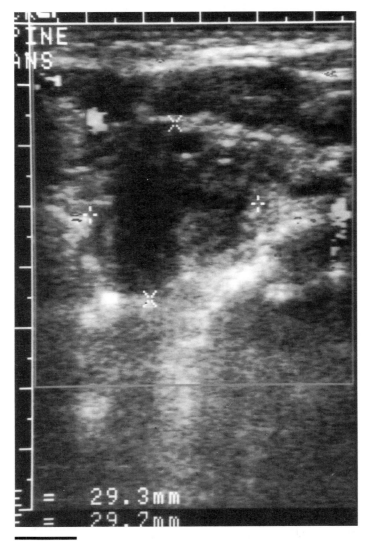

FIGURE 4.

Ultrasound examination of the retropharyngeal space in a child with a retropharyngeal abscess.

patients in this study had a CT scan interpreted as showing abscess. Ultrasonography identified only three out of the ten as having abscesses. In the three patients who had US evidence of abscess, intraoperative US guided surgical drainage. Two additional children with CT evidence of abscess, but US examination showing only adenopathy, underwent US guided NA of the retropharyngeal mass, and no pus could be aspirated. Ultrasonography correctly identified retropharyngeal adenitis/cellulitis in seven children, whose infections all resolved with antibiotic therapy alone.[13] In a series of 12 children,[14] US was able to differentiate abscess from adenopathy/cellulitis. Intraoral US was recently used to identify peritonsillar abscess in 12 patients.[15]

It would appear that if CT or MRI are not available, or if the CT or MRI findings are not clear regarding the presence of an abscess versus cellulitis/adenopathy, US is indicated to aid in the diagnosis. Finally, US appears to be useful for intraoperative localization of abscesses.[12, 16]

AIRWAY MANAGEMENT FOR HEAD AND NECK SPACE INFECTIONS

A key point in children with head and neck space infection is maintenance of a stable airway, which may be accomplished when necessary by endotracheal intubation or tracheostomy. If trismus or soft tissue edema preclude endotracheal intubation, tracheostomy is necessary. Establishment of an artificial airway in a child with a tenuous airway should be strongly considered before the child depletes all of his or her respiratory reserve or progresses to complete obstruction that will precipitate a more risky emergency tracheostomy. In extreme circumstances, cricothyroidotomy may be required. Securing the airway by initial endotracheal intubation or with a rigid bronchoscope prior to tracheostomy is recommended. However, unsuccessful attempts at intubation may also precipitate acute airway obstruction and, thus, tracheostomy under local anesthesia has occasionally been performed. A nasopharyngeal or oral airway may be useful as a temporizing measure in selected cases.

SUPERFICIAL FASCIA OF HEAD AND NECK

Consisting of the subcutaneous tissue, the superficial fascia of the head and neck contains fat and covers the superficial muscles of the head and neck.

DEEP FASCIA OF NECK

SUPERFICIAL LAYER OF DEEP CERVICAL FASCIA

Distinct from the superficial fascia of the neck as it is a deeper structure, the superficial or anterior layer of the deep cervical fascia (DCF) arises from the vertebral spinous processes and ligamentum nuchae on both sides of the neck. It then travels between and encircles the trapezius, sternocleidomastoid, and omohyoid muscles, and then passes anterior to the strap muscles. Attached to the hyoid bone superiorly, it splits below to attach to both surfaces of the sternum, creating the suprasternal space (of Burns).

MIDDLE LAYER OF DEEP CERVICAL FASCIA

Anterolaterally, the middle, pretracheal, or visceral layer of the DCF is continuous with the superficial layer of the DCF at the lateral borders of the strap muscles. It then passes posterior to the strap muscles and anterior to the trachea and thyroid gland, hence the name pretracheal fascia. Next, it travels posteriorly to envelop the pharynx and esophagus, hence the name visceral fascia. The middle layer of the DCF is continuous with the buccopharyngeal fascia. Superiorly, the middle cervical fascia fuses with the hyoid bone and thyroid cartilage. Inferiorly, it travels deep to the sternum extending into the superior mediastinum.

POSTERIOR LAYER OF DEEP CERVICAL FASCIA

The posterior or prevertebral layer of the DCF also arises on the vertebral spinous processes and ligamentum nuchae. It then passes deep to the trapezius muscles and covers the scalene muscles, levator scapulae, longus coli, brachial plexus, and phrenic nerve. This layer also covers the vertebral column and attaches to the clavicles inferiorly. The portion of this fascia that covers the vertebral bodies and longus coli muscles is described by some authors[17, 18] as two distinct layers with a posterior prevertebral fascia and an anterior alar fascia. In contrast, contemporary head and neck anatomists describe only a single layer of prevertebral fascia with no alar fascia (personal communication, Doctors E. N. Myers and J. T. Johnson).

FASCIA OF UPPER NECK, FACE, AND HEAD

SUPERFICIAL LAYER OF DEEP CERVICAL FASCIA

Above the hyoid bone, the superficial layer of the deep DCF extends from the hyoid bone to the mandible and zygomatic arch. This fascia, which lies deep to the platysma muscle, splits to cover both surfaces of the mandible, as well as submandibular and parotid glands to form their capsules. It also covers the myelohyoid, the anterior belly of digastric, the lateral aspect of masseter, and the medial aspect of the internal pterygoid muscles.

BUCCOPHARYNGEAL FASCIA

Continuous with the visceral fascia (middle layer of DCF) covering the esophagus, the buccopharyngeal fascia covers the pharynx. It covers the buccinator muscle laterally, and attaches to the pterygomandibular raphe.

SPACES OF NECK, FACE AND HEAD. ANATOMY, CLINICAL PRESENTATION OF INFECTIONS, AND OPEN SURGICAL PROCEDURES FOR TREATMENT OF INFECTIONS

PERITONSILLAR SPACE

Located between the capsule of the palatine tonsil and the constrictor muscles, the peritonsillar (paratonsillar) space is the most common site of head and neck space infections. It extends anteriorly and posteriorly to the tonsillar pillars. Superiorly, it may extend to the level of the hard palate or torus tubarius and as low as the pyriform fossa. At Children's Hospital of Pittsburgh, 63% of 61 children with peritonsillar infection had trismus,[1] which results from extension of the infection to the lateral pharyngeal space and internal pterygoid muscle.

Children with peritonsillar space infections (quinsy) present with pain, fever, dysphagia, cervical adenopathy, and fetor oris. The hallmark is swelling of the tissues lateral and superior to the tonsil, with medial and anterior displacement of the tonsil. Displacement of the uvula may occur. The tonsils may be red, enlarged, and covered with exudate. If an abscess is present, it usually (but not always) forms at the superior pole of the tonsil.

Differentiation of peritonsillar cellulitis versus abscess is an important issue. Some abscesses may be clinically obvious, while for others, the clinical distinction is more difficult. An initial 12 hour to 24 hour trial of appropriate intravenous antibiotics is reasonable in selected patients with no evidence of abscess or complications. When extension of peritonsillar infection to adjacent deep neck spaces is suspected, CT scan is indicated. If improvement does not occur following a trial of intravenous antimicrobial agents, NA may be attempted in selected patients in order to identify an abscess. Intraoral US correctly identified 12 out of 12 peritonsillar abscesses in ten adults and two children, and was a useful guide for NA.[15]

Traditional treatment for peritonsillar abscess has been incision and drainage (I+D) through an anterior pillar incision, followed by blunt dissection into the abscess cavity with a hemostat. Interval tonsillectomy is then performed in 4 weeks to 12 weeks.[19] Some advocate immediate tonsillectomy ("Quinsy tonsillectomy", "tonsillectomy à chaud") to ensure complete drainage and to avoid a second hospitalization for interval tonsillectomy (20–24). The incidence of bleeding following Quinsy tonsillectomy in adults and children ranged from 0% to 7% with an overall incidence of 1% for 1,027 patients combined from these series.[20-24] In a study involving 55 children who underwent Quinsy tonsillectomy, no patient had postoperative or delayed bleeding.[23] In a military population,[22] there was no difference in bleeding between Quinsy and interval tonsillectomy.

In one study, 90% of 41 patients (age not specified) were successfully managed with NA of peritonsillar abscesses at the point of maximum bulging, or if the first aspiration was unsuccessful, 1 cm lower.[25] In a second series of 74 patients (adults and children) with peritonsillar infections who underwent NA of the superior, middle, and inferior peritonsillar areas, pus was aspirated in 70%. A second series of aspirations were required for seven (10%) patients on the following day.[26]

In a series of 29 children, the incidence of recurrent peritonsillar abscess and recurrent tonsillitis following peritonsillar abscess were each 7%.[27] Recurrence rates for peritonsillar abscess for all ages range from 6% to 36%, with an average of 17% for 526 patients combined from six studies.[20, 22, 24, 27-29] Rates for recurrent tonsillitis before or after peritonsillar abscess range from 7% to 50%, with an average of 28% for 345 patients combined from four studies.[20, 27-29]

Thus, in the treatment of peritonsillar abscess, Quinsy tonsillectomy,

I+D with or without interval tonsillectomy, and NA have all been shown to be safe and effective. In patients with peritonsillar abscess and significant airway obstruction or associated complications, Quinsy tonsillectomy is appropriate. If I+D or NA have failed, immediate tonsillectomy is indicated. Additionally, in patients with a prior history of recurrent peritonsillar abscess, or recurrent tonsillitis warranting tonsillectomy, Quinsy tonsillectomy should be considered, in order to avoid a second period of hospitalization and morbidity. In this last scenario, I+D with interval tonsillectomy would also be reasonable.

Needle aspiration of peritonsillar abscesses is the least invasive treatment, and is safe and effective for older, cooperative children without complications. For children with a bleeding diathesis or whose general condition is too poor to tolerate a general anesthetic, NA is the treatment of choice.

RETROPHARYNGEAL (PREVERTEBRAL, DANGER) SPACE

Superiorly, the retropharyngeal space is limited by the cranial base, and inferiorly, continues as the retrovisceral space into the mediastinum to the level of the carina. As described by Grodinsky and Holyoke[17] and cited by Hollinshead,[18] the posterior layer of the DCF is composed of two distinct layers with an anterior alar fascia, and a posterior prevertebral fascia. The space between these two layers is called the danger space, and extends from the cranial base to the diaphragm.[17] According to Grodinsky and Holyoke, the prevertebral space lies posterior to the prevertebral fascia and anterior to the vertebral bodies.

Contemporary authorities report that the terms "retropharyngeal," "danger," and "prevertebral" spaces are synonymous. In their view, this space lies between the single layer of prevertebral fascia and the buccopharyngeal fascia on the posterior wall of the pharynx. The alar layer is felt to not exist (personal communication, Doctors E. N. Myers and J. T. Johnson).

According to Grodinsky and Holyoke[17] and Hollinshead,[18] infections in the "prevertebral" space (between the vertebral bodies and the prevertebral layer of the DCF) bulge in the midline, are bilateral, and are best approached by the open surgical approach to deep neck infections as described below, rather than by the transoral approach in order to avoid the possibility of a persistent draining fistula in the pharynx with the potential for aspiration. These infections may require prolonged antimicrobial therapy for osteomyelitis or tuberculous infection of the vertebral bodies.[30]

Children with typical retropharyngeal infection present with irritability, fever, dysphagia, muffled speech or cry, noisy breathing, stiff neck, and adenopathy. Stridor and drooling may be present. In our series of 27 children with retropharyngeal infections, nine (33%) had torticollis.[1] The buccopharyngeal fascia is adherent to the prevertebral fascia in the midline, so that infections in the retropharyngeal space are unilateral. If the patient is in respiratory distress, examination should be performed in the operating room, as the child will probably require I+D or an artificial airway. In addition, the child might have supraglottitis if fever, stridor, and drooling are of sudden onset. A localized, unilateral, posterior pharyngeal swelling is usually an enlarged retropharyngeal lymph node. Generalized unilateral swelling that extends from the nasopharynx to the retroesophageal area is usually either cellulitis or an abscess.

A transoral approach is recommended for I+D of an abscess of the retropharyngeal space. The patient is intubated orally, which can be done safely by introducing the tube on the side opposite the abscess. To avoid aspiration of purulent material, the patient should be in the Trendelenburg position. The position and mouth gag for tonsillectomy are used. Before the I+D, a NA of the abscess should be obtained for Gram's stain, culture, and antimicrobial sensitivity studies, and to prevent tracheal aspiration of pus at the time of the I+D. Next, a small vertical incision is made in the lateral aspect of the posterior pharynx between the junction of the lateral one-third and medial two-thirds of the distance between the midline of the pharynx and the medial aspect of the retromolar trigone. The space is then opened bluntly to drain the abscess and avoid possible injury to vascular structures. No drain is placed. If the infection also involves the lateral pharyngeal space, drainage should be performed through an external incision through the neck, as described below in the section on the open surgical approach to deep neck space infections. Occasionally, both transoral and external neck approaches are needed. If the child has early recurrence, or does not improve rapidly following a transoral procedure, then an external approach is used.

MANDIBULAR SPACE

This space is formed by splitting of the two leaflets of the superficial layer of the DCF, attaching to the inferior border of the mandible laterally, and at the level of the mylohyoid, medially. The space is limited anteriorly by the attachment of the anterior belly of the digastric, and posteriorly by the attachment of the medial pterygoid to the mandible.

Mandibular space infections usually occur when a suppurative dental process erodes through the lingual cortex of the mandible, and creates an abscess between the mandible and the inner leaflet of fascia. This painful intraoral swelling lies more anterior than that seen during infection of the medial portion of the masticator space. There is no external facial swelling, unless the submandibular space is also involved. Mandibular space abscesses may be drained through intraoral incision along the body of the mandible.

MASTICATOR SPACE

Fat, loose connective tissue, the ramus of the mandible, the temporalis muscle, mandibular nerve, and internal maxillary artery are contained in the masticator space. Created by the splitting of the superficial layer of the DCF around the masseter and internal pterygoid muscles, this space extends anteriorly as the fascia covers the buccal fat pad and then ends as the fascia attaches to the maxilla and buccinator fascia. It ends posteriorly as the two lamina of the fascia fuse along the posterior border of the mandible. Superiorly, the medial aspect of the masticator space is limited by the origin of the temporalis muscle from the skull, and laterally, by the temporalis fascia. Medially, it extends to include the pterygopalatine fossa. Infection in the masticator space may occur medial or lateral to the mandible. The superior portion of the masticator space is sometimes referred to as the temporal space with compartments medial and lateral to the temporalis muscle.

Infections of the masticator space are usually related to dental pathology. Osteomylitis or subperiosteal abscess of the mandible may be present. The major symptom is pain along the ascending ramus of the mandible. Trismus, sore throat, dysphagia, and pain on moving the tongue are often present. Swelling is present in the retromolar trigone if the medial compartment is involved, which may be mistaken for a peritonsillar abscess. There may be swelling of the floor of the mouth and lateral pharyngeal wall. With lateral compartment infection, swelling will be seen externally.

When the lateral portion of the masticator space requires I+D, an incision is made below and parallel to the body of the mandible. The facial vein and possibly the facial artery are then identified and ligated, and elevated with the platysma, capsule of the gland, and marginal mandibular nerve. The tendon of the masseter is detached from the mandible, thus draining the lateral portion of the masticator space. Drains or packing are placed. The medial portion of the masticator space is approached by an incision medial to the ascending ramus of the mandible in the retromolar trigone.

When requiring drainage, the temporal space may be approached through preauricular or hairline incisions through the temporalis fascia to reach abscesses lateral to the temporalis muscle, or through the temporalis muscle to reach medially located abscesses. Penrose drains or packing are placed.

BUCCAL SPACE

Lateral to the buccinator muscle lies the buccopharyngeal fascia which is the medial wall of the buccal space. The skin of the cheek is the lateral boundary. Limiting the buccal space inferiorly is the lower border of the mandible. The posterior limit is the pterygomandibular raphe. The buccal space contains the buccal fat pad, Stensen's duct, and facial artery.[31]

Infections in the buccal space present with cheek swelling. There is often trismus from inflammation of the masseter muscle. There is usually little intraoral swelling. Buccal space infections may occasionally involve the maxillary sinus, orbit, preseptal orbital tissues, or cavernous sinus. Buccal space abscesses usually present subcutaneously and are drained by skin incision and blunt dissection parallel to the facial nerve branches.

CANINE SPACE

This potential space lies anterior to the canine fossa of the maxilla. There is debate as to whether it represents a true fascial space. Toothache usually precedes canine space infection. Swelling is present lateral to the nares, which may be mistaken for dacryocystitis, and drainage may occur just inferior to the medial canthus of the eye. If the infection extends inferiorly, swelling will also be present in the labial sulcus. Abscesses in the canine space may be approached by incision in the labial sulcus through the periosteum. Dissection is then performed superiorly to drain the abscess. Treatment of the dental infection is necessary.[31]

PAROTID SPACE

As the superficial layer of the DCF splits to cover the medial and lateral surfaces of the parotid gland, the parotid space is formed, which contains the periparotid lymph nodes, the facial nerve, and may contain the auriculotemporal nerve, external carotid and superficial temporal arteries, and retromandibular vein. Pain, redness, and edema over the parotid constitute the typical picture of parotid space infection. Even when an abscess is present, the thick fascia covering the gland prevents palpation of fluctuation.

Parotid space abscesses are approached by a parotidectomy type incision. The parotid fascia is detached from the tragus and sternocleidomastoid muscle and, thus, superficially incised to drain the parotid space. If necessary, the facial nerve is identified to allow drainage of abscesses that lie in the posterosuperomedial aspect of the parotid space. Intraparenchymal abscesses may be drained by blunt dissection parallel to the branches of the nerve.

OPEN SURGICAL APPROACH TO DEEP NECK SPACE INFECTIONS

Mosher's 1929 description[32] of the open surgical approach to deep pus in the neck is still useful today, with some modification, for drainage of visceral, submandibular, and lateral pharyngeal space infections, infections of the carotid sheath, and selected infections of the retropharyngeal space. Most uncomplicated retropharyngeal abscesses may be drained transorally as described above. Mosher's T-shaped incision has been modified in that the horizontal limb is slightly lower in relation to the body of the mandible, and the vertical limb omitted. After incising skin and platysma, dissection is carried out anterior to the sternocleidomastoid and posteroinferior to the submandibular gland. The fascial layers may be extremely thickened. Care is taken to avoid or ligate the facial artery during elevation of the gland. If the abscess is limited to the space of the submandibular gland, the capsule of the gland can be simply incised along its lower border for drainage, or the gland may be excised. The carotid sheath structures are identified opposite the tip of the greater horn of the hyoid bone and may require I+D. At this point, finger dissection superiorly along the carotid sheath allows drainage of the lateral pharyngeal space up to the cranial base. Blunt dissection medial to the carotid sheath in an inferior direction will allow drainage of the visceral space. Penrose type drains or iodoform packing are placed for several days and the wounds are closed loosely.

Head and neck space abscesses in any location that are obviously pointing may be managed by simple skin and subcutaneous tissue incision, evacuation of pus, and blunt or digital exploration of the abscess cavity to drain any areas of loculation. Drains or packing are then placed.

LATERAL PHARYNGEAL SPACE

Shaped like an inverted pyramid, the lateral pharyngeal (parapharyngeal) space extends from the cranial base to the hyoid bone. It lies lateral to the buccopharyngeal fascia of the pharynx, and medial to the pterygoid muscles and fascia on the medial surface of the parotid gland. Anterosuperiorly, it extends to the pterygomandibular raphe, and posteriorly to the posterior surface of the carotid sheath. The styloid process and attached fascia of the tensor veli palatini muscle, divide the lateral pharyngeal space into a prestyloid compartment containing the internal maxillary artery, maxillary nerve and tail of parotid gland, and a poststyloid compartment containing the carotid artery, internal jugular vein, cervical sympathetic chain, and cranial nerves IX-XII.

Pain, fever, and stiff neck are the usual presenting complaints seen with lateral pharyngeal space infection. Trismus is secondary to inflammation of the internal pterygoid muscle. There may be perimandibular edema. Lateral pharyngeal wall swelling is seen, which is often posterior to the tonsil. The tonsil is usually medially and anteriorly displaced. Computed tomography, MRI, or US may help differentiate abscess versus cellulitis. Airway obstruction or neuropathies may be present. When indicated, lateral pharyngeal space infections are drained by the open surgical approach described above.

CAROTID SHEATH

All three layers of the DCF contribute to the carotid sheath, which contains the carotid artery, internal jugular vein, and vagus nerve. Stiffness, swelling, and torticollis are present during carotid sheath infection. With thrombosis of the internal jugular vein, spiking ("picket fence") fevers may occur as septic emboli seed the pulmonary circulation. The open surgical approach to this deep neck space is described above.

VISCERAL SPACE

Contents of the visceral space include the thyroid gland, trachea, and esophagus. It is divided into pretracheal and retrovisceral spaces which are in continuity superiorly. Above the level where the inferior thyroid artery enters the thyroid gland, there is only one visceral compartment, surrounded by the middle layer of the DCF anteriorly, the carotid sheath laterally, and the posterior layer of the DCF. Below the level where the inferior thyroid artery enters the thyroid gland, dense connective tissue attaches the lateral aspect of the esophagus to the prevertebral layer, thus creating a pretracheal space anterior to the esophagus, and a retrovisceral space, posteriorly. The pretracheal portion extends up to where the strap muscles join the thyroid cartilage and hyoid bone, and inferiorly to the anterior mediastinum. Superiorly, the retrovisceral portion continues as the retropharyngeal space. Inferiorly, it extends to the level of the carina, and is a common pathway for neck infection to spread into the mediastinum.

Symptoms of visceral space infections include neck swelling, pain, dysphagia, and hoarseness due to glottic edema which may progress to airway obstruction. Perforation of viscera can lead to mediastinal and neck emphysema, or pneumothorax. Open surgical therapy is required as described above.

SUBMANDIBULAR SPACE INFECTIONS AND LUDWIG'S ANGINA

The limits of the submandibular space are the mucosa of the floor of the mouth and the tongue superiorly, and the superficial layer of DCF as it runs from the hyoid bone to the mandible. According to Hollinshead,[18] the sublingual space is the portion of the submandibular space that lies superior to the mylohyoid muscle, and contains the sublingual glands, the lingual and hypoglossal nerves, and a portion of the submandibular gland and duct. Contemporary anatomists divide the submandibular space into a supramylohyoid portion that is equivalent to the sublingual space, and an inframylohyoid portion that contains the structures lateral to the digastric muscle and medial to the mandible as well as the submental space, between the anterior bellies of the digastric muscles (personal communication, Doctors E. N. Myers and J. T. Johnson). The supramylohyoid and inframylohyoid portions of the submandibular space are in continuity posterior to the mylohyoid muscle.

With infection of the supamylohyoid portion, there is induration and edema of the floor of mouth and tongue. If the inframylohyoid portion is involved, induration and edema are noted inferior and medial to the mandible.

Bilateral involvement of the submandibular spaces can lead to massive edema of the tongue and floor of the mouth with posterior displacement of the tongue, which combined with trismus from involvement of the internal pterygoid muscles and possibly glottic edema, cause respiratory compromise. The involved tissues are extremely indurated. This constellation of signs and symptoms is called Ludwig's angina, and by definition, is a bilateral process. An abscess may be present, but cellulitis is sufficient to make a diagnosis of Ludwig's angina. In Ludwig's angina, release of tension is the basic surgical principle.[33] It is important, however, to look for abscesses and drain them if present. Even if imaging studies do not show an abscess, open surgical intervention is recommended in all but the exceptional mild, early case of Ludwig's angina. Early control of the airway is advised. A horizontal skin and platysmal incision is made approximately 1 cm above the hyoid bone, which may be extended to explore the space of the submandibular gland. The superficial layer of the DCF is incised vertically in the midline from the mandibular symphysis to the hyoid bone. The digastric, myelohyoid, and a variable portion of the tongue are divided in the sagittal plane to decompress the floor of the mouth. Blunt dissection between the layers of muscles laterally is useful to drain any possible abscesses. Multiple Penrose drains or packing are placed and the wounds left open. If an abscess is pointing within the oral cavity it may be drained transorally.

SPACE OF SUBMANDIBULAR GLAND

As the superficial layer of the DCF splits to form a capsule around the submandibular gland and lymph nodes, the space of the submandibular gland is formed, which lies within the inframylohyoid portion of the submandibular space. On its posteromedial surface, the fascia is perforated by the submandibular duct, which allows spread of infection above the mylohyoid muscle. This space is drained, when necessary, by the open approach described above.

SURGICAL VERSUS NONSURGICAL THERAPY FOR HEAD AND NECK SPACE INFECTIONS

Controversy exists concerning the need for, and timing of, surgical intervention in head and neck space infections. Some clinicians are advocating treating even documented abscess with a prolonged course of antimicrobial agents, without surgical drainage. One author[34] reported resolution of seven small, early, CT-documented retropharyngeal and parapharyngeal abscesses in children with intravenous antibiotics as the sole treatment. In 65 children with retropharyngeal abscesses,[35] 73% were treated with I+D, while 27% were treated medically. In another series of 17 children with retropharyngeal abscesses,[36] 82% were treated with I+D, and 18% with antibiotics alone. All had a good outcome. Antimicrobial agents are highly effective in treating most patients thought to have uncomplicated cellulitis or adenopathy, however, when patients have a compromised airway or fail to rapidly improve on antimicrobial therapy, I+D are indicated, despite the lack of evidence from imaging that an abscess is present. Continued medical treatment of children despite lack of improvement over a reasonable period (24 hours to 72 hours), puts the child at risk for catastrophic complications that can occur with these infections. In patients with documented abscesses, surgical drainage should be performed. When the imaging studies are negative or equivocal for abscess, an initial trial of medical management is appropriate. Repeating imaging studies during medical treatment can be helpful when a child is not rapidly improving, and may be positive for abscess. The most effective method to determine causative organisms, and to select antimicrobial agents, is to obtain a culture during NA or I+D, which would be indicated when an unusual organism is suspected, as in the immunocompromised patient. Needle aspiration in the awake infant or young child is not recommended and can be dangerous, but is safe for selected older children. One or two NAs plus intravenous antimicrobial agents were successful in 56% of 18 neck abscesses in 17 children.[37] Unilocular and small abscesses had a higher response rate to NA than multilocular and large ones, which often required I+D.

For abscesses associated with complications, and for those that fail NA, I+D are indicated. For uncomplicated head and neck space abscesses, the choice of intravenous antibiotics alone versus NA or I+D plus intravenous antibiotics, is left to the clinical judgement of the clinician, although I+D are strongly recommended.

COMPLICATIONS OF HEAD AND NECK SPACE INFECTIONS

Complications such as airway obstruction during the course of a head and neck space infection are potentially fatal and require an open surgical approach. An intrathoracic complication during the course of a head and neck space infection requires consultation with a chest surgeon. A sentinel bleed from the pharynx or ear may be a harbinger of arterial erosion and massive hemorrhage. Arteriography may be indicated to identify the bleeding vessel if there is sufficient time for this examination. Obtaining access to the great vessels for ligation is critical in this situation. Thrombosis of the internal jugular vein is characterized by spiking fevers, chills, and facial and orbital swelling, with evidence of septic emboli in the pulmonary, and occasionally the systemic circulation. The diagnosis of internal jugular vein thrombosis may be made on the basis of the typical clinical picture plus evidence of thrombosis using CT with contrast,[38] US,[39] or MRI with flow sensitive pulse sequences. Arteriography and venography are unnecessarily invasive for most cases of internal jugular vein thrombosis, because the CT and MRI are reliable and safer (personal communication, Dr. H. Curtin). Internal jugular vein thrombosis may require systemic anticoagulation, ligation or possible excision of the vein.[39]

An abscess may rupture into the airway causing asphyxiation, pneumonia, lung abscess, or empyema. Inflammatory torticollis with cervical vertebral subluxation requiring cervical traction and fusion has been reported to occur during head and neck space infections.[40] Neuropathies may complicate lateral pharyngeal space infections.[41, 42] It is the clinician's responsibility to prevent complications by making a rapid diagnosis and by delivering effective and timely medical and surgical interventions.

REFERENCES

1. Ungkanont K, Yellon RF, Weissman JL et al: Deep neck infections in infants and children: The Pittsburgh experience. *Otolaryngol Head Neck Surg* 112:375–382, 1995.
2. Asmar BI: Bacteriology of retropharyngeal abscess in children. *Pediatr Infect Dis J* 9:595–597, 1990.
3. Brook I: Microbiology of abscesses of the head and neck in children. *Ann Otol Rhinol Laryngol* 96:429–433, 1987.
4. Alvi A: Mycobacterium chelonae causing recurrent neck abscess. *Pediatr Infect Dis J* 12:617–618, 1993.
5. Zangwill KM, Jamilton DH, Perkins BA et al: Cat scratch disease in Connecticut: epidemiology, risk factors, and evaluation of a new diagnostic test. *N Engl J Med* 329:8–13, 1993.
6. Behrman, R, Vaughan V, Nelson W (eds): *Nelson Textbook of Pediatrics*, 13th ed. Philadelphia, WB Saunders, 1987, pp 529, 632, 638–639, 710–711.
7. Reinhardt JF, Johnston L, Ruane P et al: A randomized, double-blind comparison of sulbactam/ampicillin and clindamycin for the treatment of aerobic and aerobic-anaerobic infections. *Rev Infect Dis* 8(suppl 5):S569–S575, 1986.
8. Retsema JA, English AR, Girard A et al: Sulbactam/ampicillin in vitro spectrum, potency, and activity in models of acute infection. *Rev Infect Dis* 8(suppl 5):S528–S534, 1986.
9. Syriopoulou V, Bitsi M, Theodoridis C et al: Clinical efficacy of sulbactam/ampicillin in pediatric infections caused by ampicillin-resistant or penicillin-resistant organisms. *Rev Infect Dis* 8(suppl 5):S630–S633, 1986.
10. Haug RH, Wible RT, Lieberman J: Measurement standards for the preverte-

bral region in the lateral soft-tissue radiograph of the neck. *J Oral Maxillofac Surg* 49:1149–1151, 1991.

11. Weber AL, Baker AS, Montgomery WW: Inflammatory lesions of the neck, including fascial spaces—evaluation by computed tomography and magnetic resonance imaging. *Isr J Med Sci* 28:241–249, 1992.

12. Glasier CM, Stark JE, Jacobs RF et al: CT and ultrasound imaging of retropharyngeal abscesses in children. *Am J Neuroradiol* 13:1191–1195, 1992.

13. Ben-Ami T, Yousefzadeh DK, Aramburo MJ: Pre-suppurative phase of retropharyngeal infection: Contribution of ultrasonography in the diagnosis and treatment. *Pediatr Radiol* 21:23–26, 1990.

14. Kraus R, Han BK, Babcock DS: Sonography of neck masses in children. *Am J Radiol* 146:609–613, 1986.

15. Haeggstrom A, Gustafsson O, Engquist S: Intraoral ultrasonography in the diagnosis of peritonsillar abscess. *Otolaryngol Head Neck Surg* 108:243–247, 1993.

16. Lewis GJS, Leithiser RE, Glasier CM et al: Ultrasonography of pediatric neck masses. *Ultrasound Quarterly* 7:315–335, 1989.

17. Grodinsky M, Holyoke E: The fasciae and fascial spaces of the head, neck and adjacent region. *Am J Anat* 63:367, 1938.

18. Hollinshead W (ed): *Anatomy for Surgeons*, 3rd ed, vol I. Philadelphia: Harper and Row, 1982, pp 269–289.

19. Paparella MM, Shumrick DA, Meyerhoff WL et al (eds): *Otolaryngology*, 2nd ed, vol. III. Philadelphia: WB Saunders Co, 1980, pp 2272–2273.

20. Beeden AG, Evans JNG: Quinsy tonsillectomy-a further report. *J Laryngol Otol* 84:443–448, 1970.

21. Grahne B: Abscess tonsillectomy. *Arch Otolaryngol Head Neck Surg* 68:332–336, 1958.

22. McCurdy JA: Peritonsillar abscess: A comparison of treatment by immediate tonsillectomy and interval tonsillectomy. *Arch Otolaryngol Head Neck Surg* 103:414–415, 1977.

23. Richardson KA, Birck H: Peritonsillar abscess in the pediatric population. *Otolaryngol Head Neck Surg* 89:907–909, 1981.

24. Templer JW, Holinger LD, Wood RP: Immediate tonsillectomy for the treatment of peritonsillar abscess. *Am J Surg* 134:596–598, 1977.

25. Herzon FS: Permucosal needle drainage of peritonsillar abscesses. *Arch Otolaryngol Head Neck Surg* 110:104–105, 1984.

26. Schechter GL, Sly DE, Roper AL et al: Changing face of treatment of peritonsillar abscess. *Laryngoscope* 92:657–659, 1982.

27. Holt GR, Tinsley PP: Peritonsillar abscesses in children. *Laryngoscope* 91:1226–1230, 1981.

28. Herbild O, Bonding P: Peritonsillar abscess: Recurrence rate and treatment. *Arch Otolaryngol Head Neck Surg* 107:540–542, 1981.

29. Nielsen VM, Greisen O: Peritonsillar abscess. I. Cases treated by incision and drainage: A follow-up investigation. *J Laryngol Otol* 95:801–807, 1981.

30. Battista RA, Baredes S, Krieger A: Prevertebral space infections associated with cervical osteomyelitis. *Otolaryngol Head Neck Surg* 108:160–166, 1993.

31. Topazian R, Goldberg M (eds): *Management of Infections of the Oral and Maxillofacial Regions*. Philadelphia: WB Saunders, 1981, pp 196–199.

32. Mosher H: The submaxillary fossa approach to deep pus in the neck. *Trans Am Acad Opthalmol Otolaryngol* 34:19–36, 1929.

33. Tschiassny K: Ludwig's angina—a surgical approach based on anatomical and pathological criteria. *Ann Otol Rhinol Laryngol* 56:937–945, 1947.

34. Brodsky L, Belles W, Brody A et al: Needle aspiration of neck abscesses in children. *Clin Pediatr* 31:71–76, 1992.

35. Broughton RA: Nonsurgical management of deep neck infections in children. *Pediatr Infect Dis J* 11:14–18, 1992.
36. Thompson JW, Cohen SR, Reddix P: Retropharyngeal abscess in children: A retrospective and historical analysis. *Laryngoscope* 98:589–592, 1988.
37. Morrison JE, Pashley NRT: Retropharyngeal abscesses in children: A 10-year review. *Pediatr Emerg Care* 4:9–11, 1988.
38. Merhar GL, Colley DP, Clark RA et al: Computed tomographic demonstration of cervical abscess and jugular vein thrombosis. *Arch Otolaryngol Head Neck Surg* 107:313–315, 1981.
39. Bach MC, Roediger JH, Rinder HM: Septic anaerobic jugular phlebitis with pulmonary embolism: Problems in management. *Rev Infect Dis* 10:424–427, 1988.
40. Bredenkamp JK, Maceri DR: Inflammatory torticollis in children. *Arch Otolaryngol Head Neck Surg* 116:310–313, 1990.
41. Langenbrunner DJ, Dajani S: Pharyngomaxillary space abscess with carotid artery erosion. *Arch Otolaryngol Head Neck Surg* 94:447–457, 1971.
42. Varghese S, Hengerer AS, Putam T: Neck abscess causing Horner's syndrome. *N Y State J Med* 82:1855–1856, 1982.

Index